BASIC PRINCIPLES
OF COMPUTED
TOMOGRAPHY

BASIC PRINCIPLES OF COMPUTED TOMOGRAPHY

by
Carlisle Lee Morgan, M.Phil., Ph.D., M.D.
Attending Radiologist
Henrico Doctors' Hospital
Richmond, Virginia

formerly
Picker Scholar in Academic Radiology of the James Picker Foundation
and
Co-Director of Computed Body Tomography and Clinical Ultrasound
Duke University Medical Center
Durham, North Carolina

with a contribution on Computer Theory and Applications *by*
Michael D. Miller, M.S., Ph.D., M.D.
Attending Radiologist
Elliot Hospital
Manchester, New Hampshire

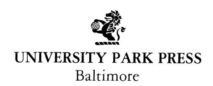

UNIVERSITY PARK PRESS
Baltimore

UNIVERSITY PARK PRESS
International Publishers in Medicine and Human Services
300 North Charles Street
Baltimore, Maryland 21201

Copyright © 1983 by University Park Press

Typeset by Maryland Composition Company
Manufactured in the United States of America by The Maple Press Company

All rights, including that of translation into other languages, reserved. Photomechanical reproduction (photocopy, microcopy) of this book or parts thereof without special permission of the publisher is prohibited.

Library of Congress Cataloging in Publication

Morgan, Carlisle Lee
Basic principles of computed tomography.

Includes index.
1. Tomography. I. Miller, Michael D. II. Title.
RC78.7.T6M67   1983   616.07'57   82-23757
ISBN 0-8391-1705-1

Contents

About the Author / vii
Preface / ix
Acknowledgments / xi

CHAPTER 1
Introduction to Tomography / 1
Conventional Tomography (Sectional Roentgenography)
Computed Tomography: Background and Development
References and Suggested Readings

CHAPTER 2
**Principles of Computed Tomography:
Combined Translational-Rotational Scanning Systems** / 19
Basic Radiological Physics
Introduction to Computed Tomography
Translational-Rotational Systems: The First Generation
Translational-Rotational Systems: The Second Generation
Additional Concepts and Fundamentals
   of Computed Tomography
References and Suggested Readings

CHAPTER 3
Purely Rotational Scanning Systems / 51
A Purely Rotational Scanning Geometry
Rotating Tube and Detector Array:
   The Third Generation
Rotating Tube and Fixed Detectors:
   The Fourth Generation
Comparison of Third and Fourth Generation Scanners
References and Suggested Readings

CHAPTER 4
Computer Theory and Applications / 69
by Michael D. Miller
Computers: Background and Development
Hardware
Software
Computer Applications in Computed Tomography
References and Suggested Readings

CHAPTER 5
Theory and Techniques of Reconstruction / 107

Reconstruction Techniques
Back-Projection
Iteration
Analytical Methods
Comparison between Iterative and Analytical Techniques
Reconstruction Techniques for Divergent Beams
References and Suggested Readings

CHAPTER 6
The Image Display / 125

The Synthesized Image
Display Monitor: The Cathode Ray Tube
Basic Image Presentation and Manipulation
Computer Graphics and Measurements
Contrast Enhancement
Filtering
Hard Copy
References and Suggested Readings

CHAPTER 7
A Practical Computed Tomography System / 157

The CT System: Component Parts
Scanning Parameters
Environmental Requirements
References and Suggested Readings

CHAPTER 8
Image Quality, Resolution, and Dosage / 175

Image Clarity (Visibility) in Radiography
Spatial Resolution in Computed Tomography
Contrast Resolution and Noise in Computed Tomography
Patient Dosage in Computed Tomography
Accuracy and Reliability of CT Numbers
CT Phantoms
References and Suggested Readings

CHAPTER 9
Further Applications of Computed Tomography and Other Tomographic Techniques / 213

Further Applications of Computed Tomography
Other Tomographic Techniques
References and Suggested Readings

APPENDIX I
Artifacts / 275

APPENDIX II
Mathematics of Reconstruction / 291

APPENDIX III
Comparative Features of CT Units / 298

Glossary / 311
Index / 337

About the Author

Carlisle Lee Morgan received his undergraduate degree in physics magna cum laude from Villanova University in 1966. He received the M.Phil. degree in physics in 1968 and a Ph.D. in atomic physics in 1971, both degrees from Yale University. He attended the University of Miami School of Medicine and received the degree of M.D. in 1973.

Dr. Morgan then interned in internal medicine at Duke University Medical Center and was a resident in diagnostic radiology there until 1976, when he was named Co-Director of Body Computed Tomography and Diagnostic Ultrasound at Duke, a position he held until 1979. During that time he also served as Assistant Professor of Radiology and was named by the James Picker Foundation as a Picker Scholar in Academic Radiology.

From 1979 until 1982 Dr. Morgan served as an Attending Radiologist at St. Mary's Hospital in Richmond, Virginia. He is now an Attending Radiologist at Henrico Doctors' Hospital in Richmond.

In addition to several earlier publications in physics, Dr. Morgan has authored numerous articles in the field of diagnostic radiology, and particularly in the areas of computed tomography and ultrasound. He is a member of several scientific and professional societies, including the American College of Radiology, the American Roentgen Ray Society, the Radiological Society of North America, the American Institute of Ultrasound in Medicine, the Richmond Radiological Society, the Richmond Academy of Medicine, and the Medical Society of Virginia.

*To my children
Eva, Alexander, and Ursula*

Preface

The purpose of this book is to provide a description of the basic principles of computed tomography. The book is primarily directed to physicians and to medical imaging personnel, and the language and style of the text have been selected accordingly by the author. The basic approach is descriptive and explanatory, rather than mathematical or technical. The emphasis is on the presentation of fundamental ideas and methods in an easily understood fashion. This presentation is reinforced by the use of practical examples from popular commercial instruments. Background radiation physics, radiologic technology, and computer theory are interwoven into the text and explained in a simplified manner. Numerous diagrams and figures are used to illustrate basic concepts throughout the book.

The historical background, developments, and innovations involving CT are both significant and interesting. However, it is important to view CT from the general perspective of medical imaging, in particular as one method of tomographic or cross-sectional imaging. For this reason other tomographic techniques are described, and their similarities and differences with computed tomography discussed.

Any technology is the result of an evolutionary process involving the accumulated efforts and experiences of many individuals. The roots of CT lie within radiation physics, medical imaging, and computer science. The author has attempted to elucidate these relationships throughout the book as well as to provide some historical flavor to the text. The evolution of CT is detailed in earlier chapters with emphasis on concepts and methods that retain their validity and importance throughout different technical innovations.

Included in the book is an introduction to computers which describes their history and development, logic theory and circuits, computer hardware and software, and computer applications in CT and other fields.

The theory and techniques of image synthesis and reconstruction are presented. The significance and methods of image display and manipulation also are described. To provide an even more realistic background, the author analyzes a complete CT system using as an example a widely used commercial system.

The concepts of image quality and resolution are outlined for conventional radiography with emphasis on important image parameters. This provides a language which is used to develop the concepts of image quality and resolution in CT. Radiation dosage and its measurement are also discussed.

The extension of the clinical applications of CT is described in computed radiography, multiplanar reconstruction, dynamic imaging, high resolution studies, radiation therapy, and gated and dual energy studies. Related tomographic imaging modalities are described, including conventional tomography, ultrafast scanning, emission CT, ultrasound, nuclear magnetic resonance, and microwave imaging. This permits a better understanding of the role of CT within the framework of tomographic imaging modalities.

Scan artifacts, the mathematics of image reconstruction, and comparative features of CT units are incorporated as appendices. A glossary of terms used in CT, other tomographic imaging modalities, and computer technology is also included at the end of the book.

The author has attempted to present realistic examples, including specific data for different commercial units, throughout the book. The data were obtained from scientific articles, technical manuals, and published company specifications as well as through the courtesy of numerous individuals who willingly supplied information. Because of the constant changes and innovations in the field, the data should be regarded as representative specifications illustrating a particular method. These data are obviously subject to change; however, the author feels that even approximate values for different instruments and parameters may be helpful in understanding and appreciating the technology.

C.L.M.

Acknowledgments

There are many individuals to whom I owe acknowledgment, either directly or indirectly, for their help or contribution to this effort.

My friend and former colleague Dr. Michael D. Miller wrote the chapter on computer theory and applications and has reviewed the rest of the book. His support has been especially helpful and meaningful.

Dr. Fearghus O'Foghludha, Chief of Radiation Physics at Duke University Medical Center, was kind enough to review several of the initial chapters and offer advice and encouragement in the early part of this effort.

Almost all of the drawings throughout this book are the work of Robert Margulies of the Department of Audiovisual Education at Duke University Medical Center. His talent has significantly enhanced this work. The ultrasound drawings are the effort of Mr. Stanley Wain of Medical Multimedia.

Some of the early photography for this book was initially done by the Department of Audiovisual Education at Duke University Medical Center. Most of the photographic work, especially in the middle and later chapters, is the effort of the Medical Media Services of St. Mary's Hospital, Richmond. Special credit goes to W. C. Sleeman, III, of St. Mary's for the photography.

I would like to acknowledge the support of former colleagues and technologists at St. Mary's Hospital. I would also like to acknowledge the support I received from the James Picker Foundation as a Picker Scholar during my earlier career in academic radiology.

Dr. Gopala Rao, Chief of Radiation Physics at the Medical College of Virginia, reviewed the section on radiation therapy planning.

Early typing efforts from Mrs. Jackie Wright of the Department of Radiology at Duke University Medical Center helped to get this book started. My secretaries at St. Mary's Hospital labored patiently through multiple drafts of each chapter. I would especially like to thank Dee Dee Vice and Valerie Potts for their tireless typing efforts.

Representatives of numerous companies have provided information for this book. These include the Compagnie Generale de Radiologie (CGR Medical Corporation); Elscint, Inc.; EMI Medical, Inc.; General Electric Medical Systems; Omnimedical; Pfizer Medical Systems, Inc.; Philips Medical Systems, Inc.; Picker Corporation, Searle Medical Systems, Siemens Corporation, Technicare Corporation, Toshiba Medical Systems, and Varian.

Individuals whom I would particularly like to acknowledge for supplying technical information regarding their units include Dr. Robert Ledley, developer of the ACTA Scanner; H. Froger of CGR; Dr. R. P. Schwenker of the DuPont Company; Moshe Avnet, John Cassese, and Ben Noy of Elscint; Diane Kurtz, Terry Moore, and Dr. Promod Haque of EMI; Laura J. Ash, Leslie Lewin, Edwin Robbins, and John Roughton, and Drs. S. M. Blumenfeld and Jeffrey DiSantis of General Electric Medical Systems; Michael P. Garippa and John F. O'Brien of Omnimedical; Dr. David G. Hill of Pfizer

Medical Systems; H. Eerdmans and Dr. Tommie J. Morgan of Philips Medical Systems; Dr. Donald O. Elliott, John J. Barni, and Robert Tahaney, of the Picker Corporation; Craig Burch and Herman E. Derrington of the Siemens Corporation; Richard F. Borrelli, Russell Hannan, Dennis Hegler, Mark A. Jernigan, and Raymond A. Schulz of Technicare Corporation; John F. O'Malley of Toshiba Medical Systems; and Lynn Hamilton of Varian.

I have attempted to give the reader a representative presentation of specific technical parameters for many commercially available CT units. The constant updating of present systems, introduction of new units, withdrawal from the marketplace by several CT manufacturers, and transfer or sale of particular CT unit models among companies has made it difficult to maintain completely up-to-date information on all possible units. Not all units are described in this book. However, it is hoped that the data presented are reasonably complete and relevant, at least from a historical and developmental perspective. As the purpose of this book is a presentation of the basic principles of CT, not a complete exposition of all the technical specifications for every CT unit, the reader should consult up-to-date technical brochures for any company or specific unit.

I have a special debt to those individuals who have contributed so much to the development and/or exposition of CT. These include Drs. Rodney A. Brooks, Allan M. Cormack, Giovanni Di Chiro, Godfrey N. Hounsfield, Peter M. Joseph, Robert Ledley, Edwin C. McCullough, William H. Oldendorf, J. Thomas Payne, Michel M. Ter-Pogossian, and Leslie M. Zatz. Their work and their writings have contributed greatly to my own education in CT and are reflected in this book.

I am particularly grateful to Drs. Brooks, Cormack, Di Chiro, Hounsfield, and Oldendorf as well as Drs. W. Dennis Foley, E. Ralph Heinz, and Perry Sprawls for allowing me to use illustrations from their work.

I would especially like to acknowledge the help and encouragement of my editor at University Park Press, Mrs. Ruby Richardson, a fine lady and personal friend. The efforts of Michael Treadway, production editor at University Park Press, are also gratefully acknowledged.

I would also like to acknowledge for Dr. Miller both Joan Marineau and Jackie Cloutier for their help in preparing the manuscript for Chapter 4 on computer theory and applications.

C.L.M.

CHAPTER 1
INTRODUCTION TO TOMOGRAPHY

CONVENTIONAL TOMOGRAPHY
(SECTIONAL ROENTGENOGRAPHY)

History and Development
Principles of Conventional Tomography
Types of Conventional Tomography
   Linear Tomography
   Pluridirectional Tomography
   Axial Transverse Tomography
Limitations of Conventional Tomography

COMPUTED TOMOGRAPHY:
BACKGROUND AND DEVELOPMENT

Oldendorf's Experiment
Early Emission Computed Tomography—Kuhl and Edwards
Cormack's Work
Hounsfield and the Development of the EMI Scanner
Ledley and the ACTA Whole Body Scanner
Awards

REFERENCES AND SUGGESTED READINGS

CONVENTIONAL TOMOGRAPHY (SECTIONAL ROENTGENOGRAPHY)

History and Development

The word "tomogram" is derived from the Greek words *tomos*, a cutting (section), and *gramma*, a writing. Conventional tomography or sectional roentgenography is a method for taking sectional roentgenograms in which "by giving the x-ray tube a curvilinear motion during exposure synchronous with the recording plate but in the opposite direction, the shadow of the selected plane remains stationary on the moving film while the shadows of all other planes have a relative displacement on the film and are therefore obliterated or blurred" (Stedman's). Alternative terms for this technique include planigraphy, stratigraphy, laminagraphy, body section radiography, zonography (thick section tomography), and noncomputed tomography. The medical usefulness of tomography rests on the ability to localize objects within the body and the capability of identifying and delineating structures within a body section without undesired interference or overlap from objects outside the section of interest.

Tomography was first attempted by Karol Mayer, a Polish radiologist, in 1914. He imaged the heart on a chest radiograph while simultaneously blurring the rib shadows by moving the x-ray tube back and forth during the x-ray exposure. All of the structures were blurred, but the heart, being farther from the tube than the posterior ribs, was less blurred.

The Italian radiologist C. Baese applied in 1915 for a patent on a unit in which an x-ray tube and a fluoroscopic screen would be linked so that there was a proportional, reciprocal motion between them. This could be used for localizing foreign bodies such as bullets by adjusting the position of the focal plane within the patient until the relative motion of the foreign object was stopped, thereby isolating it in the focal plane. This is the principle of tomoscopy.

In 1921, a French physician, André-Edmund-Marie Bocage, applied for a patent on a machine in which both the x-ray tube and the photographic film were moved reciprocally and proportionally. This patent was a forerunner of the present tomographic devices. However, it was not constructed until 1938. Bocage outlined the principles for three different types of tomography units including: 1) a fixed fulcrum system with a linear tube-film movement in which the tube was beneath the object and the film above it (the opposite situation from most devices now used), 2) a pluridirectional device with circular and spiral motions, and 3) a device to perform tomography of a curved surface, which served as a forerunner to pantomography. Bocage emphasized the need for keeping the ratio of the tube-object distance to the object-film distance constant to avoid unequal magnification of structures within the focal section, which would result in distortion within the focal plane. He also emphasized the use of a grid to eliminate scattered radiation and was the first to suggest the possibility of axial transverse tomography.

The French physicians F. Portes and M. Chausse applied for a French patent in 1922 for deep radiation therapy on a device similar to Bocage's second model. In 1927 the German radiologist E. Pohl applied for and received a German patent for a tomographic device.

Jean Kieffer, an American radiologic technologist, while recuperating from tuberculosis conceived a method of tomography that would permit radiographic imaging of his own mediastinum. His initial concepts were outlined in a patent application in 1929.

During this entire period, each investigator worked independently and without knowledge of the related activities of others. In addition, none of the work to this time had led to an actual working tomographic unit. The next phase of historical development of tomography resulted in the successful development and actual use of tomographic devices in the 1930s.

The Italian physician Alessandro Vallebona developed a device, which he described in a publication in 1930, in which the x-ray tube and photographic film were stationary and the patient was rotated in the x-ray beam on a platform. Only those structures in the central axis of rotation of the film remained in focus. This is actually the basic principle of "autotomography" as it is used in modern applications. In 1933, Vallebona also developed a tomographic unit in which the x-ray tube and film were rotated.

B. G. Ziedses des Plantes, a Dutch physician, developed concepts of body section radiography in 1921 and 1922 but did not publish his work until 1931. He emphasized that the way in which the tomographic method was conceived could highly influence its further technical development. Although impressed by the optical analogy of the microscopic image formed by refraction and restricted to a very shallow section (ideally a plane) within an object, he knew that the extremely small wavelength of x-rays precludes refracting or bending x-rays with lenses, as can be done with visible light (optical radiation). He suggested, however, that the results obtained in a microscope could be imitated by moving the tube and the film during the exposure (Figure 1.1). He finally developed a unit in which the x-ray tube and film tray were mounted at opposite ends of a jointed parallelogram. These could be moved synchronously in parallel planes, circles, or spirals. Thus, he introduced pluridirectional as well as linear tomography. Ziedses des Plantes also introduced simultaneous (multisection) tomography in 1931, air encephalography with tomography in 1934, and lipiodol-myelography with tomography in 1934.

Another Dutch radiologist, D. L. Bartelink, developed a fixed-fulcrum device utilizing a sinusoidal movement, which he described in 1932. Initially, J. Robert Andrews (1936), felt that "This method is not quite so practical as that of Vallebona's." With modern knowledge and experience from tomographic units, however, it is becoming accepted that the geometric characteristics of fixed-fulcrum systems are more favorable that those of adjustable-fulcrum systems.

G. Grossmann studied the mathematical and geometric basis of tomography in depth and employed a device he called the "tomograph" in which the x-ray tube and film rotated through arcs and the central ray of the tube was directed at all times to the center of the film. His work was published in 1935. He demonstrated geometrically that overlying shadows could be more completely eliminated by a spiral tube motion than by a circular motion. However, he emphasized the considerable increase in exposure time and radiation for the spiral motion compared to the circular, and for the circular movement compared to a plain film. His efforts at the time provided a simple and economical approach to tomography.

In 1936, Andrews of the Cleveland Clinic and Robert J. Stava of the Picker Corporation collaborated in the construction of the first American tomographic unit. Soon afterwards, Kieffer with the help of Sherwood Moore constructed a unit which they called the laminagraph at the Mallinckrodt Institute.

The technique of axial transverse tomography was developed by the radiologic technologist William Watson. An axial transverse tomogram is a roentgenogram in which a section of the body located at

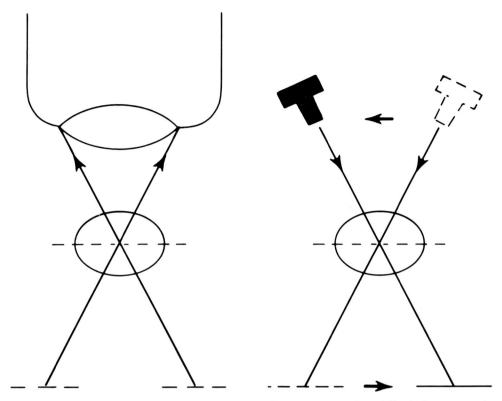

Figure 1.1. An analogy between an optical microscope and a moving x-ray tube and film during tomography.

right angles to the coronal and sagittal planes is imaged. That is, it is perpendicular to the longer vertical axis of the body. Watson described the principles of axial transverse tomography in 1936 and published the material relating to this work in 1939.

The initial workers recognized that the pluridirectional movements were superior to linear ones in achieving a more complete blur of structures outside the plane of interest (the focal plane or tomographic plane). A tomographic device permitting a number of orientational motions, developed by Raymond Sans and Jean Porcher in 1949, attracted the attention of Jean Massiot, who manufactured a model of this unit on an industrial scale. It was given the commercial name Polytome. This unit was presented to the public initially in 1951. A hypocycloidal motion was eventually incorporated in this unit, which has become one of the best known and most successful pluridirectional tomographic units developed. In addition to further modifications of the Polytome, additional pluridirectional units have been developed, in particular the Stratomatic, which was developed in 1970 by the CGR Benelux Company of Belgium, and which features a spiral motion. These units usually have the capability for linear tomography, as well as the circular and elliptical pluridirectional motions.

Principles of Conventional Tomography

The purpose of conventional tomography is the detailed radiographic display, without distortion, of structures lying in a focal plane within the body. To achieve this end, the radiographic shadows from structures outside of this focal plane are deliberately blurred. A conventional tomogram is thus composed of two parts: the image of the body section in focus and the superimposed blur from structures above and below this focal plane. The basic components of the conventional tomographic system are the x-ray tube, the x-ray film, and a rigid connection (for example, a rod) between them. The connection ensures synchronous movement of the tube and film in opposite directions through an angle θ about a point termed the fulcrum, as illustrated in Figure 1.2 for two simple approaches. Figure 1.2A demonstrates a rectilinear motion of the tube and film; in Figure 1.2B the tube and film move through an arc.

The tomographic angle or arc is the angle θ through which the tube and film move. It is this angle, rather than the absolute distance through which the tube travels, that influences the degree of blurring and thereby determines the effective thickness of the focal section.

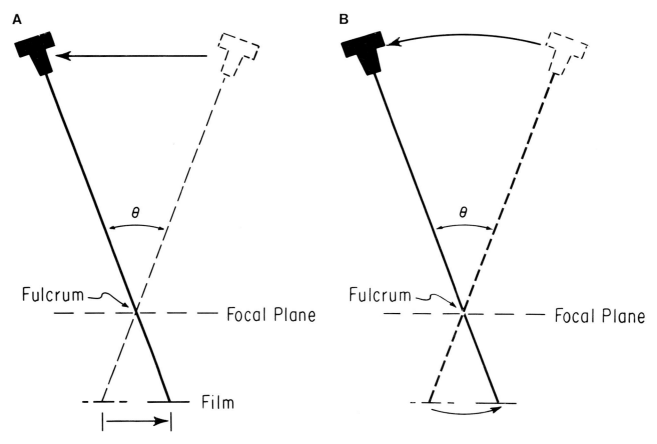

Figure 1.2. Synchronized rectilinear (A) and curvilinear (B) motion of the x-ray tube and film through the tomographic angle θ. The fulcrum is the pivotal point about which rotation occurs, and it determines the position of the focal plane. In both A and B, the central ray of the x-ray beam is shown.

The fulcrum determines the position of the plane that will be in focus. Points lying above or below this plane will be blurred. The fulcrum may be fixed or adjustable. In a fixed fulcrum system the patient is moved up or down on an adjustable table until the desired section of interest is at the level of the fulcrum. In an adjustable fulcrum system, the fulcrum is moved to the level of the plane or section which is to be imaged, the table remaining stationary.

The tomographic principle is illustrated in Figure 1.3. As the tube and film travel, all points outside the focal section are blurred; that is, the image point on the film representing an object point outside of the focal section does not remain stationary on the film but changes its relative position. Thus, the image of an object point that lies outside of the focal plane is a blur, not a point. However, an object point that lies within the focal plane always retains its same image position on the film during the movement, so that this object point is reproduced on the image as a point.

The focal thickness is the depth of the section that remains in focus on the tomogram. Although theoretically the focal plane is truly a plane, without thickness or depth, in practice a layer or section about the focal plane undergoes sufficiently little blurring to be considered as comprising a focal section. Rather than an abrupt cutoff, there is gradual increase in blurring for planes lying outside of the focal plane. Because of this gradual transition in blurring, the section thickness (cut thickness) may be defined in terms of the minimal perceptible blur. The actual thickness of the section that is in focus is inversely proportional to the tomographic angle through which the connecting rod swings; that is, the larger the tomographic angle, the thinner the corresponding section. This is illustrated in Figure 1.4. This relationship is also illustrated in Figure 1.5, which demonstrates a hyperbolic relationship between section thickness and tomographic angle. For practical purposes, it can be considered that the section thickness does not significantly change for angles greater than 10°, al-

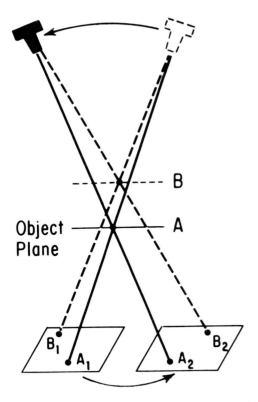

Figure 1.3. The tomographic principle. A point lying in the focal plane A will retain its relative image position on the film during the synchronous tomographic motion. A point lying outside of the focal plane, for example in plane B, will have its image position shifted during the tomographic motion.

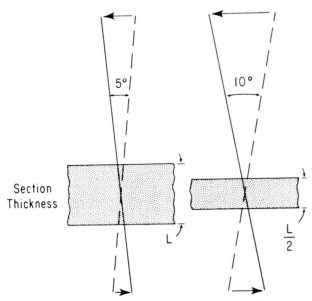

Figure 1.4. A larger tomographic angle results in a thinner section. In this example, increasing the angle from 5° to 10° results in a halving of the section thickness. The shaded slab representing a section thickness lies within a much thicker slab of tissue in each case.

though the blurring of objects outside of this focal plane does continue to increase with a larger tomographic angle.

The width of the blur is the distance along the focal plane over which the image of an object point is spread out on the film. Several factors influence this blurring. The width of the blurring is directly proportional to the tomographic angle; that is, doubling the tomographic angle doubles the width of the blur. In addition, the farther away a given object is from the focal plane, the greater the degree of blurring. Thus, there is only minimal blurring of objects immediately contiguous to or outside the focal plane, whereas structures which lie far from this plane are maximally blurred.

Points undergo more blurring if they are located farther away from the film. In particular, if two points are equally spaced away from the focal plane but on opposite sides of the focal plane, the point farther from the film will be blurred more than the point closer to the film.

Structures outside the focal plane whose long axes are perpendicular to the direction of the movement of the x-ray tube and film are maximally blurred or effaced. However, those structures whose axes lie parallel to the direction of movement of the tube and film will not be blurred. That is, when the longitudinal axis of a structure lies parallel to the direction of motion of the tube, no blurring occurs along the central axis, but rather the central axial portion of the structure in question is merely elongated.

This last consideration points to the important feature that, for ideal blurring of structures outside of the tomographic plane, the central ray of the x-ray beam, or as it is frequently termed, the obscuring ray, should at various times in the cycle originate from an infinite number of directions, so that the long axis of all structures to be blurred would at some time be perpendicular to this obscuring ray, resulting in a uniform blurring. Failure to achieve this results in elongated unblurred images from structures outside the focal plane, which are referred to as parasitic shadows. The general statement may be made that the most significant single factor influencing the quality of a tomogram is the spatial direction of the tube-film obscuring movement.

This last principle can be described more analytically by the law of tangents, first described by Ziedses des Plantes in 1932 and illustrated in Figure 1.6. A radiographic image is formed by the differential attenuation of x-rays passing through different tissues of various thicknesses and absorbing properties. The differential attenuation produces a variation in grayness on the film. By itself this is not an

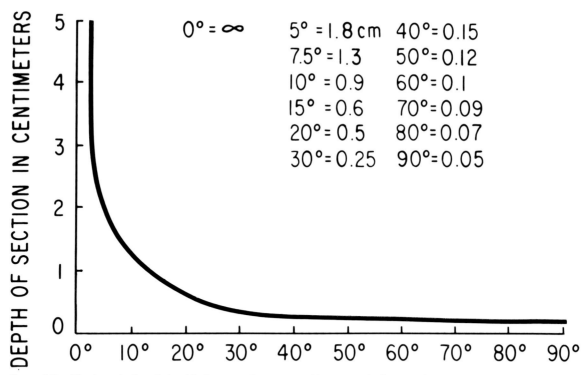

Figure 1.5. The hyperbolic relationship between the tomographic section thickness and tomographic angle is illustrated. The decrease in section thickness with increasing tomographic angle is greatest for small angles and more gradual for larger angles.

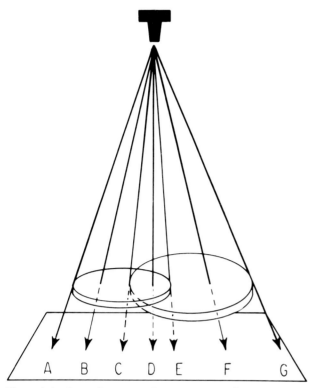

Figure 1.6. Law of tangents. Rays *A, C, E,* and *G*, which pass tangentially to object borders, are the primary image-forming rays. Rays *B, D,* and *F* are responsible for differences in grayness.

image. The portions of an object that are tangential to the x-ray beam record the border or marginal shadows that actually represent the image-forming elements of the radiograph. Essentially the steepest contrast gradients at the tangential margins of the structure are recorded. Other rays passing through the object merely create less abrupt differences in the grayness of the film. The same degree of grayness may be produced when the x-rays have passed through a large thickness of material having a low attenuation, or through a thin section of tissue having a high attenuation, and such differences in properties and thicknesses will not show up. It is the tangential margins which allow delineation of the shapes and sizes of the objects through which the beam has passed. Therefore, the tomographic movement that will provide the most complete image of the elements in a focal plane is that in which the central ray experiences the greatest number of tangential occurrences. To increase the number of tangential occurrences, the central ray should undergo as many changes in direction as possible.

Any conventional radiographic system can cause subject magnification (Figure 1.7). It can be noted from the illustration that the greater the ratio of object-film distance to tube-film distance, that is, the farther away the object is from the film for a fixed

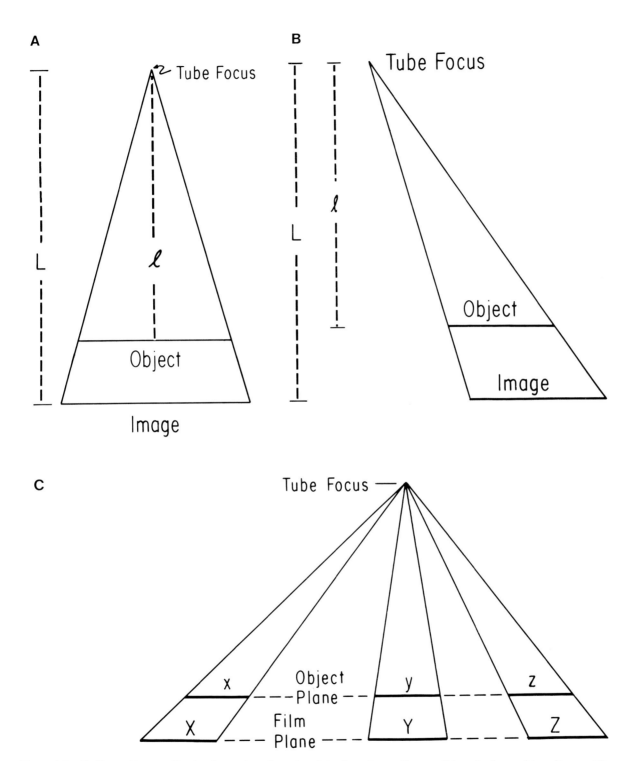

Figure 1.7. Radiographic magnification is equal to the ratio of the focus-image distance (L) to the focus-object distance (ℓ). This is valid whether the object is in the path of the central ray of the x-ray tube (A) or in the path of an oblique ray (B). Thus, in C the magnifications X/x, Y/y, and Z/z are all equal even though the x-ray path lengths are different. Distortion (unequal magnification of different parts of an object) occurs when different parts of an object are at different distances from the film.

Introduction to Tomography

tube-film distance, the more magnification the object undergoes. (Tube–film distance refers to the tube focus–film or tube focal spot–film distance.) Magnification is defined as the ratio of the image size to the object size, and from geometric considerations it is equal to the ratio of the tube focal spot-film (tube-film) distance to the tube focal spot-object (tube-object) distance (Figure 1.7). Magnification occurs in conventional tomography as in routine radiographic procedures. It may be minimized by keeping the object as close to the film as possible or by keeping the tube-film distance as great as possible. Distortion arises when there are unequal magnifications of different parts of an object. In plain film radiography this occurs when different structures within an object are not equally distant from the film. In tomography, distortion can arise as a result of unequal magnification of structures located within different portions of the focal plane, and magnification for all points projected in the focal plane should be the same throughout the entire system.

Types of Conventional Tomography

Conventional tomography may be classified according to the manner in which the x-ray tube and photographic film move during the tomographic process. The major types of conventional tomography are linear, pluridirectional, and axial transverse.

Linear Tomography In linear or unidirectional tomography, the x-ray tube and film move synchronously so that the central ray of the x-ray beam moves in a single plane (usually the vertical). In a linear tomographic system, the x-ray tube and film may move in either a rectilinear or a curvilinear fashion. Rectilinear motion implies that the x-ray tube and the film each move in a straight line (see Figure 1.2A). This movement can be described as plane-parallel. For curvilinear motion, the x-ray tube and film both move in an arc within a given plane (see Figure 1.2B).

A rectilinear system can be readily adapted to a standard x-ray table and is thus cheaper. However, the straight line motion of tube and film requires more moving parts, including slip joints at both ends of the connecting rod. These may suffer significant wear and shaking, and soon go out of adjustment. A curvilinear system requires fewer moving parts and is less likely to get out of adjustment. However, this method requires a special table and tube, resulting in significantly greater expense.

Despite the strong indications by many of the initial workers that complex tomographic motions were necessary to achieve more complete blurring, most of the early units that were developed and manufactured were of the linear type. Linear tomographic equipment is relatively inexpensive compared to pluridirectional devices, and the time needed to perform a single tomogram is relatively short. Thus, the patient is not required to hold his or her breath for an undue period of time, and the radiation dose per tomographic cut is generally less than in a pluridirectional unit. However, the restriction of the tomographic motion to a single linear motion results in a great variation in the blurring of objects outside the tomographic plane. Specifically, whereas structures whose longitudinal axes are perpendicular to the linear motion of the tube and film are maximally blurred, no blurring occurs for those structures whose longitudinal axes are parallel to the direction of tube movement. This accounts for the complete blurring of ribs on a conventional linear tomogram of the chest. Similarly, it accounts for the residual streaking of bronchovascular marks, which are longitudinal on the tomograms, as well as for streaking of longitudinal structures in the thoracic spine and the sternum. The streaks or residual lines are referred to as parasitic streaks.

This variation in blurring with the angle that the longitudinal structure of an object makes relative to the direction of tube motion suggests that the linear tomogram does not actually form an image of a true section plane. It rather images a layer or section of varying thickness, the ultimate shape of which depends on the orientation of elements outside the presumed plane of focus to the obscuring ray.

Pluridirectional Tomography In pluridirectional tomography the x-ray tube and film synchronously undergo more complex motion. The kinds of motion include circular, ellipsoidal, sinusoidal, hypocycloidal, and spiral. These are illustrated in Figure 1.8. The tomographic angle again determines the section thickness, and this angle is measured in degrees from the extremes of the tube motion (Figure 1.9). The more complex motions require greater path length for the tube and the film. This in turn requires a greater time to complete the tomogram, and therefore usually leads to a greater dose of radiation.

The purpose of these more complex tomographic motions is to produce more uniform blurring of structures outside the tomographic section. The complexity of the spatial movement of the tube and film essentially ensures that all tangential borders of an object will be viewed by the central or obscuring ray from multiple directions. Thus, the orientation of the structure becomes less important. In particular, at some point in its motion the tube and film will be perpendicular to the longitudinal axis of a structure, thus ensuring more complete blurring of this struc-

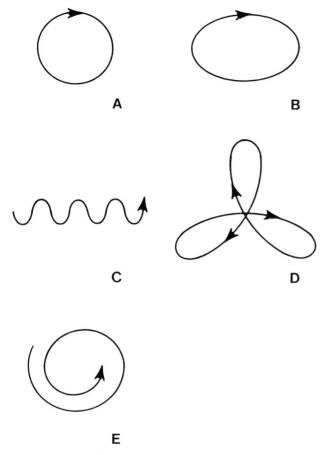

Figure 1.8. Pluridirectional tomography. Circular (*A*), elliptical (*B*), sinusoidal (*C*), hypocycloidal (*D*), and spiral (*E*) motions are indicated.

ture. Parasitic streaks are therefore reduced. The more complex motions also guarantee a final tomographic section of more uniform section thickness.

Disadvantages of the pluridirectional tomographic techniques include the greatly increased cost, the greater time to perform the tomogram, and the greater radiation dose. The greater time to perform the tomograms is particularly bothersome in the chest, where breath holding is necessary.

Another significant disadvantage is the appearance of phantom images, which are produced by the blurred margins of structures outside of the focal plane. These are most likely to occur with a circular tomographic motion or when the tomographic angle is relatively narrow. With a narrow angle, objects outside the focal plane are only minimally blurred, and their borders may remain distinct. These phantom images are of two types: the first results from the superimposition of blur margins of regularly recurring structures outside the focal section; the second type results when the blurred image of a dense structure outside the focal plane apparently simulates a less dense structure within the focal plane. An example of the first type of phantom image may be produced by bone trabeculae, teeth, or ribs. An example of the second type of phantom image may be seen when blurring of a bony structure outside the focal plane results in what appears to be a soft tissue density within the focal plane.

Axial Transverse Tomography In axial transverse tomography (also referred to as transverse axial tomography, TA tomography, or TAT) the tissue cross-section that is imaged is oriented perpendicularly to both coronal and sagittal planes. It is a transverse section as opposed to the coronal or sagittal

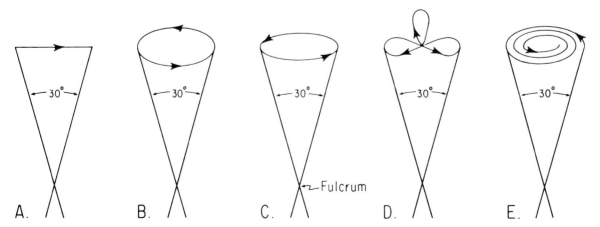

Figure 1.9. A 30° tomographic angle is illustrated for linear (*A*), circular (*B*), elliptical (*C*), hypocycloidal (*D*), and trispiral (*E*) motions.

Introduction to Tomography   9

sections described thus far. The technique is illustrated in Figure 1.10. The x-ray tube is oriented so that its central ray is directed through the patient and onto the film at an acute angle. The patient sits upright in a rotating chair. The x-ray film is placed horizontally on a table, which rotates in synchrony with the patient's chair. During the tomographic procedure, the x-ray tube remains stationary while both the patient and film rotate in the same direction and at the same velocity. Structures within the tomographic plane are the only ones which remain in sharp focus on the film during rotation. The smaller the angle between the central ray and the plane of the film, the thinner the transverse section. A grid is also placed over the film and remains stationary while the film rotates. The grid lines are blurred by the relative motion of the film and the grid.

In this system, structures close to the film are also close to the x-ray source, and structures farther from the film are farther from the x-ray source. Thus the ratios of the tube-film distance to tube-object distance are constant for all structures in the focal section. Magnification is thus equal for all structures, preventing distortion of the image.

Limitations of Conventional Tomography

Specific limitations associated with linear and pluridirectional tomography, respectively, have already been described in this chapter. However, there are several important general limitations of all conventional tomographic techniques.

In dissecting a conventional tomographic image into its two components, namely, the image of the focal plane of interest and the blur resulting from structures outside of the tomographic section, only the image component is of interest. In addition to the formation of parasitic streaks or phantom images, background blurring decreases the contrast between tissue structures in the focal plane. The blur component represents irradiated tissue that is not imaged and which detracts from the image quality of the focal plane. To achieve imaging of a specific focal plane, it is necessary to irradiate all the tissue above and below this pertinent section. This happens in plain films also but is worse in tomography, whether linear or pluridirectional, because of the increased exposure time and the greater tissue thickness in oblique x-ray paths. Therefore, the dose is high for one tomographic section, and when multiple tomographic sections are performed the resulting dose can be quite significant.

Conventional tomography does not increase or enhance natural contrast; in fact, it decreases it. Indeed, in conventional tomography it is advisable that there be a significant degree of contrast. Like conventional radiography, conventional tomography is not able to distinguish between different nonfatty soft tissues without the use of contrast-accentuating substances. Specifically, the contrast differences are the natural ones between air, fat, nonfatty soft tissues, and bone. Thus, in conventional tomography it is necessary to have a significant degree of natural contrast, as between bone or air and soft tissue, or to inject contrast media, which are concentrated in certain organs, to distinguish between different soft tissue structures and delineate their borders. Since conventional tomography does not increase natural contrast but merely blurs overlying structures, the visibility of different structures in a particular body section may be enhanced, but contrast between structures is not. This inability to distinguish between and delineate different soft tissue structures is probably the greatest single limitation in conventional radiography and tomography.

As in other radiographic techniques, the problem of unwanted magnification occurs with conventional tomography. Only certain tomographic motions are allowed if distortion is to be avoided. Even with these correct tomographic motions, however, there will be a difference in the magnification of structures in different focal planes. This difference will depend upon the ratio of the x-ray tube focus—

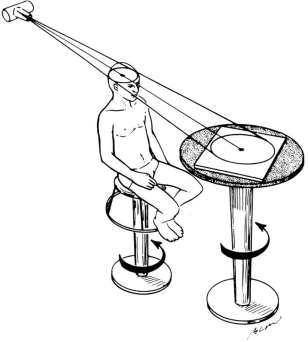

Figure 1.10. Axial transverse tomography. This is a conventional tomographic analog to computed tomography.

film distance to the x-ray tube focus—focal plane distance.

Although axial transverse tomography has found some limited use, it has not achieved widespread popularity. As in other forms of conventional tomography, it is not able to delineate the different soft tissue structures within a body slice.

The undesired irradiation of tissue structures outside of the focal section of interest adds a significant amount of radiation exposure to the patient in conventional tomography. Finally, the deleterious effect of the overlying blur superimposed on the tomographic images is also an important limitation to conventional tomography.

COMPUTED TOMOGRAPHY: BACKGROUND AND DEVELOPMENT

The fundamental concept underlying the technique of computed tomography is the capability of reconstructing or synthesizing a cross-section of the internal structure of an object from multiple projections of a collimated beam of radiation passing through the object. The technique has been variously described as transverse axial tomography, computerized transverse axial tomography, computer-assisted tomography, computerized tomography, reconstruction tomography, and computed tomography. The technique is not limited, however, to transverse cross-sections, since cross-sections in other planes can be synthesized either by scanning in these planes or by secondary reconstruction techniques using transverse cross-sectional data. Although the computer is indispensable in practice, it is not essential to the theory of the technique, and in early work reconstructed tomograms were achieved without computers. The term "reconstruction tomography" may thus be the most general basic description, but the term "computed tomography" has gained the most widespread acceptance. Computed tomography also developed historically into separate modes called transmission and emission computed tomography. In the former, the projections are obtained by measuring the transmission of an externally located x-ray beam passing through the body. In the latter, the projections are obtained from measurements of internal gamma radiation from the body resulting from the positron or direct gamma decay of radioisotopes within the body. This book deals primarily with transmission computed tomography, although some description of emission computed tomography is given in Chapter 9. A more recent historical and technical evolution is the development of nuclear magnetic resonance (NMR) tomography, which is based on the distribution of natural or artificially introduced magnets in the body (see Chapter 9).

The mathematical basis for reconstruction of an object from multiple projections through the object dates back to the work of the Austrian mathematician J. Radon, working in gravitational theory in 1917. Radon demonstrated mathematically that a two- or three-dimensional object could be replicated from the infinite set of all its projections. The physical application of the concept of reconstruction of multiple projections was utilized by R. N. Bracewell (1956) when he reconstructed a map of solar microwave emissions from data obtained by measuring the radiation in a series of ribbon-like strips crossing the solar surface. Biological applications of this technique were first utilized in electron microscopy in the reconstruction of complex biomolecular structures from a series of transmission micrograms taken at different angles. The methods of reconstruction were developed by DeRosier and Klug (1968), Gordon, Bender, and Herman (1970), Gilbert (1972), and Smith, Peters, and Bates (1973).

The early pioneering work in the medical application of image reconstruction was performed independently by Oldendorf (1961), Kuhl and Edwards (1963, 1968), and Cormack (1963, 1964).

Oldendorf's Experiment

William H. Oldendorf, an American neurologist from Los Angeles, carried out experiments based on principles similar to those later used in computed tomography. His work was an attempt to overcome obstacles imposed by the bony calvaria in the imaging of the brain.

Oldendorf's experimental apparatus is schematically diagrammed in Figure 1.11. Two concentric rings of iron nails were embedded in a plastic block measuring $10 \times 10 \times 4$ cm. Near the center of the rings another iron nail and an aluminum nail of identical diameter were also embedded within the plastic block, 1.5 cm apart. The outer concentric rings of iron nails comprised a dense boundary analogous to the skull. The centrally located nails were the objects whose locations and radiodensities were to be determined and were equivalent to the brain. Only the portions of the nails above the upper surface of the plastic block were examined.

The model was placed on a toy HO gauge flatcar, which was in turn mounted on a 22-cm long section of HO track. A clock motor pulled the flatcar with the model along the track at a rate of 80 mm per hr. The entire apparatus was placed on a phonographic turntable which was rotated at 16 rpm. A collimated beam of gamma rays from an ^{131}I source was directed

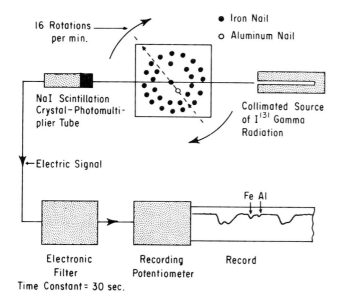

Figure 1.11. Schematic diagram of Oldendorf's experimental apparatus. The model is slowly (80 mm per hr) translated along the dashed line as indicated while simultaneously rotating (16 rpm). A collimated gamma ray beam passed through the model to a detection system using a sodium iodide crystal with a photomultiplier tube. The signal is then processed. (Modified and reproduced with permission from: Oldendorf, W. H. Isolated flying spot detection of radiodensity discontinuities—Displaying the internal structural pattern of a complex object. IEEE Transactions on Biomedical Engineering 8:68–72, 1961.)

through the axis of rotation of the turntable at a level 1 cm above the surface of the plastic block. After passing through the model, the transmitted beam was detected by a sodium iodide scintillation crystal and photomultiplier. The results were counted by a rate meter with a time constant of 30 s.

During operation, the centrally located iron and aluminum nails traveled linearly through the center of rotation of the turntable pulled along by the moving flatcar. If the turntable was not rotating, the central nails could be identified only if the outer rings of the nails were removed (Figure 1.12). With the outer nails in place, details of the central nails were completely obscured by noise from the peripheral nails (Figure 1.13). Thus, a linear scan alone is not sufficient for acquiring internal detail when there is a significant background attenuation of radiation that is not uniform.

However, if the centrally located nails travel slowly through the center of rotation of the turntable while it is rotating, the relative position and radiation attenuation of the central nails can be determined (Figure 1.14). Any nail not at the center of rotation of the turntable will interrupt the beam at twice the rotational frequency (since each nail will pass into and out of the beam twice during a single turn). The relatively more rapid variations in the transmitted beam intensity which result from these interruptions contribute a high frequency noise. Simultaneously, the translation of the central nails through the center of rotation causes a relatively slow variation in the transmitted beam. This slow variation represents a low frequency signal that can be separated from the high frequency noise and which identifies the relative position and radiation attenuation of the central nails.

Information was obtained in this manner only along one line passing through the center of rotation. Additional lines of information would require shifting the model relative to the center of rotation. Since a single pass required 1 hr, obtaining multiple lines through a two-dimensional structure would require an enormous time, and there was no appropriate means of storage for the data. In addition, the radiation dose was impractical for medical usage. How-

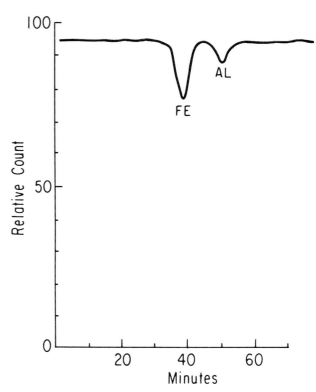

Figure 1.12. Oldendorf's experiment. The model is linearly translating through the collimated gamma ray beam. The central iron nail (brain) can be detected if the turntable is stationary only when the outer rings of nails (skull) are removed. (Reproduced with permission from: Oldendorf, W. H. Isolated flying spot detection of radiodensity discontinuities—Displaying the internal structural pattern of a complex object. IEEE Transactions on Biomedical Engineering 8:66–72, 1961.)

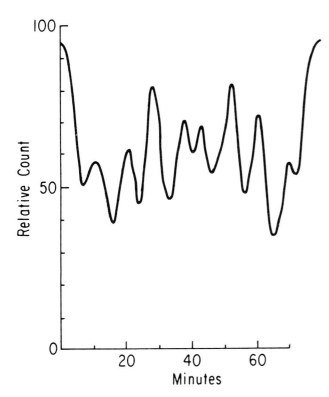

Figure 1.13. The Oldendorf model is linearly translating through the collimated gamma ray beam, but the turntable is not rotating. With the outer rings of nails in place, the central nails are obscured by noise associated with the noise generated by the outer rings. (Reproduced with permission from: Oldendorf, W. H. Isolated flying spot detection of radiodensity discontinuities—Displaying the internal structural pattern of a complex object. IEEE Transactions on Biomedical Engineering 8:66–72, 1961.)

ever, this experiment was the first published attempt at the medical application of reconstruction.

Early Emission Computed Tomography—Kuhl and Edwards

David E. Kuhl and Roy Q. Edwards in 1963 introduced transverse body section imaging by isotope scanning, subsequently further developing and refining the technique referred to as emission computed tomography. A sequence of tangential scans at regular angular intervals was performed with two opposing radiation detectors (Figure 1.15). Thus, any gamma ray emitting structure in the cross-section was scanned and viewed from multiple different directions. Summation of these multiple linear image projections was first performed by constant exposure of a film to a thin line of light moving across the face of a cathode ray tube with a speed and orientation corresponding to the detectors' line of view. Tangential scans were performed at 24 different angles (every 7.5°). This pattern of linear translation followed by a discrete rotation differed from Oldendorf's scanning technique of continuous rotation with a concurrent slow translation. These 24 separate exposures, each corresponding to a view seen by detectors at a different angle, were effectively summated together on film using an open camera shutter technique. In 1968, Kuhl and Edwards reported a process of digital summation in which the image of the transverse section was represented as a square matrix of 10,000 picture elements, each of which represented the average number of counts in a particular matrix or picture element.

The work of Kuhl and Edwards represents pioneering accomplishments in the development of emission and transmission computed tomography.

Cormack's Work

Allan M. Cormack, born in South Africa and educated in nuclear physics at Cambridge University, was

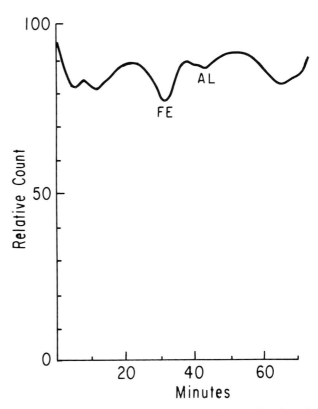

Figure 1.14. The Oldendorf model is linearly translating through the gamma ray beam. The outer rings of nails are in place about the central nails. With the turntable rotating, the relative position and radiation attenuation of the central nails (FE, AL) can be determined. (Reproduced with permission from: Oldendorf, W. H. Isolated flying spot detection of radiodensity discontinuities—Displaying the internal structural pattern of a complex object. IEEE Transactions on Biomedical Engineering 8:66–72, 1961.)

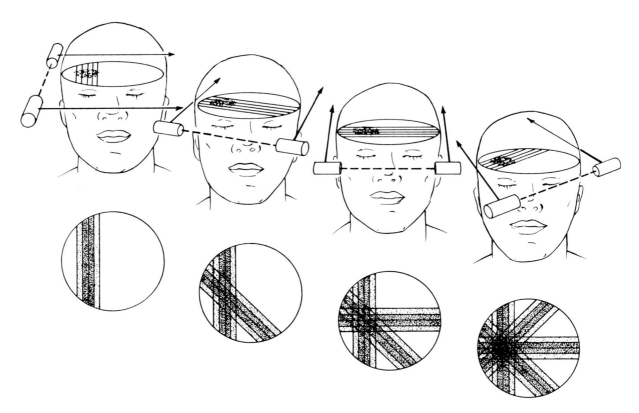

Figure 1.15. Emission computed tomography, introduced by Kuhl and Edwards. A tomographic image based on the distribution of a radioisotope is formed by the summation of successive linear scans across the section of interest. The individual linear scans differ by angular incrementations.

a member of the physics department at the University of Capetown in 1955 when the hospital physicist at the Groote Schuur Hospital resigned. As the only nuclear physicist in Capetown, Cormack was asked to spend 1½ days a week at the hospital attending to the use of isotopes for the first half of 1956.

While observing the planning of radiotherapy treatments, Cormack became aware of the value of knowing the distribution of x-ray attenuation coefficients of tissues in the body. This distribution would have to be obtained by external measurements. It also became obvious to him that this information would be useful for making diagnostic tomograms. During a sabbatical to the Cambridge Electron Accelerator at Harvard University in late 1956, Cormack derived a mathematical theory for image reconstruction. After returning to South Africa in 1957, he tested his theory with a laboratory simulation. In this experiment, a disk 5 cm thick and 20 cm in diameter was scanned using a ^{60}Co radiation source (7 mCi) to produce gamma rays with energies of 1.17 and 1.33 MeV. The gamma ray beam was collimated by a 15-cm lead shield with a circular hole in it. The overall width of the gamma ray beam was 7 mm. A Geiger counter was used as a detector. The disk consisted of a central cylinder of purealuminum, 1.13 cm in diameter, surrounded by an aluminum alloy annulus with an inner diameter of 1.13 cm and an outer diameter of 10.0 cm. This was surrounded in turn by a wooden (oak) annulus with an inner diameter of 10.0 cm and an outer diameter of 20.0 cm. The disk was translated through the gamma ray beam in 5-mm steps.

Because of the circular symmetry, the absorption profile from one scan was sufficient, since linear scans obtained in any other angle through the model would be the same. The attenuation coefficients were calculated for aluminum and wood from the experimentally obtained projection data using Cormack's reconstruction techniques.

Later in 1957, Cormack moved to the United States, becoming a member of the physics department at Tufts University. There he refined the reconstruction techniques to allow the determination of a variable attenuation coefficient in the absence of circular symmetry. In 1963 he repeated his experiment with similar equipment, but using a nonsymmetrical phantom of aluminum and plastic (lucite). An outer ring of aluminum represented the skull, the lucite inside this ring represented soft tissue, and two aluminum disks within the lucite represented tumors. This phantom is illustrated in Figure 1.16. The ratio of the attenuation coefficient of aluminum to that of lucite is about 3 to 1. In the hope of attracting the attention of those doing emission scanning using positron-emitting isotopes, the ratio was chosen to be about equal to the concentration of radioisotope in abnormal tissue compared to normal tissue. The gamma ray beam was collimated to 5 mm. Twenty-five linear scans were performed at 7½° angular intervals through a total of 180°.

The two experiments were published in 1963 and 1964, respectively. In his Nobel Lecture, Cormack remarked that "There was virtually no response. The most interesting request for a reprint came from the Swiss Centre for Avalanche Research. The method would work for deposits of snow on mountains if one could get either the detector or the source into the mountain under the snow!"

Cormack's pioneering work, the combination of multiple discrete measurements of the x-ray attenuation along different paths and the manipulation of this data with complex mathematical and computational technique to produce an anatomical image, is the basis of transmission computed tomography. All of these earlier works, however, were greatly limited by the time and difficulty in performing the necessary calculations. The development of more sophisticated computers with miniaturization and decreased cost for calculational purposes provided the technical breakthrough which allowed practical development of computed tomography to progress in medical imaging.

Hounsfield and the Development of the EMI Scanner

Godfrey N. Hounsfield at the Central Research Laboratories of EMI, Ltd., in England developed the first head scanner based on x-ray transmission computed tomography. In 1967, while investigating pattern recognition techniques, Hounsfield became aware that there were many areas where large amounts of information could be made available, but because of the inefficient techniques used for retrieval much of this potential information was lost. He deduced, independently of Cormack, that from measurements of x-ray transmissions taken from all possible directions through a body it would be possible to reconstruct the internal structure of a body. It seemed to Hounsfield, as it had to Cormack, that a tomographic approach was the most convenient form. Any three-dimensional body could be divided into slices. Each slice could then be examined by passing x-ray beams through it and then reconstructed from the transmitted x-ray data.

Preliminary calculations by Hounsfield indicated that it would be possible to measure the absolute values of the x-ray attenuation coefficients in a slice with an accuracy of .5%, nearly 100 times better than by conventional methods. This accuracy was helped by using detectors which were far more sensitive than photographic film.

Tests were performed on a computer in 1967 to prove that the mathematical solution could work. The British Department of Health then encouraged Hounsfield to test the practical feasibility of the technique.

The first laboratory machine was built on a lathe bed. An electric motor drove the lead screw in steps. The specimen was rotated in 1° steps at the end of each linear scan. In these initial efforts using a low intensity americium gamma source, the machine required 9 days to produce a picture. The computer required 2½ hr to process the readings. A total of 28,000 simultaneous equations had to be solved by the computer, which was programmed in **FORTRAN**. Unfortunately, the accuracy was only 4%.

The method of interpolation between picture points was then modified. The scanning time was reduced by using a higher intensity conventional x-ray tube to produce a finely collimated beam and a crystal detector with a photomultiplier that was mechanically aligned to scan through the brain. The accuracy then approached .5%, and scanning time was reduced to 9 hr.

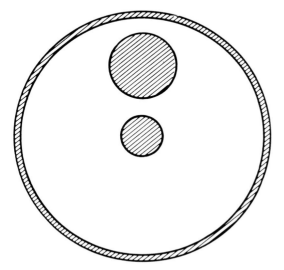

Figure 1.16. Cormack's nonsymmetrical phantom. Hatched areas are aluminum. The unhatched area inside the aluminum ring is lucite and that outside the ring is air. (Reproduced with modification by permission of the Journal of Applied Physics and A. M. Cormack.)

A faster and more sophisticated machine was built, beginning in August 1970. Scanning time was reduced to 4¼ min. Data processing time was decreased to 20 min (after completion of the scan) and subsequently decreased further to several minutes following the incorporation of a minicomputer into the system. The patient's head was positioned within a water bag in the scanner to eliminate abrupt changes in x-ray attenuation going from air to the head. The scanning motion consisted of 180 synchronous linear translations of the x-ray source and detector, each new translation or projection being obtained after a 1° rotation.

In conjunction with James Ambrose, a consultant radiologist at Atkinson Morley's Hospital, Hounsfield demonstrated a tumor in a preserved specimen of human brain. The first machine for clinical trials was installed at Atkinson Morley's Hospital in 1971. Units were first installed in the United States at the Mayo Clinic and at the Massachusetts General Hospital in 1973.

Ledley and the ACTA Whole Body Scanner

Robert S. Ledley and his staff at the National Biomedical Research Foundation, an affiliate of the Georgetown University Medical Center, built the first whole body scanner, which they introduced in 1974. The unit was called the ACTA (Automatic Computerized Transverse Axial) scanner. This unit was capable of examining every part of the human body. The water bag that had been incorporated into the first head scanner was eliminated in the body scanner. Developments in the mathematics of the reconstruction process permitted the use of a new method of image reconstruction, or algorithm, based on a technique called convolution. An image could be displayed almost immediately after the scanning was completed. In addition, a larger matrix was used to display the body sections. One complete scan was capable of producing pictures of two adjacent cross-sections.

The principles and techniques related to these early computed tomographic units are described in the next chapter.

Awards

In 1972 Hounsfield received the MacRobert Award, presented by the Council of Engineering Institutions for successful technological innovation contributing to the national prestige and prosperity of the United Kingdom. In 1975 Hounsfield and Oldendorf shared the Albert and Mary Lasker Award for Clinical Research, and in 1979 Cormack and Hounsfield shared the Nobel Prize in Physiology or Medicine for their contributions to the development of computed tomography.

REFERENCES AND SUGGESTED READINGS

Conventional Tomography

Andrews, J. R. Planigraphy. I. Introduction and history. American Journal of Roentgenology 26:575–587, 1936.

Andrews, J. R., and Stava, R. J. Planigraphy. II. Mathematical analyses of the methods, description of apparatus, and experimental proof. American Journal of Roentgenology 38:145–151, 1937.

Brecker, R., and Brecker, E. The Rays: A History of Radiology in the United States and Canada, Chap. 19, pp. 258–263. Williams & Wilkins, Baltimore, 1969.

Christensen, E. E., Curry, T. S., and Dowdey, J. E. An Introduction to the Physics of Diagnostic Radiology, 2nd Ed., Chap. 18, pp. 249–267. Lea & Febiger, Philadelphia, 1978.

Crysler, W. E. Tomoscopy and related matters. American Journal of Roentgenology 109:619–623, 1970.

Kieffer, J. T. The laminagraph and its variations: Applications and implications of the planigraphic principles. American Journal of Roentgenology 39:497–513, 1938.

Kieffer, J. T. Analysis of laminagraphic motions and their values. Radiology 33:560–585, 1939.

Littleton, J. T. A visual examination of laminagraphic systems. American Journal of Roentgenology 91:1153–1162, 1964.

Littleton, J. T. A phantom method to evaluate the clinical effectiveness of a tomographic device. American Journal of Roentgenology 108:847–856, 1970.

Littleton, J. T. Tomography: Physical Principles and Clinical Applications. Williams & Wilkins, Baltimore, 1976.

Littleton, J. T., Rumbaugh, C. L., and Winter, F. S. Polydirectional body section roentgenology. A new diagnostic method. American Journal of Roentgenology 89:1179–1193, 1963.

Littleton, J. T., and Winter, F. S. Linear laminagraphy. A simple geometric interpretation of its clinical limitations. American Journal of Roentgenology 95:981–991, 1965.

Moore, S. Body-section radiography. Radiology 33:605–614, 1939.

Sprawls, P. The Physical Principles of Diagnostic Radiology, Chap. 21, pp. 271–284. University Park Press, Baltimore, 1977.

Stedman's Medical Dictionary, 23rd Ed. Williams & Wilkins, Baltimore, 1976.

Ziedses des Plantes, B. G. Body-section radiography: History, image formation, various techniques and results. Australasian Radiology 15:57–64, 1931.

Computed Tomography

Ambrose, J. Computerized transverse axial scanning (tomography). Part II. Clinical application. British Journal of Radiology 46:1023–1047, 1973.

Bracewell, R. N. Strip integration in radio astronomy. Australian Journal of Physics 9:198–217, 1956.

Bull, J. History of computed tomography. In T. H. Newton and D. G. Potts (eds.), Radiology of the Skull and Brain: Technical Aspects of Computed Tomography, Vol. 5, pp. 3835–3849. C. V. Mosby, St. Louis, 1981.

Cormack, A. M. Representation of a function by its line integrals, with some radiological applications. Journal of Applied Physics 34:2722–2727, 1963.

Cormack, A. M. Representation of a function by its line integrals, with some radiologic applications. II. Journal of Applied Physics 35:2908–2913, 1964.

Cormack, A. M. Reconstruction of densities from their projections, with applications in radiological physics. Physics in Medicine and Biology 18:195–207, 1973.

Cormack, A. M. Early two-dimensional reconstruction (CT scanning) and recent topics stemming from it. Nobel Lecture, December 8, 1979. Journal of Computer Assisted Tomography 4:658–664, 1980.

DeRosier, D. J., and Klug, A. Reconstruction of three dimensional structures from electron micrographs. Nature 217:130–134, 1968.

Di Chiro, G., and Brooks, R. A. The 1979 Nobel Prize in Physiology or Medicine. Journal of Computer Assisted Tomography 4:241–245, 1980.

Gilbert, P. Iterative methods for the three-dimensional reconstruction of an object from projections. Journal of Theoretical Biology 36:105–117, 1972.

Gilbert, P. F. C. The reconstruction of a three-dimensional structure from projections and its application to electron microscopy. II. Direct methods. Proceedings of the Royal Society of London 182:89–102, 1972.

Gordon, R., Bender, R., and Herman, G. T. Algebraic reconstruction techniques (ART) for three-dimensional electron microscopy and x-ray photography. Theoretical Biology 29:471–481, 1970.

Hounsfield, G. N. Computerized transverse axial scanning (tomography): Part I. Description of system. British Journal of Radiology 46:1016–1022, 1973.

Hounsfield, G. N. Historical notes on computerized axial tomography. Journal of the Canadian Association of Radiologists 27:135–142, 1976.

Hounsfield, G. N. Computed medical imaging. Nobel Lecture, December 8, 1979. Journal of Computer Assisted Tomography 4:665–674, 1980.

Kuhl, D. E., and Edwards, R. Q. Image separation radioisotope scanning. Radiology 80:653–661, 1963.

Kuhl, D. E., and Edwards, R. Q. Reorganizing data from transverse scans of the brain using digital processing. Radiology 91:975–983, 1968.

Ledley, R. S., Di Chiro, G., Lussenhop, A. J., and Twigg, H. L. Computerized transaxial x-ray tomography of the human body. Science 186:207–212, 1974.

McCullough, E. C., Baker, H. L., Houser, O. W., and Reese, D. F. An evaluation of the quantitative and radiation features of a scanning x-ray transverse axial tomograph: The EMI scanner. Radiology 111:709–715, 1974.

New, P. F. J., and Scott, W. R. Historical background. In Computed Tomography of the Brain and Orbit (EMI Scanning), Chap. 1, pp. 3–6. Williams & Wilkins, Baltimore, 1975.

New, P. F. J., Scott, W. R., Schnur, J. A., Davis, K. R., and Taveras, J. M. Computerized axial tomography with the EMI scanner. Radiology 110:109–123, 1974.

Oldendorf, W. H. Isolated flying spot detection of radiodensity discontinuities—Displaying the internal structural pattern of a complex object. IEEE Transactions on Bio-Medical Electronics, Volume BMW 8:68–72, 1961.

Oldendorf, W. H. The quest for an image of brain: A brief historical and technical review of brain imaging techniques. Neurology 28:517–533, 1978.

Oldendorf, W. H. The Quest for an Image of Brain. Raven Press, New York, 1980.

Radon, J. On the determination of functions from their integrals along certain manifolds. Gerichte über die Verhandlungen der königlich Sächsischen Gesellschaft der Wissenschaften zu Leipzig. Mathematisch-Physiche Klasse 69:262–277, 1917.

Smith, P. R., Peters, T. M., and Bates, R. H. T. Image reconstruction from finite numbers of projections. Journal of Physics. A. Mathematical, Nuclear and General 6:361–382, 1973.

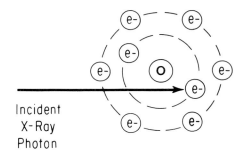

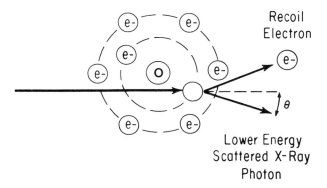

Figure 2.3. The Compton effect. An electron in the atom recoils but receives only part of the energy of the incident x-ray photon. The incident photon is scattered out of its original path, carrying away a lower energy than previously. The Compton effect occurs in loosely bound electrons, that is, those in outer (low energy) shells or in the inner shells of smaller atoms where the binding energy is considerably less than the incident photon energy.

The Compton effect was first observed and explained in the early 1920s by the American physicist Arthur Holly Compton, who received the Nobel Prize in Physics for this work in 1927.

Several general rules, which can be demonstrated mathematically, describe the end results of a Compton interaction:

1. The greater the angular deviation (the angle θ) of the deflected photon, the greater the fraction of the incident photon energy that is transferred to the electron.
2. Compton interactions are more probable for lower energy photons; probability decreases with higher energy.
3. The smaller the energy of the incident photon, the more likely the photon is to undergo a greater angular deflection.
4. The larger the energy of the incident photon, the greater is the absolute amount of energy and the fraction of the incident energy that is transferred from the photon to the electron at any given angle θ of photon scatter.
5. Even at a maximum angular deflection of 180°, the photon will not transfer all of its energy to the electron.

Following a Compton interaction, a positive ion, a "recoil" or Compton electron, and a scattered photon result. The "recoil" or Compton electron always goes in a generally forward direction (or 90° sideways in the limiting case, so that its range of deflection is from 0° through 90°). The scattered photon may be deflected through any angle from 0° to 180°.

The probability for a Compton interaction depends upon the electron density of the material, that is, the number of electrons per gram of material, or

$$\text{probability} \sim \text{electron density}. \qquad (2.6)$$

The Compton interaction does not depend upon the atomic number Z of the material. A Compton interaction becomes somewhat less likely with increasing energy, but the energy dependence is not nearly as dramatic as it is with the photoelectric effect.

Most of the incident photon energy is retained by the deflected photon. The deflected photon then leaves the point of interaction and may undergo another collision or exit directly from the patient. If it undergoes another Compton interaction, still only a small portion of the photon energy is actually absorbed, the rest of the energy remaining with the deflected photon, which usually exits the patient. Thus, the radiation dosage or energy absorbed by the patient is considerably less than the photoelectric effect. However, the lack of any dependence upon the atomic number provides little contrast enhancement between the different tissues. Since the difference between the electron density of different tissues does not usually vary dramatically, the difference in x-ray attenuation by the Compton effect is attributable as much or more to differences in the effective thickness (actually the thickness times the density in grams per cubic centimeter) of the tissues which the x-ray beam traverses. Furthermore, the scattered radiation that is produced and which exits the patient has two disadvantages: it constitutes a health hazard for anyone near the patient, as during fluoroscopy, and it transmits a large amount of scattered radiation to the film, which results in film darkening without concomitant information. A positive feature of the Compton effect, however, is the relatively low radiation dosage that the patient receives.

Attenuation of an X-Ray Beam As a parallel monochromatic or monoenergetic x-ray beam (one with a single energy or wavelength common to all the photons of the x-ray beam) passes through a substance of uniform density and atomic number, it is attenuated in an exponential fashion according to the equation

$$I = I_0 e^{-\mu x}, \qquad (2.7)$$

where I_0 is the incident radiation intensity (the energy passing through a unit area in a unit time), I is the intensity of the radiation after traveling a distance x through the substance, e is the natural exponent, and μ is the linear attenuation coefficient (Figure 2.4). The linear attenuation coefficient is a function of the x-ray beam photon energy, the atomic number, and the electron density of the substance.

The meaning of exponential attenuation is as follows: if the intensity after traveling a distance x_0 through the substance is equal to $.5I_0$, or .5 of the incident intensity, then after traveling a distance $2x_0$ the energy is reduced to $.5 \times .5\ I_0$, or .25 of the incident intensity (Figure 2.5). That is, each equal thickness of the substance attenuates the x-ray beam by an equal fraction or percentage. The thickness x_0 of a substance that reduces the x-ray beam intensity by one-half is called the half-value layer, or half-value thickness. The half-value layer is a function of both the substance itself and the keV or photon energy of the beam.

Equation 2.7 is actually only an approximation for two reasons. First, as discussed earlier, the attenuation of an x-ray beam is due to absorption by the photoelectric effect and absorption and scattering by the Compton effect. Each effect contributes its own exponential attenuation to the total attenuation; that is

$$I = I_0 e^{-(\mu_p + \mu_c)x} \qquad (2.8)$$

where μ_p is the linear attenuation coefficient due to the photoelectric effect and μ_c the linear attenuation

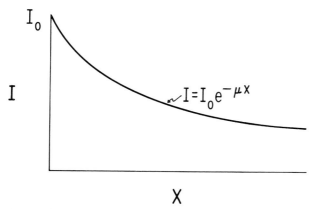

Figure 2.4. Attenuation of the intensity I (energy per unit area) is exponential and characterized by an x-ray attenuation coefficient μ, which is dependent upon the nature of the attentuating material and the kV or x-ray photon energy.

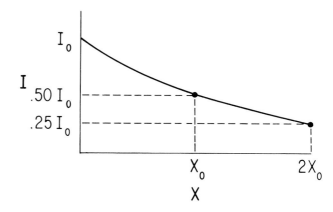

Figure 2.5. The half-value layer x_0 is the thickness of a material needed to attenuate half the incident x-ray energy.

coefficient for the Compton effect. As discussed previously for a monochromatic x-ray beam, μ_p is strongly dependent on the atomic number Z of the substance ($\sim Z^3$) and on the photon energy of the beam $\left(\sim \dfrac{1}{(\text{keV})^3}\right)$. The Compton contribution depends on electron density, not atomic number. Its dependence on keV is also less.

In addition, Equations 2.7 and 2.8 both assume a monochromatic (single energy) beam. In practice, x-ray beams are not monochromatic but polychromatic (containing a range of energies). The most nearly monochromatic x-ray sources are associated with radioactive isotopes and not with x-ray tubes. Each different energy component in a polychromatic beam is exponentially attenuated with its own attenuation coefficient in a given material. Since the softer x-rays or lower energy photons are absorbed preferentially compared to higher energy photons (due to greater photoelectric absorption), the remaining penetrating capability of the beam increases as it passes through a material. The x-ray beam is said to become harder. Another way of stating this is that the half-value thickness becomes larger as a function of distance into the substance. The effect may be reduced by prehardening the beam by initially filtering it, usually through a few millimeters of aluminum, removing many of the softer x-rays before the beam enters the substance. Polychromaticity of the x-ray beam is an intrinsic property of the production mechanism with x-ray units. To further enhance the homogeneity of the beam, the kilovoltage of the x-ray tube may be smoothed by the use of three phase generators followed by ripple filters.

Thus, Equation 2.7 is best approximated in practice for a well filtered beam and at relatively low or high values of keV where either the photoelectric or Compton effect greatly predominates. The attenuation as a function of tissue density and average atomic number is illustrated in Figure 2.6.

In computed radiography it is more convenient to think in terms of the number of photons N that will pass through the small portion of the body being irradiated during the time of a single measurement. In this case, Equation 2.7 takes the form

$$N = N_0 e^{-\mu x} \qquad (2.9)$$

where N_0 is the incident number of photons, N is the number of photons after a given path length x, and μ is the linear attenuation coefficient for the substance. As described, $\mu = \mu_p + \mu_c$.

If the density or the atomic number of the substance is not homogeneous along the path of the x-ray beam, then the object may be divided into small elements, each characterized by its own linear attenuation coefficient (Figure 2.7).

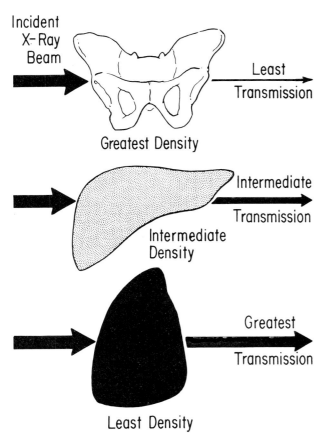

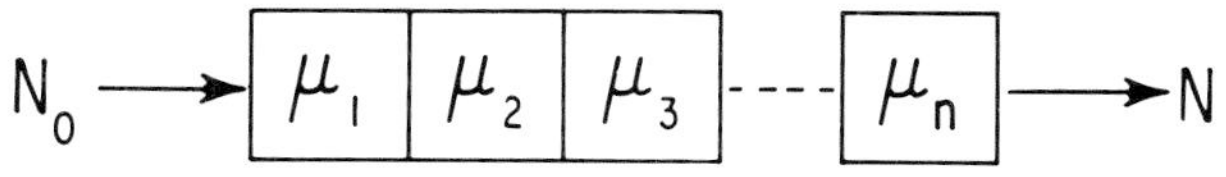

Figure 2.7. N_0, initial incident photons are attenuated by each portion or small volume of material through which the incident x-ray beam passes. Each subvolume is characterized by its own specific x-ray attenuation coefficient.

INTRODUCTION TO COMPUTED TOMOGRAPHY

Requirements for Computed Tomography

The purpose of CT is the reconstruction or synthesis of an image that faithfully reproduces the internal anatomy of a transverse cross-section (or slice) of the body (Figure 2.8). A large quantity of data is collected which represents the attenuation of a finely collimated x-ray beam passing at multiple angles through all points within the particular cross-section being imaged. This assembly of data is processed by a computer. Incorporated within the computer program is an algorithm, or procedure for reconstructing an image of the slice by performing a series of mathematical operations which may be repetitive. The final product is an array of numbers, each of which represents the linear x-ray attenuation coefficient in a small volume element within the appropriate tissue slice. Appropriate display devices can then portray each of these small volume elements in some shade of gray or color related to its attenuation coefficient. The composite of all these volume elements represents the image of the anatomical cross-section.

The significant features that permit the acquisition of data and reconstruction of these data into a synthesized cross-sectional image by CT are: 1) a finely collimated or pencil x-ray beam, which greatly reduces scatter to the detector system and which permits serial measurements of x-ray attenuation by individual small cores of tissue; 2) very sensitive signal-to-noise detectors, which allow small (.5–5%) differences in the attenuation of the x-ray beam through the various cores of tissue to be detected and recorded; 3) detectors which can be "refreshed" and used nearly continuously for multiple different measurements of x-ray beam intensity; 4) an algorithm included within the computer program for handling the large quantity of data acquired through the scanning procedure and reconstructing these data into a synthesized image; 5) a computer which processes the data by performing calculations specified by the algorithm in order to determine the linear x-ray attenuation coefficient for each separate volume ele-

Figure 2.6. Denser materials are characterized by a greater attenuation of the incident x-ray beam for a given thickness of material and therefore a larger decrease in the intensity of the transmitted beam.

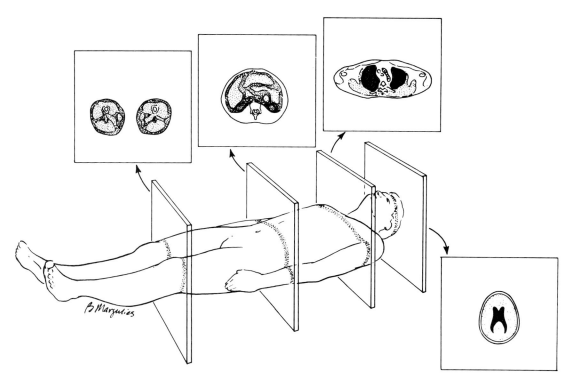

Figure 2.8. True tomographic images should demonstrate single sections of desired thickness through the body or head without interference or loss of detail from adjacent sections.

ment within the tissue slice; 6) a display system which allows the attenuation coefficients to be portrayed in varying shades of gray. There should be an accompanying photographic system for making hard copy images. In addition, the display image should be continuously variable so that the gray scale features may be altered to enhance their potential diagnostic features. Each of these requirements is discussed in detail below.

The Matrix, the Pixel, and the Voxel

A matrix can be defined as a rectangular array of elements arranged in rows and columns (Figure 2.9). Each element (or address or location) in the matrix will have a number associated with it. The matrix itself has no physical dimensions. The term matrix size denotes the number of rows and columns. For example, an 80 × 120 matrix is one with 80 rows and 120 columns. A square matrix is a special case in which the number of rows is equal to the number of columns. The total number of elements is equal to the number of rows multiplied by the number of columns, and is 9,600 for an 80 × 120 matrix.

An alternative concept is that a matrix is formed by arrays of equally spaced horizontal and vertical lines which are combined to form a cross-hatched grid (Figure 2.10). Again, the matrix does not itself have physical dimensions. The intersecting grills form individual matrix elements. The size of the matrix is the number of elements in a column multiplied by the number of elements in a row. If these are equal, the matrix is a square. Since the vertical

14	6	17	-12	28	17
-1	-8	0	2	-9	-41
72	6	18	13	12	17
-6	-8	42	7	9	43
-4	3	-20	-2	-17	18
-28	33	5	-14	2	83

Figure 2.9. A square matrix of numbers (number of columns equals number of rows).

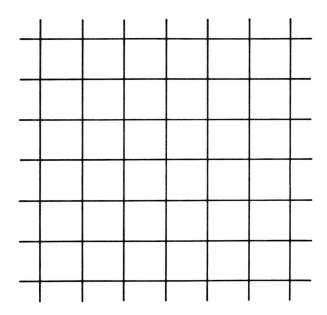

Figure 2.10. Horizontal and vertical arrays superimposed to form a matrix grid.

and horizontal lines are equally spaced, each element has the form of a square. The individual elements are termed pixels (short for picture elements; Figure 2.11).

The two definitions can be related to each other by supposing that each square element in a matrix grid is associated with or represented by a number (Figure 2.12).

A matrix grid can be superimposed on a tissue cross-section or slice (Figure 2.13). Each element or pixel of the matrix represents or covers a small portion of the total tissue cross-section. If a matrix of a given size (e.g., 320 × 320) is superimposed on a

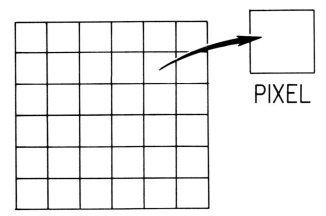

Figure 2.11. A single element or pixel of the grid characterized by its area and position in the grid. The individual pixels shown are all square and equal in area.

14	6	17	-12	28	17
-1	-8	0	2	-9	-41
72	6	18	13	12	17
-6	-8	42	7	9	43
-4	3	-20	-2	-17	18
-28	33	5	-14	2	83

Figure 2.12. With each pixel in this matrix grid is an associated number.

cross-section of fixed area (e.g., 48 × 48 cm), then each pixel represents a small area within the cross-section (e.g., 1.5 × 1.5 mm, obtained by dividing 48 cm × 48 cm by 320). This is illustrated in Figure 2.14. Since the tissue slice has a finite thickness or depth (Figure 2.15), it can be thought of as composed of individual volume elements, termed voxels (Figure

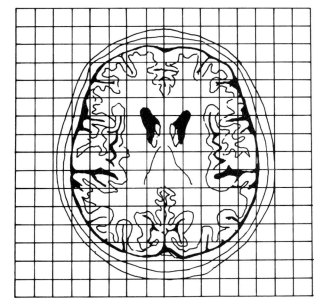

Figure 2.13. The matrix grid can be superimposed on an anatomical cross-section. The location of each pixel now corresponds to a specific small area of the cross-section.

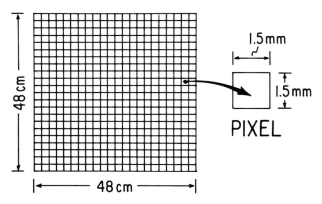

Figure 2.14. The area of the matrix grid and the number of elements in the grid together determine the area of each pixel.

2.16). Each voxel is seen to be a small box whose cross-sectional area corresponds to that of a pixel and whose depth corresponds to the tissue slice thickness (Figure 2.17). The purpose of computation in CT is the calculation of the linear x-ray attenuation coefficient associated with each of these voxels and optimum display of this information.

The Table and Gantry

In all units the patient is placed on a table or bed that is mechanically aligned in a large scanning gantry which contains the x-ray tube and detectors (Figure 2.18). The tube and detector must be maintained in perfect alignment. Within the gantry, there is a central aperture (or tunnel) through which the table and patient can be advanced. A plane through the middle of this aperture and parallel to the gantry represents the scanning plane. Many units allow a certain amount of angulation of this plane relative to the horizontal axis or table bed. This angulation of the scanning plane from the vertical is typically up to 20° (Figure 2.19). This allows scanning of off-axial planes through the patient. In addition, further obliquity of the scanning plane away from an axial or transverse plane may be obtained by positioning the patient obliquely within the scanner. For example, coronal sections through the head can be obtained by extension of the head with appropriate tilting of the gantry (Figure 2.20). With relatively larger gantry apertures, the patient's body may be placed in an oblique position, allowing scanning planes to be obtained that are at significant obliquities to the transverse plane. Particularly in pediatric patients, it may be possible to obtain near coronal or sagittal planes directly by appropriate positioning of the patient within a large aperture.

A portion of the area of the aperture represents the field of view, or the area that is to be reconstructed. A particular unit may allow areas of different sizes to be reconstructed within the aperture. In the case of a relatively small head within a relatively large aperture, it is desirable not to spend time and computational effort or experience a loss of resolution in reconstructing the region outside of the head.

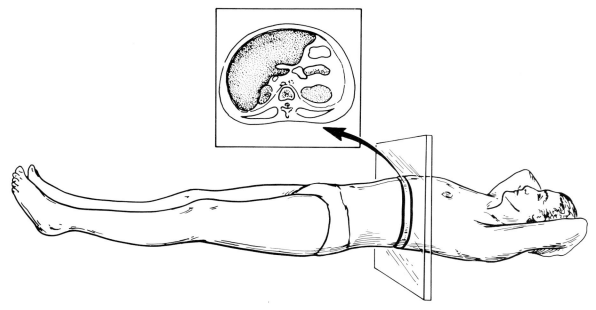

Figure 2.15. An anatomical cross-section which is imaged will have a finite thickness. A section or slice of zero thickness would not contain any tissue to attenuate x-rays.

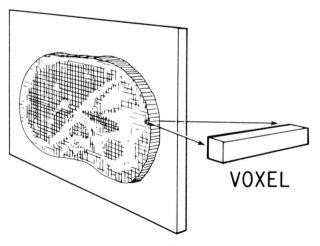

Figure 2.16. Allowing for its thickness or depth, an element of the matrix grid has a volume. The volume element or voxel has an area corresponding to a pixel and a depth which is the thickness of the tissue cross-section.

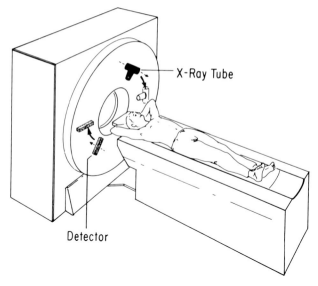

Figure 2.18. The motions of the x-ray tube and detector in the gantry are shown.

Generations of Scanners

The term "generation" is used in CT to describe successively commercially available types of scanners utilizing different modes of scanning motion and x-ray detection. More specifically, each generation is characterized by a particular geometry of scanning motion, scanning time, shape of the x-ray beam, and detector system. No single one of these features bestows a definite superiority on one generation in comparison to the others.

The first generation, typified by the original EMI Mark I head scanner and the first whole body scanner, the ACTA scanner, utilizes a single pencil x-ray beam and a single scintillation crystal-photomultiplier tube detector for each tomographic slice (Figure 2.21A). After a single linear motion or traversal of the x-ray tube and detector, during which time 160 x-ray attenuation or detector readings are typically taken, the x-ray tube and detector are rotated through 1° and another linear scan is performed. This is repeated typically 180 times.

A second generation of devices was developed to shorten the scanning time by gathering data more quickly. In these units a modified fan beam in which

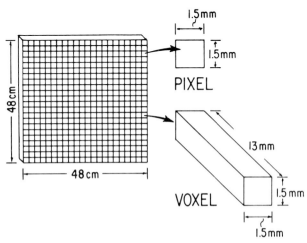

Figure 2.17. The voxel size (1.5 × 1.5 × 13 mm) is illustrated for a 320 × 320 element matrix for a cross-sectional area of 48 × 48 cm and a thickness of 13 mm.

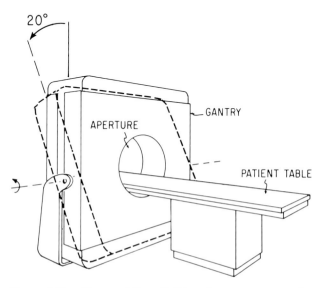

Figure 2.19. The capability of tilting the gantry to examine oblique cross-sections is illustrated. Here the tilt is 20°.

Translational-Rotational Systems   29

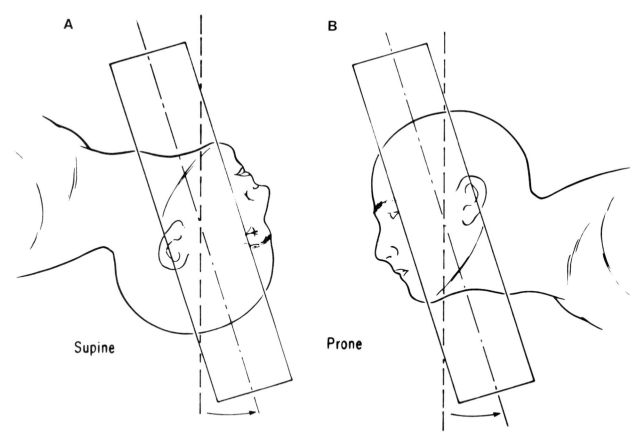

Figure 2.20. A coronal section may be obtained with the patient in either the supine (*A*) or prone (*B*) position by extension of the patient's head and appropriate tilting of the gantry.

anywhere from three (Technicare Delta 50 and Delta 100 series) to 52 (Elscint Exel 905) individual collimated x-ray beams and an equal number of detectors are used. Individual beams resemble the single beam of a first generation scanner. However, a collection of from three to 52 of these beams contiguous to one another allows multiple adjacent cores of tissue to be examined simultaneously (Figure 2.21*B*). The configuration of these contiguous cores of tisue resembles a fan, with the thickness of the fan material determined by the collimation of the beam and in turn determining the slice thickness. Because of the angular difference of each beam relative to the others, several different angular views through the body slice are being examined simultaneously. Superimposed on this is a linear translation or scan of the tube and detectors through the body slice. Thus, at the end of a single translational scan, during which time 160 readings may be made by each detector, the total number of readings obtained is equal to the number of detectors times 160. The angular rotation can be significantly larger than with a first generation unit, up to as much as 36°. Thus, the number of distinct

rotations of the scanning apparatus can be significantly reduced, with a coincidental reduction in scanning time. By gathering more data per translation, fewer translations are needed.

To obtain even faster scanning times it is necessary to eliminate the complex translational-rotational motion of the first two generations. Third generation scanners therefore use a much wider fan beam. In fact, the angle of the beam may be wide enough to encompass most or all of an entire patient section without a linear translation of the tube and detectors. As in the first two generations, the detectors, now in the form of a large array, are rigidly aligned relative to the x-ray beam, and there are no translational motions at all. The tube and detector array is synchronously rotated about the patient through an angle of 180–360° (usually 360°; Figure 2.21*C*). Thus, there is only one type of motion, allowing a much faster scanning time to be achieved. After one rotation, a single tomographic section is obtained. Scanning times with this type of apparatus may be as rapid as 2–3 s. The close spacing of the detectors, which may number from 288 (Philips To-

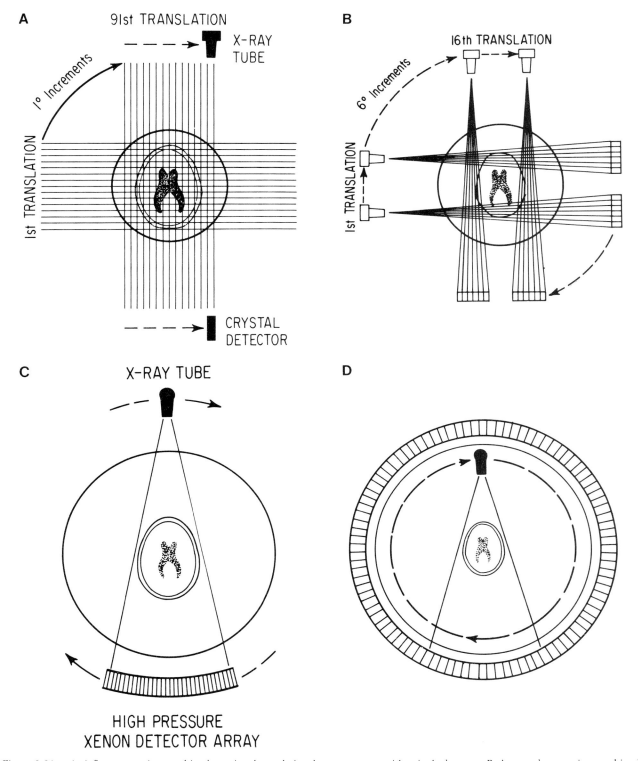

Figure 2.21. *A*, A first generation combined rotational-translational scan sequence with a single detector. *B*, A second generation combined rotational-translational scan sequence with multiple detectors. *C*, A third generation scan sequence in which the x-ray tube and detectors (typically high pressure gas cells) both rotate about the patient. *D*, A fourth generation scan sequence in which there is a circle of fixed detectors and a rotating x-ray tube.

moscan 300) to 1,024 (CGR Ce 10000) in an array, necessitates, however, the use of a different type of detector system than is used in the other scanners. Typically, high pressure inert gas ionization chambers have been used for the detection of the x-ray beam intensity. Another approach (Siemens Somatom 2) uses an array of small closely spaced cesium iodide (CsI) crystals with photodiodes to provide amplification.

Fourth generation scanners feature a wide fan beam similar to the third generation scanner. As before, the x-ray tube rotates through 360° without having to make any translational motions. However, unlike in the other scanners, the detectors are not aligned rigidly relative to the x-ray beam. In this system only the tube rotates. A large ring of detectors, typically from 360 (Picker Synerview 300) to as many as 2,400 (Pfizer PZ-2400) are fixed in an outer circle in the scanning plane (Figure 2.21D). The necessity of rotating only the tube, but not the detectors, allows potentially faster scanning time, as little as 1 s (Picker Synerview 300 and Synerview 600). In addition, the wider spacing between the x-ray detectors permits the utilization of the scintillation crystal-photomultiplier tube detectors that are also used in the first and second generation scanners.

TRANSLATIONAL-ROTATIONAL SYSTEMS: THE FIRST GENERATION

The original EMI Mark I head scanner and the ACTA 0100 (later marketed as the Pfizer 0150) total body scanner represent the first generation scanning units, which are characterized by a combination of alternate translational and rotational motions in the scanning sequence and the use of a single detector per slice for data acquisition. The concepts and mechanics typifying these units are described in detail, since the principles underlying these scanners are common to the later generations.

The X-Ray Tube

Combined translational-rotational systems generally utilize a fixed anode tube operating at a typical maximum kilovoltage (kVp) of 90–140 kV (100–140 for the Mark I and 90–120 for the ACTA). Figure 2.22 demonstrates that electrons emitted from the hot cathode are attracted by a high potential to the anode of the x-ray tube. It is this difference in electrical potential or kilovoltage that is responsible for attracting the electrons to the anode. Most of the energy (about 99%) generated in an x-ray tube in this kilovoltage range is emitted as heat. However, the accelerated electrons when striking the anode cause

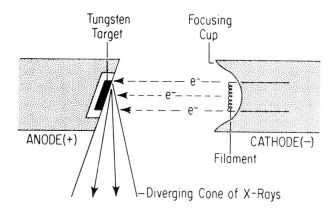

Figure 2.22. A fixed anode x-ray tube. Electrons (e^-) are accelerated through a potential difference (kVp) and strike a tungsten target, causing x-rays to be emitted.

the emission of both characteristic radiation, related the atomic properties of the tungsten anode, and bremsstrahlung (braking radiation), which is related to the fundamental electrical interaction between the incident negative electrons and the positive nuclei of the tungsten atoms. In translational-rotational units, the anode tube is fixed or stationary and the same surface of the anode is constantly being struck by the electrons. The inclination of the anode results in the selection of x-rays emitted primarily in the direction of the exit port of the tube (Figure 2.22). It also reduces the effective focal spot of the tube so that the x-ray beam is foreshortened in the direction from which it exits from the tube, and thus the beam appears to originate from a smaller area than that bombarded by electrons (Figure 2.23). In a conventional radiographic system, the x-rays diverge from a source or focus of small area in the form of a cone (Figure 2.22). In a CT unit, however, collimation of the x-ray beam at the exit assures a pencil-like configu-

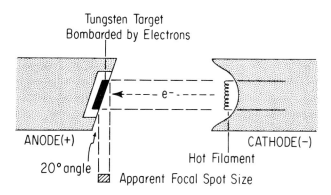

Figure 2.23. The apparent focal spot size of the tube, or area from which the x-ray photons emerge, is less than the area of the target because of the obliquity of the target to the incident electrons.

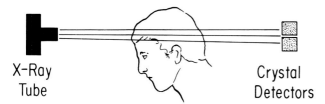

Figure 2.33. The use of one x-ray tube and two adjacent detectors to image two cross-sections simultaneously.

cores (Figure 2.34). The ACTA 0100 could make 160 or 320 such measurements during a linear translation. The resulting information of the x-ray intensity striking the detector was converted into an electrical signal, which was then digitized (converted from an analog or continuous form into a discrete form that can be handled by the computer) and stored. The location of the tissue cores as well as the electrical signals corresponding to the transmitted x-ray intensities were stored in the computer. At the end of a single linear translation, 160 or 240 discrete pieces of data were accumulated by the Mark I and either 160 or 320 pieces of data by the ACTA 0100. The entire apparatus was then rotated through 1° and the linear translational sequence was again performed. This was done for a total of 180 step rotations for the Mark I or the ACTA 0100. If 160 readings are obtained during a linear translation, then at the completion of the scan a total of 160 times 180 total pieces of data have been accumulated (Figure 2.35; see Figure 2.21A). The ACTA also had a 2° rotation mode, which reduced the scan time and patient ra-

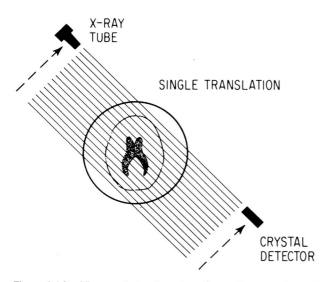

Figure 2.34. The translational motion of a single x-ray tube and detector. Measurements of the x-ray attenuation through multiple tissue cores are obtained and stored.

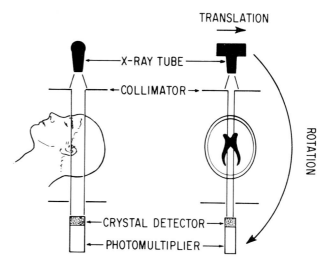

Figure 2.35. Two different views illustrating the rotation of the x-ray tube and detector in a cross-sectional plane.

diation dose by half, but yielded half as many measurements.

During each linear translation, the detector constantly intercepted the x-ray beam from the continuously emitting, stationary anode x-ray tube. The time interval during which the x-ray signal or photomultiplier output current was integrated into a single discrete measurement was predetermined by the computer program. For the ACTA 0100 this measurement interval was 4–5 ms.

TRANSLATIONAL-ROTATIONAL SYSTEMS: THE SECOND GENERATION

The second generation of CT units is characterized by a combination of translational and rotational motions in the scanning sequences and the use of a modified x-ray fan beam in conjunction with a group or array of anywhere from three to 52 detectors. The modifications of the x-ray beam and detector system allow the x-ray signals or data to be collected more rapidly. The individual detectors in the array perform simultaneous measurements of the x-ray transmission through multiple different cores of tissue. These tissue cores are adjacent to one another, but at different angular orientations, so that the collection of tissue cores examined during a single measurement forms a fan coinciding with the x-ray fan beam. Each detector in the array will examine the tissue cross-section at a different angle than the other detectors during a single translation or traversal.

For example, six detectors each collect a full set of data at six different angular orientations in one linear translation. A first generation unit would require six different translations, each separated by an angular rotation (typically 1°) to accumulate these data. Thus, the unit with six detections does not need to perform as many translations as a first generation unit, and the rotational increments between the translations can be significantly larger. Larger numbers of detectors permit more rapid data accumulation per translation, and thus fewer translations (and so fewer discrete rotations) are required.

Second generation scanners may be designated as dedicated head units (head only) or as total body scanners capable of examining the torso or the head.

The X-Ray Tube

A stationary anode tube that continuously emits x-rays is employed, just as in the first generation. Oil cooling is most commonly used. A heat exchanger, using cold water, may be utilized to remove heat from the recirculating oil. The anode-to-cathode voltage is in the range of 100–140 kV, more commonly 120–140 kV. The tube current is generally about 25–40 mA. The anode-cathode axis of the tube is typically in the plane of the image section, as in first generation units.

Collimation

After leaving the x-ray tube, the beam is collimated into a fan beam, which is further subdivided into multiple pencil beams, the number of such pencil beams being equal to the number of detectors. There is additional collimation at the detectors.

Each pencil beam is rectangular in cross-section. In the Pfizer 0200 FS, the width ranges from 1.0–1.5 mm, with a variable thickness of 5, 8, or 13 mm. As an example, the Pfizer 0200 FS collimators are constructed of an aluminum base, tungsten apertures, and tantalum sides. Tantalum, with an atomic number of 73 and a density of 16.65 g/cc, is 30–40% more dense than lead and has about the same atomic number; it therefore provides more x-ray absorption than lead.

The Detector System

Scintillation crystals and photomultipliers are used for the detector system in second as in first generation units. EMI second generation scanners (CT 1005, CT 1010, CT 5005, and EMI 7020) utilize sodium iodide, whereas the Pfizer 0200 FS uses calcium fluoride as detecting elements. Other second generation units (Elscint Exel 905; Omni 4001; Picker Synerview 120; Technicare Delta 50, Delta 50 FS, Delta 25 and Delta 100 series; and Toshiba TCT-35A) have all employed bismuth germanate (BGO) scintillation crystal detectors. Bismuth germanate has the desirable characteristics of high efficiency and no afterglow.

Increasing the number of detectors to as many as 52 increases the rate at which data samples are collected and decreases the time required for scanning. The type and number of detectors used to obtain a single slice and the fastest scan time available for different second generation commercial units are listed in Table 2.1. The table also indicates the number of slices obtained per scan as well as whether the unit is a dedicated head scanner or a total body scanner. Additional information on these units is given in Appendix III.

An additional detector, not used for data sampling, may also be incorporated as a reference detector.

Table 2.1. Features of selected second generation CT units

Company/model	Dedicated head (H) or total body (B) scanner	Type of detectors	Number of detectors per slice	Number of slices per scan	Fastest scan time (s)
Elscint Exel 905	B	BGO[a]	52	1	5.3
EMI CT 1005	H	NaI	8	2	60
EMI CT 1010	H	NaI	8	2	60
EMI CT 5005	B	NaI	30	1	20
EMI 7020	B	NaI	30	1	20
Omni 4001	H	BGO	3	2	120
Pfizer 0200 FS	B	CaF_2	30	1	19
Picker Synerview 120	B	BGO	41	1	12
Technicare Delta 50	B	BGO	3	2	120 (H) 150 (B)
Technicare Delta 50 FS	B	BGO	12	2	15 (H) 18 (B)
Technicare Delta 25	H	BGO	7	2	80
Technicare Delta 100 series	H	BGO	3	1 or 2	120
Toshiba TCT-35A	H	BGO	8	1	105

[a] BGO, bismuth germanate.

Number of Slices per Scan

Several units have the capability of obtaining two slices or sections during a single scanning sequence (Table 2.1).

Scanning Sequence

The scanning sequence for a second generation unit with a six-detector array was illustrated in Figure 2.21B). Six different angular orientations are examined in each linear translation. After completion of a translation, there is a 6° angular incrementation of the x-ray tube and detectors. The incremental angle of rotation is approximately equal to the fan angle. Another translational motion is then performed, and data are obtained for six additional angular orientations. This is repeated through approximately 180° of rotation. In this example, scanning through 180° would require 30 translations and 15 angular incrementations.

The number of data samples obtained is equal to the number of detectors times the number of measurements per detector during a translation times the number of translations. The same number of data samples could be obtained by doubling the number of detectors and halving the number of translations (with a concomitant decrease in the number of angular incrementations).

ADDITIONAL CONCEPTS AND FUNDAMENTALS OF COMPUTED TOMOGRAPHY

The Ray, the Ray-Sum, and the Profile

Definitions for the First Generation Units

Ideally, a ray represents a straight line path (ray-path) from the x-ray tube to the detector through the tissue slice (Figure 2.36). Practically, a ray encompasses that portion of the x-ray beam travelling from the tube to the detector (Figure 2.37). In the first generation the ray includes all of the beam within a core of tissue between the x-ray tube and the detector examined

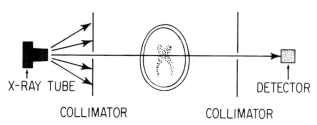

Figure 2.36. Theoretically, a ray is a single straight line path of an x-ray beam. It has no cross-sectional area.

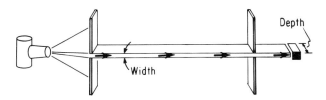

Figure 2.37. In practice, a ray does have an area, that of the x-ray beam measured by a single detector.

during a single measurement (a single data sample or integrated signal from the transmitted x-ray beam).

A ray-sum is the total x-ray attenuation, as measured by the detector, of a ray as it passes from the x-ray tube through the tissue slice to the detector (Figure 2.38). The value of the ray-sum is the result of the summated attenuations by each voxel through which the ray passes. The measured value of the ray-sum is thus related to the summated values of the linear attenuation coefficients in each of the voxels in the path of the ray. The ray-sum may be regarded as a single x-ray signal or data sample. A ray-sum is obtained or measured for each ray during a translation.

A profile is the collection of ray-sums accumulated during a single linear translation in a first generation scanner. Each translation results in the acquisition of a new profile. A profile is also referred to as a view or a projection.

The total number of data samples or measurements obtained during a scan is given by the following equation:

$$\text{total number of data samples} = \text{number of translations} \times \text{number of data samples per translation}. \quad (2.10)$$

Since the number of translations is equal to the number of profiles, and the number of data samples per

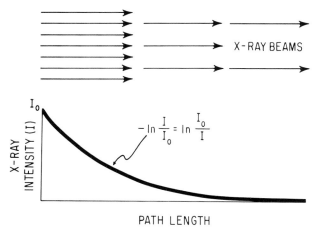

Figure 2.38. The ray-sum is a measurement of the x-ray beam attenuation.

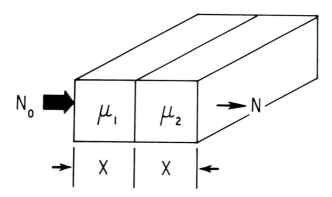

Figure 2.39. Each voxel is characterized by a different x-ray attenuation coefficient μ related to the attenuation of the x-ray beam, or incident photons, passing through the volume of the voxel.

translation is equal to the number of rays per translation (or equivalently the number of rays per profile), Equation 2.10 may be rewritten:

$$\text{total number of data samples} = \text{number of profiles} \times \text{number of rays per profile}. \quad (2.11)$$

Mathematical Illustration for the First Generation The attenuation of N_0 x-ray photons passing through a voxel with a linear attenuation coefficient μ_1 will result in N transmitted photons by Equation 2.9:

$$N = N_0 e^{-\mu_1 x},$$

where x is the voxel width or pixel dimension. If the ray then passes through a second voxel with linear attenuation coefficient μ_2 (Figure 2.39), the number N of transmitted photons will be

$$N = (N_0 e^{-\mu_1 x}) e^{-\mu_2 x} = N_0 e^{-(\mu_1 + \mu_2)x}. \quad (2.12)$$

For 160 successive voxels (Figure 2.40), each with its own attenuation coefficient, the number N of transmitted photons will be

$$N = N_0 e^{-(\mu_1 + \mu_2 + \cdots + \mu_{160})x}. \quad (2.13)$$

Considering the attenuation of two rays in both the vertical and horizontal directions for four voxels (Figure 2.41):

$$\begin{aligned} N_1 &= N_0 e^{-(\mu_1 + \mu_2)x} \\ N_2 &= N_0 e^{-(\mu_3 + \mu_4)x} \\ N_3 &= N_0 e^{-(\mu_1 + \mu_3)x} \\ N_4 &= N_0 e^{-(\mu_2 + \mu_4)x} \end{aligned} \quad (2.14)$$

For a larger array (Figure 2.42) an even greater number of equations will be obtained.

$$\begin{aligned} N_1 &= N_0 e^{-(\mu_{1,1} + \mu_{1,2} + \cdots + \mu_{1,160})x} \\ N_2 &= N_0 e^{-(\mu_{2,1} + \mu_{2,2} + \cdots + \mu_{2,160})x} \\ &\vdots \\ N_{160} &= N_0 e^{-(\mu_{160,1} + \mu_{160,2} + \cdots + \mu_{160,160})x} \\ N_{161} &= N_0 e^{-(\mu_{1,1} + \mu_{2,1} + \cdots + \mu_{160,1})x} \\ &\vdots \\ N_{320} &= N_0 e^{-(\mu_{1,160} + \mu_{2,160} + \cdots + \mu_{160,160})x} \end{aligned} \quad (2.15)$$

If the attenuation of oblique rays (those other than the horizontal and vertical rays) is examined, then the number of equations can exceed the total number of voxels. Since the number of unknowns (the individual linear attenuation coefficients μ in each voxel) is equal to the number of voxels, the equations can be solved for the linear attenuation coefficients of the different voxels.

The ray-sum can be defined mathematically as

$$-\ln(N/N_0) = (\mu_1 + \mu_2 + \cdots + \mu_n)x$$
$$= \ln(N_0/N), \quad (2.16)$$

where μ_1 through μ_n are the linear attenuation coefficients of each voxel through which the ray has passed, ln the natural logarithm, N_0 the number of

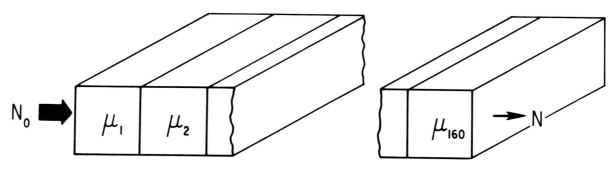

Figure 2.40. Multiple voxels, each characterized by an attenuation coefficient μ.

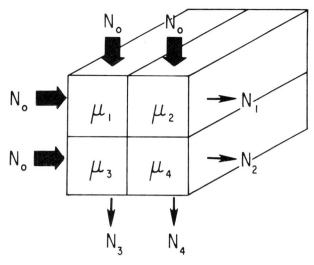

Figure 2.41. The incident photons are attenuated differently along the various paths the x-ray beam traverses. This is determined by the number and attenuation coefficients of the voxels in each path.

incident photons, N the number of transmitted photons, and x the voxel width or pixel size. The quantity $\ln(N_0/N)$, or equivalently $\ln(I_0/I)$, where I_0 and I represent the incident and transmitted x-ray intensity, respectively, along the ray, is measured by the detector. Therefore, knowing the measured values of all the ray-sums, the linear attenuation coefficients can be calculated for all the voxels.

In the first generation unit with a single detector per slice, the profile is the continuous graph or curve of values representing the ray-sums over a single linear traversal of the tube and beam as it scans through the patient once (Figure 2.43). After a rotation of the tube and beam through approximately 1° a second series of ray-sums or another profile or projection is obtained.

Definitions for Second Generation Units A ray is defined in exactly the same way in the second generation units as in the first generation. Theoretically, the path from the x-ray tube to each detector defines a different ray-path and ray. Practically, the ray encompasses that portion of the x-ray beam traveling from the tube to a single detector. It includes all of the beam within the core of tissue between the x-ray tube and a single detector examined during a

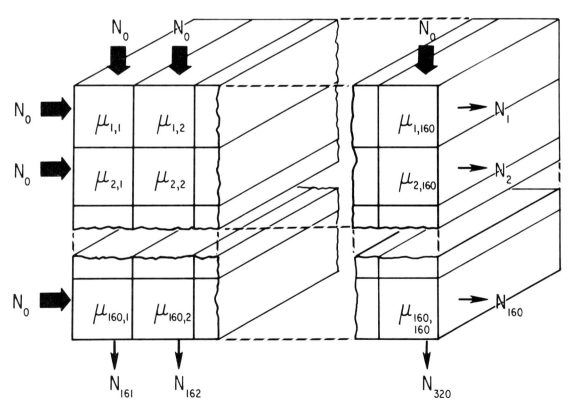

Figure 2.42. Multiple measurements are made as the x-ray beam passes through different series of voxels. This is illustrated for a 160 × 160 array of voxels.

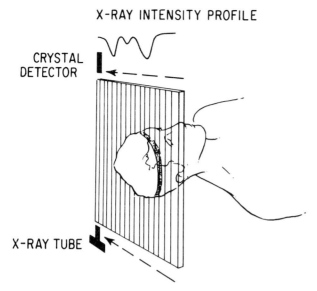

Figure 2.43. The profile is the curve or series of x-ray transmission measurements made through different cores of tissue in a single linear traverse.

single measurement (a single data sample or integrated signal from the transmitted x-ray beam).

A ray-sum is defined as for first generation units as the experimentally measured total x-ray attenuation of a ray. A profile in second generation units is the collection of ray-sums (data samples) accumulated by one detector during a single translation. Thus, during a translation the number of profiles obtained is equal to the number of detectors. Another translation results in the accumulation of a new set of profiles equal in number to the number of detectors. The total number of profiles is therefore equal to the number of detectors times the number of translations. By this definition, a profile is simply the collection of measurements or data samples obtained by one detector at one angle, and it is equivalent to the definition of a profile for first generation units.

The total number of data samples or measurements obtained is given by the equation:

total number of data samples =
number of data samples per translation × (2.17)
number of translations,

or, equivalently,

total number of data samples =
number of data samples per detector per translation ×
number of detectors × (2.18)
number of translations.

The number of data samples per detector per translation is equivalent to the number of rays per detector per translation, or the number of rays per profile. The product of the number of detectors times the number of translations is equal to the total number of profiles accumulated during the scan, as previously discussed. Therefore, Equation 2.18 can be rewritten as:

total number of data samples =
number of rays per profile × (2.19)
number of profiles.

In first generation units only the central ray within the x-ray beam is used. The single detector is aligned to be perpendicular to this central ray. In second generation units, rays that are oblique with respect to the central ray are also used. The number of such rays transmitted through the patient is determined by the beam-forming or entrance collimation. The detectors at the ends of the array intercept the more obliquely oriented rays, that is, those rays at the greatest angle with the central ray.

The fan angle used for the x-ray beam is determined not only by the number of detectors but also by the angular spacing between the detectors, that is, the angle between the rays intercepted by adjacent detectors. The incremental angle of rotation between successive translations usually approximates the fan angle of the x-ray beam. If the rotational increment were significantly greater than the fan angle, measurements or data samples would not be obtained for those angular orientations that had been bypassed.

For the Delta 50 scanner there are three detectors with a diverging or fan angle of 2° between the three collimated pencil beams. After each linear translation, the x-ray tube and detectors undergo a 3° angular incrementation. A total of 60 translations are performed over 180°.

In the Pfizer 0200 FS there are 30 detectors. The incremented angle of rotation between translations is 20°, and this approximates the fan angle. Nine translations and eight rotations are performed in scanning through 180°.

The Elscint Exel 905 has 52 detectors with an angular spacing of .7° between adjacent detectors. The total fan angle is approximately 36°. Five linear translations are performed at angular increments of about 36°, for a 180° scan.

Computer Reconstruction

Each piece of data measuring the x-ray transmission through a single core of tissue or the ray-sum is converted into an electrical signal by the scintillation crystal and photomultiplier detector system. This electrical signal, which is proportional to the transmitted x-ray intensity or ray-sum and which may vary continuously, is converted into a digital signal by an analog-to-digital converter, which transforms a continuous signal of varying amplitude into one made up of discrete, equal amplitude pulses. The spacing of these pulses describes the numerical data encoded by the amplitude of the analog signal. The data are stored within the computer memory and then, following an algorithm for performing computations, processed by the computer to yield the value of the x-ray attenuation coefficient in each individual voxel. The central role of the computer is illustrated in Figure 2.44, which presents a schematic diagram of a CT system.

The unique feature of CT that differentiates it from other diagnostic imaging modalities is the use of the computer in the actual reconstruction or synthesis of the final image. The use of the computer in diagnostic radiology is not new. Previously, however, the computer was used either in an ancillary role or in attempting to obtain further diagnostic information through computer-assisted interpretation of images already obtained by more conventional techniques. In CT, by contrast, the role of the computer is central and essential in the formation of the image. The information collected in the scanning process is formulated so that it might serve as input to the computer. The rapid computational capabilities of the computer are used to reconstruct a final diagnostic image from the input data by means of an algorithm that instructs the computer on how to manipulate the large amount of input data. In theory, the process of reconstruction tomography does not require a computer, but without the computer, it would not be practical to derive the final images.

The final product of this computer synthesis is a series of numbers, arrayed in a matrix form, each of which represents the linear attenuation coefficient expressed as an integer, called a CT number, in the corresponding voxel or volume element of the section that was scanned. As such, the data can be stored on devices such as magnetic disks or tapes. These are convenient methods of retaining the data for storage, retrieval, and further data manipulation. However, it is necessary to portray the image in a more conventional visual form in terms of a varying gray scale.

The CT Number

The linear attenuation coefficient is generally expressed as a decimal number. For example, that of water is about .19 cm^{-1} at an effective energy of 73 keV. However, this is not a particularly meaningful form to most physicians. For this reason, it has been found very convenient to express the attenuation coefficient in terms of an integer or whole number. This number is called the CT number, and is defined in the following way:

$$\text{CT number} = \frac{\mu_{\text{substance}} - \mu_{\text{water}}}{\mu_{\text{water}}} \times K \quad (2.20)$$

where K is a scale factor set as a matter of convention to equal either 500 or 1,000. This equation converts all the attenuation coefficients into integers, where the baseline or reference value of zero is assigned to the linear attenuation coefficient of water for the particular kilovoltage of the x-ray beam utilized. CT numbers that are negative in value imply an attenuation coefficient less than that of water; those that are positive imply an attenuation coefficient greater than water. Two scale factors or values of K have been utilized. The original EMI units used a constant of 500; other units have adopted a constant of 1,000. The former system is called the EMI or old Hounsfield scale and is illustrated in Figure 2.45. The factor of 1,000 is associated with the new Hounsfield system shown in Figure 2.46. Fat generally has a value of about -40 in EMI units and -80 in new Hounsfield units. The soft tissue structures of the brain and body generally have values ranging from 15–40 EMI units. Values significantly above 50 EMI units usually imply the presence of calcification. Lung tissue, because of

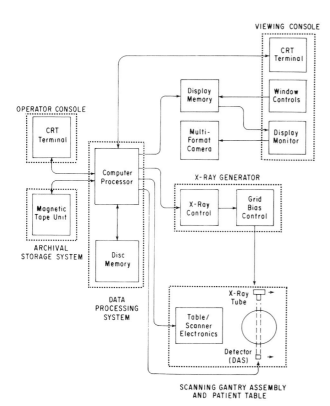

Figure 2.44. A schematic diagram of a computed tomography system. The diagram illustrates the central role played by the computer.

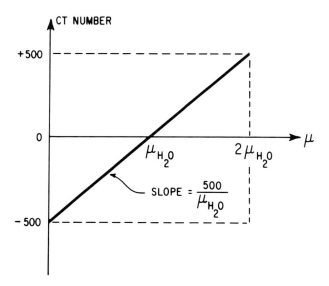

Figure 2.45. The relationship of CT numbers to the x-ray attenuation coefficient coefficient μ in old Hounsfield or EMI units.

the great amount of air it contains, usually has values in the range of -200 to -500 EMI units. Dense bone usually has values of from $+200$ to $+500$ EMI units.

The original ACTA scanner utilized a different CT number system or scale with a range of 0–2,048. This scale has been abandoned in favor of the scale described in Equation 2.20, with K set at either 500 or 1,000; in more recently manufactured units, 1,000 is most frequently used as the scale factor.

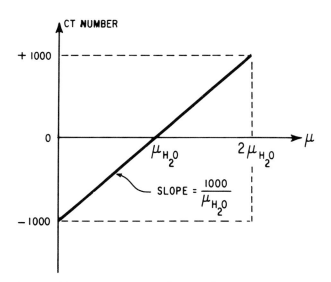

Figure 2.46. The relationship of CT numbers to the x-ray attenuation coefficient μ in new Hounsfield units.

Beam Hardening

When a homogeneous or uniformly dense object is irradiated with a monoenergetic beam of x-rays (that is, a beam in which all the x-ray photons have the same energy), the attenuation in a given thickness is always the same, irrespective of how much substance has already been traversed. However, x-ray beams used in medical diagnosis are not monochromatic but polychromatic. They contain a significant proportion of low energy x-rays, which are preferentially absorbed as the x-ray beam is transmitted. The average energy of the remaining beam thus becomes higher, and the beam more penetrating or "harder." Thus, there is relatively more absorption (and hence attenuation) of the x-ray beam on the entrance side of the object than on the exit side, causing the object to appear less dense (i.e., more transparent and less attenuating to x-rays) on the exit side of the beam.

Hardening can introduce a "cupping" artifact in the CT numbers (Figures 2.47 and 2.48). There are several ways in which this effect can be corrected. Addition filtration of the x-ray beam can be used to eliminate many of the low energy (softer) x-rays before they strike the patient. The water bag used in the original EMI Mark I scanner provided additional filtration of this kind. Other corrections can be made

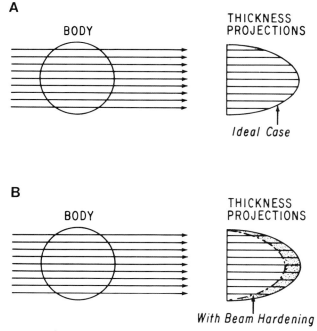

Figure 2.47. A, Ideal case of the thickness projection of a circular cross-section. B, The real situation where hardening of the x-ray beam (selective attenuation of the lower energy photons) causes cores of tissue of greater length to attenuate x-ray photons less per unit path distance as the path length increases.

Basic Principles of Computed Tomography

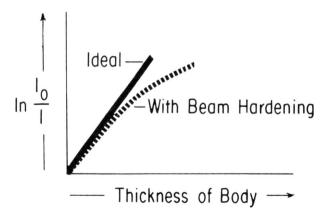

Figure 2.48. The change in apparent body thickness with uncorrected beam hardening as opposed to the ideal situation where there is no beam hardening.

utilizing the computer itself. The detector output can be "linearized" by introducing a mathematical correction based on the observed attenuation of the x-ray beam. Reference readings can be made when the x-ray beam is not passing through the object being scanned, and these readings can be used to correct the data for beam hardening.

Sampling and Data Acquisition

During the continuous translation of the x-ray tube and detector in a single linear traversal, the x-ray beam is continuously passing through the patient and striking the detector. However, measurement of the transmitted x-ray beam intensity is done only over a very short interval (for example, 4–5 ms in the ACTA scanner). During this time, the total transmitted beam energy that is detected is amplified and stored in the computer as the value of the ray-sum or transmitted x-ray beam for that measurement. For an approximate linear translational velocity for the tube and detector of about 330 mm per s, the center of the photon beam will have moved 1.6 mm during this measurement. Thus, the actual width of the tissue through which the pencil beam has passed at some time during a single measurement will actually be greater than the width of the collimator (Figure 2.29). This potential loss in resolution can be compensated by sampling at closer intervals, narrower collimation

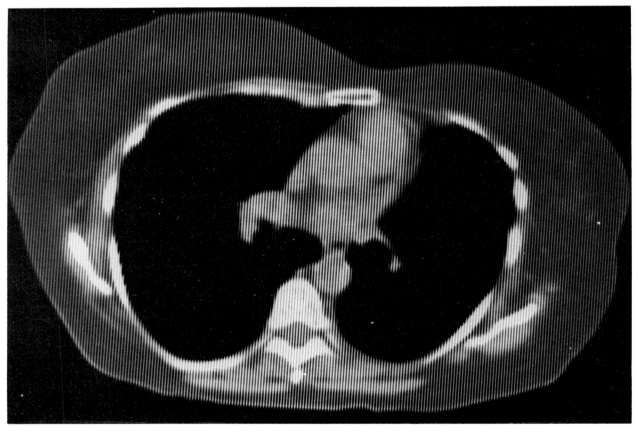

Figure 2.49. CT image of the thorax: negative mode.

of the beam, and smaller detector aperture (exit collimation to the detector).

The Gray Scale Window

In conventional radiography an abrupt transition from black to white with very few intervening shades of gray is referred to as a short gray scale and is associated with high contrast. A large number of shades of gray with a very gradual gradation from black to white indicates a long gray scale or relatively low contrast. Both radiographic techniques and the film itself contribute to the gray scale or contrast.

In CT the contrast can be significantly altered by adjustment of the assignment of the gray scale to the different CT numbers. Even the polarity of the final image is optional in CT. The image can be displayed as a negative, analogous to conventional radiography, with the bones portrayed as white and the aerated lung as black (Figure 2.49), or it can be displayed as a positive, with the bones portrayed as black and the aerated lung as white (Figure 2.50). It is an accepted convention to display the image as a negative. However, bone detail is often better displayed in a positive mode.

The CT window refers to the range of CT numbers in which the pixel elements having these CT numbers are assigned some shade of gray, but not black or white. In other words, it is the gray scale range of the image. The window width may be made large or small. Specifically, a large window width indicates that there is a relatively long gray scale range, or a large block of CT numbers that will be assigned some value of gray. Thus, the transition zone between the lower CT numbers portrayed as black and the higher CT numbers portrayed as white will be large. A narrow window width implies that the transition from black to white will take place over a relatively few CT numbers (Figure 2.51).

The window level is defined as the center of the gray scale. That is, it determines the CT number that will be assigned the medium gray shade. If it is centered at a higher CT number, such as that in bone, then structures like the lungs and soft tissues having lower CT numbers will be seen as dark gray or black in a negative display mode. Conversely, if the window level is set at a lower CT number, such as that in lung, then the soft tissues and bones will appear light gray to white in a conventional negative display

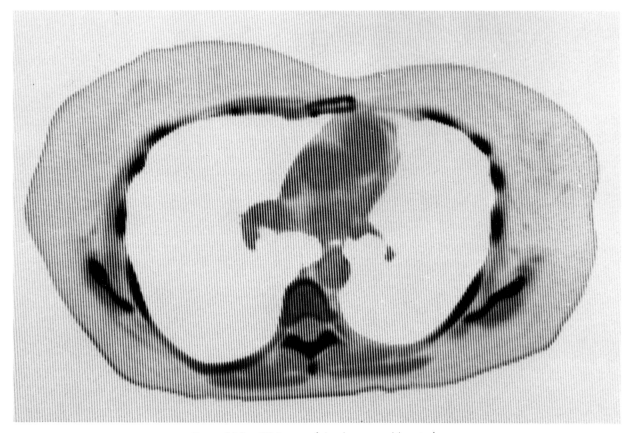

Figure 2.50. CT image of the thorax: positive mode.

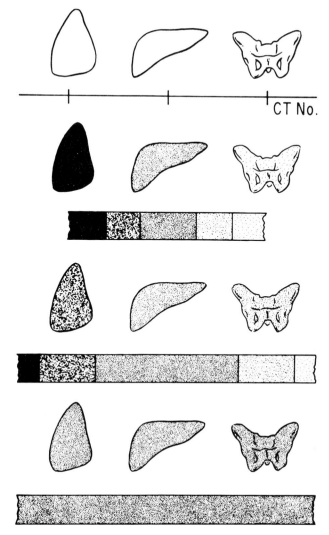

Figure 2.51. The change in the gray tone of different organs having widely different CT numbers with variation in window width.

mode. If the window level is centered at an intermediate CT number (e.g., zero), the soft tissues will appear in the middle of the gray scale, the bones will appear light gray or white, and the lungs dark gray to black (Figure 2.52).

Both the window level and width are easily adjusted by the operator to optimize the appearance of the image on the display monitor cathode ray tube. This should be done in conjunction with appropriate settings of brightness and contrast to optimize visualization of the gray scale.

If it is necessary to look at a large range of CT numbers on one image, as in the chest, then a wide gray scale is appropriate. However, if subtle changes in the density or x-ray attenuation of an organ are sought, such as might be seen in metastatic lesions within the liver, then a narrow CT window would be appropriate. If lung detail is desired, then it is probably helpful to assign a window level that is relatively low and centered in the range of lung parenchyma. If, on the other hand, bone is to be examined in detail, the window level should be centered in bone.

The significant advantages of this capability to manipulate the gray scale are that the operator has some ability to compensate for what might otherwise be for technical reasons a less than optimal image. In addition, multiple different images of the same slice can be obtained with optimal rendering of different body tissues merely by changing the window settings. If the hard copy or film image is lost, another image can be made if the computer data composed of the matrix of CT numbers have been stored.

A CT scale based on new Hounsfield units and illustrating the relationship of the window width and level is shown in Figure 2.53.

The Partial Volume Effect

Because of the finite thickness of the collimated x-ray beam, a tissue slice rather than a plane is imaged. Because of the finite thickness of the slice, a voxel may encompass more than one kind of tissue. The actual linear x-ray attenuation coefficient or CT number calculated for this voxel will actually be an average for the different tissues included within the slice, weighted by their relative contribution to the x-ray attenuation in the voxel. This is referred to as the partial volume effect, or volume averaging. The partial volume effect has significant clinical consequences in measuring tissue x-ray attenuation. For a reliable estimate of the CT number, it is necessary to look at voxels completely within the tissue whose CT number is to be measured. This is illustrated in Figure 2.54 for a kidney containing both a cystic and a solid mass.

The Image Display

In conventional radiographic procedures, the final image is made on the photographic film during the actual process of taking the image. All the information collected is present on the film. Should inappropriate radiographic techniques be used or difficulties occur in the processing of the film, the quality of the final image will suffer. A film might be overexposed or underexposed. Although varying the transmitted light through the film may offer some aid in viewing, the final film image is fixed and cannot be changed. In particular, it is frequently difficult to achieve optimal image quality in the lung, soft tissues, and bone simultaneously. Thus, multiple exposures

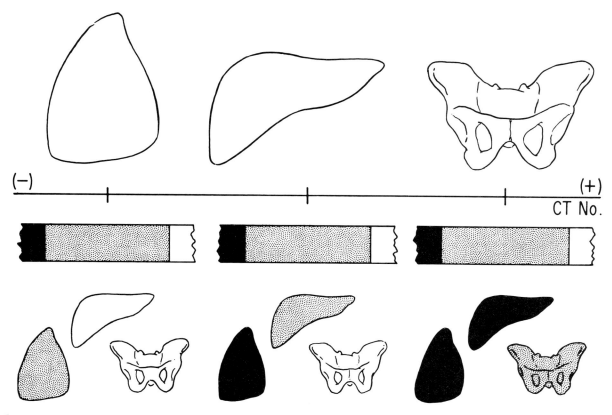

Figure 2.52. The change in the gray tone of different organs having widely different CT numbers with changes in the window level.

of the same area may be needed, as in an extremity for bone and for soft tissue detail.

The CT image does not suffer from these limitations. The basis for the image is the matrix of CT numbers representing the individual voxel linear attenuation coefficients. These data can be stored temporarily or permanently. In either form, the data are available for image display and manipulation. The final image can be displayed on a monitor or on hard copy (film), which is photographed from a monitor. The two-dimensional presentation can be thought of as a matrix of the array of different pixels. Each pixel can be assigned a shade of gray corresponding to the CT number of the corresponding voxel. However, the operator may vary the gray scale assignment of CT numbers to optimize the image for a specific organ or body tissue. Perhaps the nearest analogy in diagnostic imaging to this capability is the use of postprocessing techniques in ultrasonography, which permit emphasis of different echo levels in an image after it has been formed.

An advantage of viewing the image directly on the cathode ray tube monitor is that changes in the window settings can be made during the viewing and measurements can be performed. However, it is certainly not practical to review all previous scans from the monitor, since this would entail locating each scan on a magnetic tape or disk. Thus, a hard copy image is necessary.

Initially, Polaroid film was utilized for hard copy. Polaroid has the great advantage that the image can be made into hard copy almost immediately and without necessitating the use of a darkroom or developing process. However, there are several distinct disadvantages. Polaroid is relatively expensive. In addition, the image is a reflected one and may not be viewed through a viewbox. Finally, Polaroid images usually significantly shorten the gray scale, making the subtle changes in the gray more difficult to discern, particularly at the extreme light and dark ends of the scale.

More commonly, the monitor image is photographed on radiographic film to obtain a transparent hard copy, which is examined on viewing boxes. The most common technique of printing this hard copy is by a multiformat film imager. This typically allows four to six images to be recorded on a standard 8 × 10 inch piece of radiographic film, or alternatively

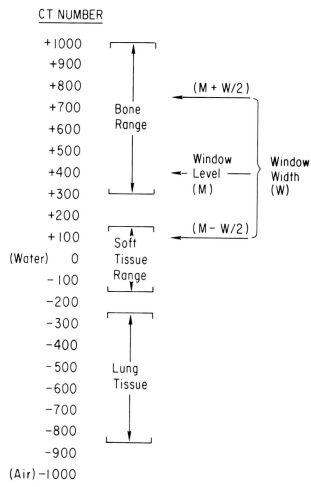

Figure 2.53. CT scale using new Hounsfield units.

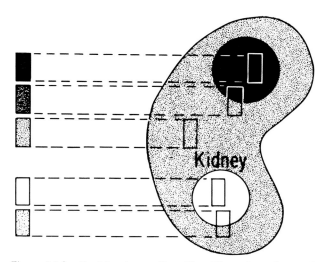

Figure 2.54. Partial volume effect. The CT number of a voxel varies with its location in portions of an organ with different CT numbers and as different tissue sections of the organ are included in a single voxel. This can lead to an error in measuring the CT number of an organ or a mass within the organ.

four or 12 images on a 14 × 17 inch film. The quality of the transparent image is usually superior to that of Polaroid, with less abrupt contrast changes and better demonstration of subtle gradations among the gray tones in the image. The slight delay from film processing is usually more than offset by the higher quality image and significant cost savings.

REFERENCES AND SUGGESTED READINGS

Bassano, D. A., Chamberlain, C. C., Mozley, J. M., and Kieffer, S. A. Physical, performance, and dosimetric characteristics of Δ-50 whole-body/brain scanner. Radiology 123:455–462, 1977.

Brooks, R. A., and Di Chiro, G. Beam hardening in x-ray reconstruction tomography. Physics in Medicine and Biology 21:390–398, 1976.

Christensen, E. E., Curry, T. S., and Dowdey, J. E. An Introduction to the Physics of Diagnostic Radiology (in particular, Chap. 24, Computed tomography), pp. 329–366. Lea & Febiger, Philadelphia, 1978.

Freundlich, D., and Zaklad, H. Scintillation crystal-photomultiplier tube detectors. In T. H. Newton and D. G. Potts (eds.), Radiology of the Skull and Brain: Technical Aspects of Computed Tomography, Vol. 5, Chap. 118, Part XVII, Sect. II, pp. 4104–4112. C. V. Mosby, St. Louis, 1981.

General Electric Company. Introduction to Computed Tomography. General Electric Publication 4691, 1976.

Haque, P., and Stanley, J. H. Basic principles of computed tomography detectors. In T. H. Newton and D. G. Potts (eds.), Radiology of the Skull and Brain: Technical Aspects of Computed Tomography, Vol. 5, Chap. 118, Part XVII, Sect. I, pp. 4097–4103. C. V. Mosby, St. Louis, 1981.

Hill, K. R., and Joyner, R. W. Computerized x-ray tomography. Scientific Progress 62:237–262, 1975.

Hounsfield, G. N. Computerized transverse axial scanning (tomography): Part I. Description of system. British Journal of Radiology 46:1016–1022, 1973.

Hounsfield, G. N. Historical notes on computerized axial tomography. Journal of the Canadian Association of Radiologists 27:135–142, 1976.

Hounsfield, G. N. Computed medical imaging. Nobel Lecture, December 8, 1979. Reproduced in Journal of Computer Assisted Tomography 4:665–674, 1980.

Johns, H. E., Battista, J., Bronskill, M. J., Brooks, R., Fenster, A., and Yaffee, M. Physics of CT scanners: principles and problems. International Journal of Radiation Oncology, Biology Physics 3:45–51, 1977.

Ledley, R. S. Introduction to computerized tomography. Computers in Biology and Medicine 6:239–246, 1976.

Ledley, R. S., Di Chiro, G., Luessenhop, A. J., and Twigg, H. L. Computerized transaxial x-ray tomography of the human body. Science 186:207–212, 1974.

Ledley, R. S., Wilson, J. B., Golab, T., and Rotolo, L. S. The ACTA-scanner: The whole body computerized transaxial tomography. Computers in Biology and Medicine 4:145–155, 1974.

McCullough, E. C. Factors affecting the use of quantitative information from a CT scanner. Radiology 124:99–107, 1977.

McCullough, E. C., Baker, H. L., Houser, O. W., and Reese, D. F. An evaluation of the quantitative and radiation features of scanning x-ray transverse axial tomography: The EMI scanner. Radiology 111:709–715, 1974.

McCullough, E. C., and Payne, J. T. X-ray transmission computed tomography. Medical Physics 4:85–98, 1977.

McCullough, E. C., Payne, J. T., Baker, H. L., Hattery, R. R., Sheedy, P. F., Stephens, D. H., and Gedgaudus, E. Performance evaluation and quality assurance of computed tomography scanners, with illustrations from the EMI, ACTA, and Delta scanners. Radiology 120:173–188, 1976.

Marshall, C. H. Principles of computed tomography. Postgraduate Medicine 60:105–109, 1976.

New, P. F. J., and Scott, W. R. General description of the EMI scanner: Operational notes. *In* Computed Tomography of the Brain and Orbit (EMI Scanning), Chap. 2. pp. 7–22. Williams & Wilkins, Baltimore, 1975.

New, P. F. J., and Scott, W. R. Patient positioning. *In* Computed Tomography of the Brain and Orbit (EMI Scanning), Chap, 3, pp. 23–34. Williams & Wilkins, Baltimore, 1975.

New, P. F. J., and Scott, W. R. Physical considerations in computed tomography. *In* Computed Tomography of the Brain and Orbit (EMI Scanning), Chap. 4, pp. 35–53. Williams & Wilkins, Baltimore, 1975.

New, P. F. J., Scott, W. R., Schnur, J. A., Davis, K. R., and Taveras, J. M. Computerized axial tomography with the EMI scanner. Radiology 110:109–123, 1974.

Ommaya, A. L., Murray, G., Ambrose, J., Richardson, A., and Hounsfield, G. Computerized axial tomography: Estimation of spatial and density resolution capability. British Journal of Radiology 49:604–611, 1976.

Payne, J. T., and Gedgaudus, E. Basic principles of computerized tomography. *In* P. Gerhardt and G. van Kaick (eds.), Total Body Computerized Tomography. International Symposium, Heidelberg, 1977, pp. 2–9. Georg Thieme, Stuttgart, 1979.

Payne, J. T., and McCullough, E. C. Basic principles of computer-assisted tomography. Applied Radiology 103:53–60, 1976.

Pfizer Medical Systems. Principles of Scanning (M. S. Scureman), 1977.

Seidelman, F. E., and Reich, N. E. Computed tomography using the EMI scanner: Part I. The apparatus, the normal scan, and its variants. Journal of the American Osteopathic Association 75:1125–1132, 1975.

Seidelman, F. E., and Reich, N. E. Computed tomography of the total body: Part I. Technical advances, devices, and normal scans. Journal of the American Osteopathic Association 75:644–650, 1976.

Sprawls, P. The Physical Principles of Diagnostic Radiology. University Park Press, Baltimore, 1977.

Ter-Pogossian, M. M. Basic principles of computed axial tomography. Seminars in Nuclear Medicine 8:109–127, 1977.

Ter-Pogossian, M. M. Computerized cranial tomography: Equipment and physics. Seminars in Roentgenology 12:13–25, 1977.

Thompson, T. Computed tomography. *In* A Practical Approach to Modern X-Ray Equipment, Chap. 8, pp. 167–189. Little, Brown & Company, Boston, 1978.

Webster, E. W. Physics in Diagnostic Radiology. Based on a course of 11 lectures delivered to radiologists in the New England region under the auspices of the New England Roentgen Ray Society. Copyright E. W. Webster, Massachusetts General Hospital, 1972.

Zatz, L. M. Basic principles of computed tomography scanning. *In* T. H. Newton and D. G. Potts (eds.), Radiology of the Skull and Brain: Technical Aspects of Computed Tomography, Vol. 5, Chap. 109, Part XVI, pp. 3853–3876. C. V. Mosby, St. Louis, 1981.

Zatz, L. M. General overview of computed tomography instrumentation. *In* T. H. Newton and D. G. Potts (eds.), Radiology of the Skull and Brain: Technical Aspects of Computed Tomography, Vol. 5. Chap. 116, Part XVII, pp. 4025–4057. C. V. Mosby, St. Louis, 1981.

Chapter 3
PURELY ROTATIONAL SCANNING SYSTEMS

A PURELY ROTATIONAL SCANNING GEOMETRY

ROTATING TUBE AND DETECTOR ARRAY:
THE THIRD GENERATION

General Description
X-Ray Tube
Alignment of the X-Ray Tube Relative to the Gantry
Collimation and Detector Spacing
Detectors
Variations in the Third Generation
Direct Magnification (Shift)
Slip-Rings
Detectors
X-Ray Tube
A Combined Second and Third Generation Scanner

ROTATING TUBE AND FIXED DETECTORS:
THE FOURTH GENERATION

General Description
X-Ray Tube
Collimation and Detector Spacing
Detectors
Variations in the Fourth Generation

COMPARISON OF THIRD AND
FOURTH GENERATION SCANNERS

REFERENCES AND SUGGESTED READINGS

A PURELY ROTATIONAL SCANNING GEOMETRY

In the first generation computed tomographic units, the long scanning time made it difficult to eliminate artifacts occurring because of patient motion, respiration, and bowel peristalsis. Respiration and bowel peristalsis have no effects in head scanning but can cause significant artifacts in body scanning, adversely affecting image quality and sometimes making it impossible to obtain adequate images. Patient motion, as in an agitated patient, is of course very detrimental in both head and body work.

In second generation units, gross patient motion can frequently be eliminated, and many patients are able to restrain respiration for the 15–30 s usually required for scanning. However, even in these short intervals, artifacts arising from bowel peristalsis are common in the body. In addition, many ill patients cannot restrain respiration for the 15–30 s typically required for the scan. Thus, it is highly desirable to achieve faster scanning times, especially in the chest and abdomen, to reduce artifacts related to these types of motion and ensure better image quality.

To bring the scanning time much below 15–30 s it is necessary to eliminate the complex mechanical motion associated with the first and second generation scanning techniques (although one unit employing second generation translational-rotational principles, the Elscint Exel 905, has achieved a scanning time of 5.3 s). This has been achieved in both third and fourth generation scanners by employing a scanning geometry that requires only a single type of motion, namely, rotation, and eliminates the translational component of the scanning motion. These two modes of scanning and their common variations are discussed in this chapter.

ROTATING TUBE AND DETECTOR ARRAY: THE THIRD GENERATION

General Description

The x-ray tube and a curved array of detectors, typically subtending a fan or arc of about 30–40° from the x-ray tube, are mounted within the gantry in perfect alignment (Figure 3.1). The tube and detector array are usually rotated through 360° for a single scan (Figure 3.2). An abbreviated or shorter scan can be performed utilizing a 180° rotation. CT scanners using this design have been popularly referred to as third generation scanners. The number of detectors varies from 288 (Philips Tomoscan 300), 289 (General Electric CT/T 7800), and 301 (Varian V-360-3) to 504 (Omni 6000, formerly Searle Pho/Trax 4000 and EMI CT 6000), 511 (General Electric CT/T 8800), and 512 (Siemens Somatom DR2 and DR3 and Toshiba TCT-65A) to 576 (Philips Tomoscan 310) to 742 (General Electric CT/T 9800) to 1,024 (Compagnie Générale de Radiologie (CGR) CE 10000) in commercially available units using this principle. The close spacing of the detectors in the array, combined with the necessity of rotating the entire array, precludes the use of the relatively bulky scintillation crystal/photomultiplier tube combinations. Most commonly, high pressure ionization chambers filled with xenon gas are used. Alternatively, an array of small semiconductor detectors, for example, cesium iodide crystals, coupled with photodiodes (in place of photomultiplier tubes) is employed (e.g., Siemens Somatom 2).

These systems generally employ pulsed x-ray tubes (in which the x-rays are emitted in pulses of finite duration rather than continuously), although some units (Omni 6000 and General Electric CT/T 9800) use a continuously operating x-ray tube. Each detector in the array will record a signal corresponding to the quantity of x-rays it has detected during a finite measuring time. If the x-ray tube is pulsed, this is called the pulse time. The pulse time may be variable; commonly it is about 1–4 ms. In a continuously operating tube, a finite measuring time or

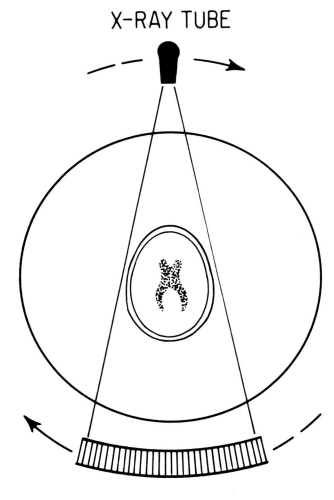

Figure 3.1. The third generation, a rotating x-ray tube and detector array. The x-ray tube is aligned to an array of high pressure xenon cells, which function as the detection system.

integration period is preselected. During this measurement time, a number of data or readings equal to the number of detectors in the array are obtained.

The set of measurements obtained at a specific angle of the fan beam detector array (ignoring the small amount of rotation during the measurement time) constitutes a view (profile or projection) in a third generation or rotating tube and detector array system. Following a fixed rotation of the tube and detector array, another set of measurements (i.e., another view) is obtained. The total number of sample data or individual measurements obtained in a single scan sequence will be equal to the number of detectors in the array times the number of measure-

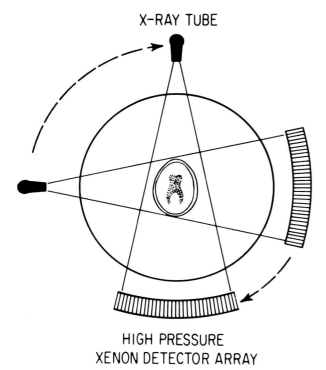

Figure 3.2. The alignment of the x-ray tube relative to the detector array is maintained as both rotate in synchrony.

ments made by each detector (the number of separate views). The number of individual data samples or measurements made by each detector (which is equal to the number of views) is related to the frequency with which measurements are made and the total time in which data samples are taken. Theoretically, the number of views collected during a scan may be increased by increasing the scanning time and/or increasing the frequency with which views are obtained. Practically, this is commonly achieved by increasing the scanning time.

Typical values for the number of views obtained as a function of time include: 500+ in 3.4 s for the CGR CE 10000; 288 views in 4.8 s and 576 views in 9.6 s for the General Electric CT/T 7800 and CT/T 8800; 372 views in 2.6 s, 600 views in 4.2 s, and 1,200 views in 8.4 s for the Philips Tomoscan 300; 233 views in 3 s, 360 views in 5 s, and 720 views in 10 s for the Siemens Somatom 2; and 300 views in 4.5 s and 600 views in 9 s for the Toshiba TCT-65A series.

The total number of data samples or measurements obtained by a third generation unit during a scan may be expressed as:

$$\begin{aligned}\text{total number of data samples} =\\ \text{number of detectors} \times \\ \text{number of data samples per detector,}\end{aligned} \quad (3.1)$$

or, equivalently,

$$\begin{aligned}\text{total number of data samples} =\\ \text{number of data samples per view} \times \\ \text{number of views,}\end{aligned} \quad (3.2)$$

since in third generation units the number of data samples or measurements per view is determined by and identical to the number of detectors, and the number of views is equal to the number of data samples or measurements by each detector.

Each individual detector intercepts a ray during a single view. A ray is defined for the third generation in an equivalent or analogous fashion to its definition for translational-rotational systems. Theoretically, it is a straight line path from the x-ray tube to the detector. Practically, it encompasses all that portion of the x-ray beam from the tube to a single detector. A view is composed of individual rays. In the third generation the number of rays in a view is equal to the number of detectors, or, equivalently, the number of data samples per view. Thus Equations 3.1 and 3.2 may also be written in the form:

$$\begin{aligned}\text{total number of data samples} =\\ \text{number of rays per view} \times \\ \text{number of views.}\end{aligned} \quad (3.3)$$

This is illustrated by the original third generation scanner, the General Electric CT/T 7800. In performing a 4.8-s scan with 289 detectors for data sampling, 288 views were obtained. The total number of measurements or data samples was 289 × 288 = 83,232. By doubling the scanning time to 9.6 s, a total of 576 views were obtained; this results in 289 × 576 = 166,464 data samples or measurements. The updated General Electric CT/T 8800 has 511 detectors for data sampling. In a 4.8-s scan, 288 views are obtained, so that 511 × 288 = 147,168 data samples or measurements are collected. For a 9.6-s scan with the CT/T 8800, the number of views is increased to 576, so that 511 × 576 = 294,336 data samples are collected.

Appendix III summarizes in tabular form many of the comparative features of different CT units.

X-Ray Tube

In a rotating tube and detector system, the x-ray tube employed is generally a pulsed tube with a rotating anode. That is, a disk anode with a bevelled edge, rotating at up to 10,000 rpm, is typically used instead of a fixed anode tube (Figure 3.3). The Omni 6000 uses a continuously operating stationary anode tube. The use of a rotating anode tube increases the actual surface area of the tungsten that is bombarded by the electron stream, so that no point on the surface of the tungsten is constantly being bombarded. As a

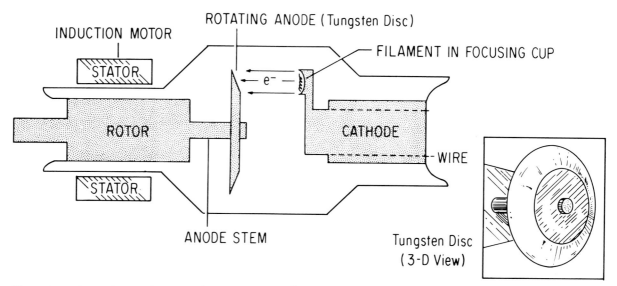

Figure 3.3. A rotation anode x-ray tube increases the effective tungsten surface area for electron bombardment, thereby permitting an increased x-ray output without overheating the tungsten target.

result, a relatively smaller portion of the tungsten can be bombarded at any given time with a higher electron beam density (although even the same electron beam density would give some gain). Thus, the output of the tube can be increased while at the same time the effective area of the beam is reduced, typically to a .6-mm focal spot size. For any pulsed tube, x-rays are radiated for a small fraction of the time of the scan.

Individual measurements or views are made during the time interval of approximately 1–4 ms in which the tube is radiating x-rays. Then there is commonly a period of approximately 12–15 ms during which the tube is not emitting x-rays.

Continuous operation of the tube is generally not used because this might lead to inefficient use of x-rays per unit of heat load, unnecessary patient radiation exposure, and an inefficient photon flux per view. There is no value in having the tube emit x-rays when no measurements are being made. Some additional benefits from this pulsing effect include elimination of a large number of time integrators within the x-ray circuit which would be needed for pulsing the detector circuitry, and the capability to recheck the electronic zeroing between pulses when no detector current is present. Also, pulsing permits the adjustment of the pulse length to the size of the patient in order to optimize the photon statistics and the point of operation of the detector response curve. The duty cycle for a pulsed x-ray tube is defined as the fraction of the time during which the x-ray tube is emitting x-rays. Typically, the tube current (electron flow from cathode to anode) ranges from 100–600 mA (General Electric CT/T 8800).

Oil is typically used for cooling the rotating anode tube in CT. Long cooling periods may be required since the tube cooling may be limited by the anode and x-ray tube housing heat capacities.

An alternative approach has been developed which uses a stationary or nonrotating anode that continuously emits x-rays. The original unit of this type was developed by Searle as the Pho/Trax 4000. Following Searle's exit from the manufacturing and marketing of CT units, this particular unit was incorporated into the EMI family of CT systems, where, following modification, it was marketed as the EMI CT 6000. After EMI's withdrawal from the CT industry, this unit was transferred to Omnimedical, where it is marketed with modifications as the Omni 6000. The anode current for this system is only 30–40 mA, similar to that in translational-rotational systems. During a scan of 5–20 s, 360, 540, or 1,080 measurements may be made by each of the 504 high pressure ionization detectors, which are arranged in a 40° arc. Thus, depending on the scan time, 360, 540, or 1,080 views may be obtained. Since the dead time of the detectors (time between measurements) is only 5% of the total scan time, measurements can be made during the 95% of the time that the patient is being irradiated. However, the time of an individual measurement may range from 9–14 ms. The advantage of this longer measurement time is that it permits the detection of a statistically significant number of x-rays, comparable to that from a pulsed rotating anode tube. Its disadvantage is that the tube and detectors may move a significant distance during this measurement integration time.

Alignment of the X-Ray Tube Relative to the Gantry

The stationary anode tubes of translational-rotational systems are usually mounted with their long axis parallel to the scanning plane (Figure 3.4). This is in contradistinction to the pulsed x-ray tubes, which are aligned with their long axis (from cathode to anode) perpendicular to the scanning plane, that is, parallel to the axis of rotation of the gantry (Figure 3.5). The principal reason for this change is to avoid the gyroscopic effect in which a torque occurs on the anode bearings if the axis of rotation of the anode is different than the axis of rotation of the entire tube as it rotates in the gantry.

In addition, orientation of the tube axis perpendicular to the scanning plane avoids nonuniformity in the fan-shaped x-ray beam resulting from consequences of the heel effect. In this effect, partial reabsorption of the x-ray beam by the anode results in the x-ray beam being less intense on the anode than on the cathode side of the tube (Figure 3.6). If the width of the fan beam were in the plane of the long axis of the x-ray tube, it would cause the portion of the beam on the anode side to be less intense than that on the cathode side. The results of this heel

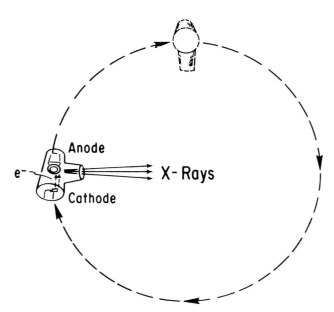

Figure 3.5. Typical x-ray alignment and motion relative to the scanning plane in a purely rotational geometry which uses a rotating anode x-ray tube. The axis of the rotating anode is parallel to the axis of the scanning plane.

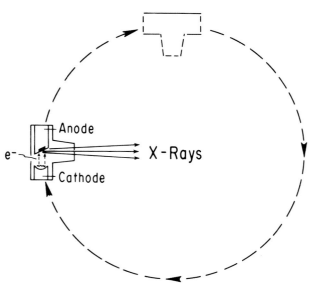

Figure 3.4. Typical x-ray tube alignment and motion relative to the scanning plane in the early combined translational-rotational units using a stationary anode x-ray tube. The anode-cathode axis is perpendicular to the scan axis and thus parallel to (actually within) the plane of the scan. The rotational motion indicated is actually performed in increments, which are interrupted by the sequential translations.

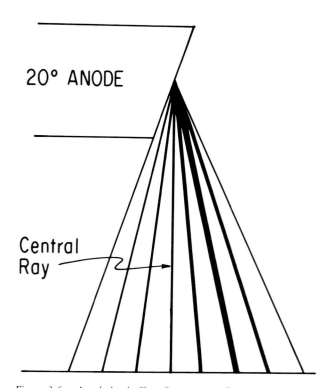

Figure 3.6. Anode heel effect. Resorption of x-ray photons close to the anode results in asymmetry of the x-ray intensity (indicated by the relative thickness of the lines in the diverging x-ray beam) with a lower intensity in the portion of the beam adjacent to the anode.

effect can be removed by calibration of the detectors without a patient in the gantry. The x-ray fluxes striking each detector element should then all be equal, and any discrepancies can be measured and corrected. However, it is always better to remove a potential problem, if possible, than to have to correct it. Positioning the tube so that its axis is perpendicular to the scanning plane means that any heel effect would only occur over the length of the detector or the thickness of the slice and would be minimal. In addition, it would equally affect all voxels at a particular radial distance from the tube.

Collimation and Detector Spacing

In the third generation fan beam system, there is an entrance collimator between the x-ray tube and the patient to shape the fan beam. Since there is virtually no spacing between the high pressure ionization cells, no exit collimator is used between the patient and the detector array. Thus, essentially the entire exit beam passes into the detectors; that is, the detectors have a geometric capture efficiency of nearly 100% (Figure 3.7). Some internal collimation inside the detectors does aid, however, in discriminating against scattered x-rays. Because of the virtual lack of spacing between detectors and the absence of exit collimation, the physical width of a detector is essentially identical to the detector aperture (the geometric aperture or slit through which x-rays must pass to enter the detector). The relatively small width of the xenon detectors (about 1.5 mm or less, e.g., in the General Electric CT/T 8800), means that this is a narrow aperture detector system.

Detectors

In a third generation unit individual detectors are very closely spaced, on the order of 1–2 mm between detector centers. Furthermore, detectors are actually rotating within the gantry with the x-ray tube. These factors preclude the use of scintillation crystal detectors with photomultiplier tubes. The crystal-photomultiplier combination, in particular the photomultiplier tubes, cannot usually be made this small and closely spaced. In addition, the weight of the photomultiplier tubes attached to a rotating system would be formidable.

An alternative detection system utilizes a high pressure inert gas, usually xenon. The x-ray beam traversing a core of tissue will strike a single detector cell and cause a quantity of ionization of the xenon gas that is linearly proportional to the intensity of the transmitted x-ray beam (Figure 3.8). Adjacent high pressure xenon cells separated by thin tungsten plates comprise the individual detectors. In the General Electric CT/T 8800, every other plate is connected to a 500-V DC power supply and attracts free electrons. The alternate plates are essentially electrically floating but are approximately at 0 V (Figure 3.9). These plates collect the ionized heavy xenon nuclei, which represent the signal current. The magnitude of the voltage within each cell is adjusted so that the electrical current collected is approximately linearly proportional to the incident x-ray beam. Although in principle the detector resembles that of a Geiger counter, the voltage is kept substantially lower so that the nonlinear avalanche effect characteristic of a Geiger counter does not occur. The xenon gas in the different cells communicates, so that the pressure is identical in all the cells. However, each cell is electrically isolated from the other cells.

It was thought that a mixture of gases might be more efficient than xenon alone, since it might be possible to trap some of the fluorescent radiation from the xenon. The efficacy of this approach was

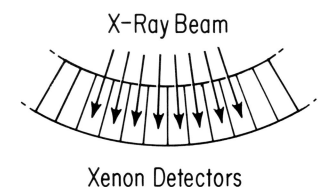

Figure 3.7. The walls between the individual high pressure xenon cells are very thin, ensuring that nearly the entire beam passes into the individual xenon cells without being intercepted by the walls.

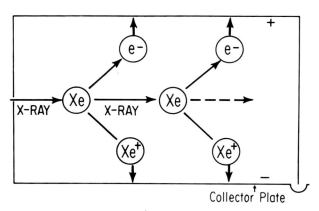

Figure 3.8. The passage of x-rays through the high pressure xenon gas cells results in the production of positive xenon ions and negative electrons. Negative electrons migrate to the positive collecting plate; positive xenon ions migrate to the relatively more negative collecting plate.

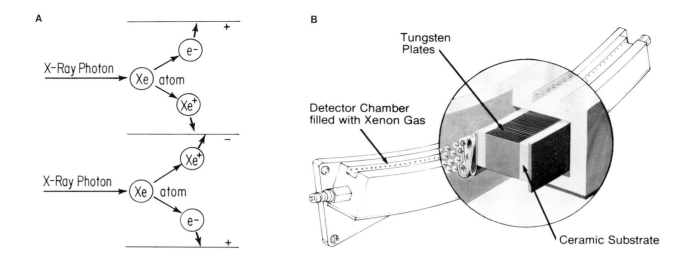
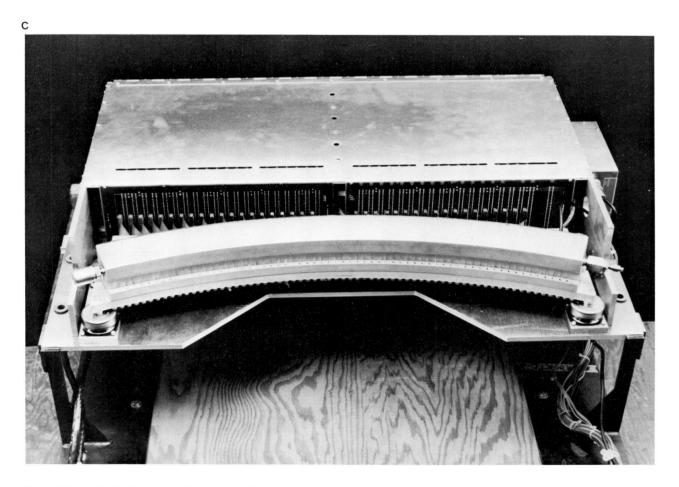

Figure 3.9. *A*, Collection of negative electrons by the positive (500 V) plates and of the positive xenon ions by the relatively negative (floating) plates is shown for two adjacent cells. *B*, Drawing of a xenon detector array (courtesy of General Electric Medical Systems). *C*, Photograph of a xenon detector with some of its associated electronic apparatus (courtesy of General Electric Medical Systems).

studied by Yaffe et al. (1977), who measured the ion current as a function of the proportion of krypton mixed with xenon for a total pressure of 5 atm. They found that, although the krypton did absorb much of the fluorescent radiation from the xenon, it was less efficient in absorbing the primary radiation. Also, since more energy was required to produce an ion pair in krypton (24.3 eV for krypton compared to 21.9 eV for xenon), there was a net reduction in yield. They concluded from their experimental results that there was no gain by the addition of krypton at 5 atm. However, theoretical calculations suggested that at pressures greater than 20 atm, where there was enough xenon for full absorption of primary photons, the addition of krypton might offer a slight yield. In fact, a mixture of xenon and krypton gases (approximately 95% xenon and 5% krypton) was employed for research purposes by Varian. However, the Varian commercial units (V-360-3, no longer manufactured) all used essentially 100% xenon at an approximate pressure of 6–8 atm.

The main disadvantage related to gas detection systems is their relative inefficiency. Because of the low density of the gases, the fraction of the incident x-ray beam that is captured and transferred into a usable signal is significantly less per centimeter thickness of gas than a corresponding scintillation crystal detection. However, these disadvantages can be overcome 1) by utilization of xenon, the heaviest of the inert gases except for radioactive radon; 2) by increasing the pressure of the xenon to 10–25 atm, thus increasing the density of the gas and the possible number of ionizing encounters that may occur with the incident x-ray beam; and 3) by making the capture chamber relatively long to increase the number of possible ionizations. With these design features incorporated, the detection efficiency of these high pressure xenon detectors approximates 60% of that of a sodium iodide detector.

The high pressure xenon detectors also demonstrate some highly desirable attributes. There is relative uniformity in the composition of the gas detectors compared to the solid-state detectors. The afterglow problems of some scintillation crystals, specifically sodium iodide, are avoided with gas detectors. Particularly important is the relatively linear response over the range of beam intensities expected.

One commercially available third generation system, the General Electric CT/T 8800, uses 4-cm-long xenon cells at a pressure of approximately 25 atm (S. M. Blumenfield, private communication). Another system, the Omni 6000, has utilized 8-cm-long xenon cells at a pressure of 10 atm. In the latter system, a decreased number of ionizing encounters because of the lower pressure is compensated in part by lengthening the chamber or path through which the x-ray passes. In addition, the longer path provides some internal collimation. However, the larger plates are more susceptible to vibrations, which introduce electrical noise.

An alternative rotating detector system utilizing an array of crystal detectors in conjunction with solid state photodiodes has been developed. An array of 520 small, closely spaced cesium iodide scintillation crystals, including eight reference detectors, is employed (Siemens Somatom 2). The photodiodes are solid-state analogs of photomultiplier tubes. A photodiode converts the light signal from a scintillation crystal into an electrical signal and then amplifies the electrical signal. This is analogous to the function of a photomultiplier tube, but the solid-state photodiode is significantly smaller in size. This permits the use of an entirely solid-state detector system featuring an array of a large number of individually small, closely spaced detector elements.

Variations in the Third Generation

There have been several significant variations or engineering modifications introduced into third generation systems.

Direct Magnification (Shift) In a fan beam geometry, the sector angle is determined by the number and size of the detectors, the collimation of the beam, and the distance of the detectors from the x-ray tube. The patient is generally placed in a position midway between the x-ray tube and the detectors. Third generation units have a relatively large sector angle, typically 30–40°. The physical width of the beam where it intercepts the patient may exceed the diameter of the particular patient cross-section that is being scanned. This most frequently occurs when the cross-section being examined is in the head or involves the body of a child. In these cases, many of the peripheral detectors are idle. In a third generation scanner, the peripheral detectors may never be utilized in collecting image data samples during an entire scan of the smaller object, although they may be used as reference detectors for calibration (Figure 3.10). These unused detectors result in a reduction of usable data for image reconstruction, with a resulting decrease in image accuracy.

One technique to overcome this problem is to shift the position of the tube and detectors relative to the cross-section being scanned. Specifically, for smaller cross-sections the entire tube and detector system may be shifted radially so that the tube is closer to the object and the detectors are farther away (Figure 3.11). Thus, the object can intercept the en-

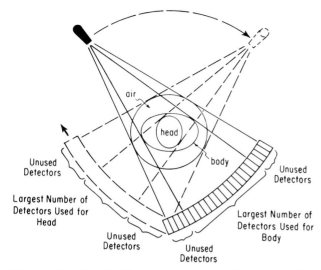

Figure 3.10. A small object may not intercept the lateral portions of the x-ray beam during the scan. The associated detectors receive a constant, unattenuated beam which conveys no information about the object scannned. These unused detectors do not collect image data samples; however, they may be used as reference detectors for calibration.

tire fan beam. This is similar to magnification in conventional radiography. By shifting or offsetting the center of rotation of the x-ray tube and detectors in such a manner that the object intercepts the entire fan beam, all the detectors can be utilized, with a resultant increase in data for reconstruction.

Slip-Rings These were initially introduced in the Varian V-360-3 unit to facilitate continuous gan-

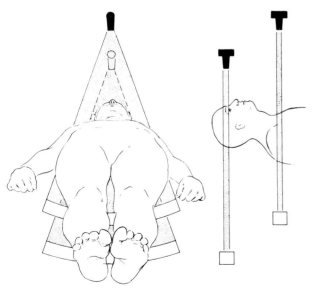

Figure 3.11. Moving the x-ray tube closer to the patient when scanning a smaller cross-section permits the entire fan-shaped beam to be intercepted by the patient; thus, the entire beam is used to gather image data.

try rotation. The slip-ring design allows both data signals and high-voltage x-ray tube power to flow between the continuously rotating gantry and the stationary CT components through electrical contacts that glide on rotating slip-rings. The slip-ring design eliminates constant cable flexing and massive gantry stop/start shock forces, as well as minimizing wear to major moving parts. Ideally, the slip-ring might facilitate gated studies and dynamic scanning.

In the Varian-360-3 the continuous gantry rotation permits scanning through more than 360°. In addition to a 3-s scan through 360° (with 360 views), a 12-s scan is available based on four complete 360° rotations, or 1,440° total (with 1,440 views). To assure that each group of 360 views collected during successive 360° rotations in a 12-s scan is independent, there is a shift by $1\frac{1}{4}$ detectors after each 360° rotation.

Detectors Two modifications have been attempted or introduced: the use of a mixture of krypton and xenon gases, and the introduction of solid-state scintillation crystal detectors, for example, cesium iodide in the Siemens Somatom 2. Both of these have been previously described.

X-Ray Tube The use of a steady operation stationary anode continuously emitting x-rays in the Omni 6000, described earlier, was initially the only exception to the otherwise uniform employment of a pulsed rotating anode tube in the third generation CT units. However, the Elscint Exel 1002, a combined second and third generation scanner described in the next section, has also employed a stationary anode x-ray tube. The more recently introduced General Electric CT/T 9800 employs a continuously operating rotating anode tube.

A Combined Second and Third Generation Scanner The Elscint Exel 1002 offers a choice between two scanning modes: a second generation translational-rotational motion and a purely rotational motion of the x-ray tube and detector array. This unit employs a 36° fan beam with 280 solid-state detectors and photodiodes for signal amplification. A stationary anode x-ray tube is used.

In the combined translational-rotational mode, five discrete translations are performed. Four individual rotational increments of 36° are required to cover 180°. This is similar to the Elscint Exel 905. However, since 280 detectors are now spaced over 36° (compared to 52 over the same angle in the Exel 905), the angular spacing between the detectors is now 36°/280 or .16°. Each detector obtains 512 readings (data samples or rays) per translation. Since there are 280 detectors, 280 views are obtained per translation, a view being the readings obtained by a single detector during a single translation. For five translations a total of 5 × 280 = 1,400 views are obtained; each view consists of 512 rays. This is the high resolution scanning mode.

In the purely rotational scan mode, more rapid scanning can be performed. The simultaneous collection of readings (ray measurements) made by the 280 detectors constitutes a single view. The number of views is determined by the frequency with which data are collected during the scanning time.

ROTATING TUBE AND FIXED DETECTORS: THE FOURTH GENERATION

General Description

An alternative design for faster scanning is one that utilizes an x-ray tube undergoing purely rotational motion in a circular path within the gantry about the patient, as in third generation devices, but in which the detectors do not rotate but rather are fixed in a larger, concentric ring within the gantry about the tube and the patient. The x-rays are collimated into a fan beam which intercepts a portion or arc of the detector ring. This is illustrated in Figure 3.12. The fan angle or subtended arc may range from 24–60°. The tube typically rotates through approximately 360° for a scan. The rotation angle may be greater than 360°, as either a fixed routine or an optional overscan. The data obtained during an overscan may be used to eliminate or compensate for patient motion between the start and finish of the scan period. When the detectors make up less than a complete 360°, the tube rotational angle is also correspondingly limited. These rotational angles are listed in Appendix III. Scanners employing this design have been called fourth generation systems. It must be emphasized that "generation" is a popular term, partly of commercial origin, and should be thought of as a general description of a scanning geometry. The term "generation," in general, should not be regarded as an indication of the superiority or obsolescence of the design of a CT system. This is particularly worth remembering with regard to third and fourth generation systems.

The number of detectors employed in fourth generation scanners has varied from 360 (Picker Synerview 300) and 424 (Technicare Delta 2005 and Delta 2010) to 600 (the AS&E, which was later marketed as the Pfizer 0500; the Pfizer/AS&E 0450; the Picker Synerview 600) and 720 (Technicare Delta 2020) to 1,088 (EMI 7070, a modified fourth generation unit), 1,200 (Picker Synerview 1200SV), and 2,400 (Pfizer PZ-2400). All of these employ solid-state detectors (scintillation crystals).

All fourth generation CT units have employed an x-ray tube with a rotating anode that continuously emits x-rays. As the tube rotates about the gantry, the detectors are constantly sensing the transmitted x-ray beam. Each detector measures a portion of the transmitted x-ray beam over a finite preselected time interval, during which a signal is built up or integrated into a data sample or measurement. This signal integration time or data collection period represents the time during which a detector intercepts and interrogates a single ray, thus accumulating a ray-sum. Representative figures for this time are .25–.9 ms for the Technicare 2000 series (the shorter figure for a high resolution 12½-cm field of view), 2.0 ms for the AS&E and the Pfizer/AS&E 0450, and .5–2.0 ms for the Pfizer PZ-2400. These successive measurement periods or signal integration times follow one another almost immediately, allowing for the recovery time, or dead time, associated with the electronics. Thus, in a fourth generation unit the patient is continuously being irradiated during the scan. Simultaneously, data are continuously being collected, except for the very brief electronic dead times. One necessary reason for having this electronic dead time, during which signal information cannot be integrated, is related to the time occupied in switching the electronic output of an analog-to-digital converter from one location in buffer memory to another. Approx-

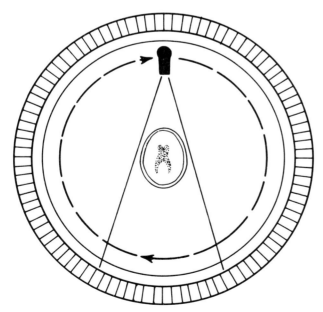

Figure 3.12. The fourth generation, a rotating x-ray tube and fixed circular array of detectors. The x-ray tube moves in a circular path, and the x-ray beam is intercepted by different detectors during the course of the tube rotation.

imate values for the electronic dead time are about 10 μs (.01 ms) for the Technicare 2000 series and 5% or less of the signal integration time for the Pfizer 0450. The order of magnitude is about 10–100 μs.

In a fourth generation unit, the set of measurements accumulated by each individual detector during a rotation of 360° or less constitutes a view. In these units, a view is also referred to as a data fan or detector fan, because the collection of rays seen by a detector in fourth generation units forms a fan with the apex at the detector.

For a rotation through more than 360° the extra information accumulated may be regarded as additional or overscan views. The redundant overscan views may be combined with the initial views taken by the same detectors to compensate for patient motion during the scan. The image can then be reconstructed from the corrected set of views. As an example, the earliest fourth generation unit, the AS&E scanner, acquires a total of 675 views. The first 600 views are collected in 360°, and the last 75 views in 40° of overscan. The 75 redundant views obtained in overscan are combined with the first 75 measured views, since these two sets of views are obtained with the same detectors.

A detector only intercepts the x-ray beam for that portion of the tube rotation during which the x-ray fan beam sweeps across the detector. During this time of data acquisition it intercepts all the rays and collects all the data samples comprising its view. One detector may complete its view before another detector begins to collect any data samples.

The total number of data samples or measurements obtained by a fourth generation unit during a scan may be expressed as follows:

$$\text{total number of data samples} = \text{number of detectors} \times \text{number of data samples per detector}. \quad (3.4)$$

Since in the fourth generation the number of views is equal to the number of detectors, and the number of data samples or measurements per view is equal to the number of data samples per detector, Equation 3.4 may be rewritten as:

$$\text{total number of data samples} = \text{number of views} \times \text{number of data samples per view}. \quad (3.5)$$

The concept of a ray is useful in fourth generation units, just as in translational-rotational systems and in third generation scanners. Again it is theoretically a straight line path from the x-ray tube to a detector; practically it encompasses that portion of the x-ray beam from the tube to a single detector. A view is composed of rays. In the fourth generation the number of rays in a view is again equal to the number of data samples obtained per view or per detector. Therefore, Equation 3.5 may be rewritten as follows:

$$\text{total number of data samples} = \text{number of views} \times \text{number of rays per view}. \quad (3.6)$$

Most of the measurements or data samples acquired by each detector are used as image data samples; however, some are used as calibration data samples. As an example, in the Picker Synerview 600 a total of 552 data samples are processed from each detector during a 48-cm (field of view), 360° scan. Of these 552 data samples, 512 are image data samples used in image reconstruction, and 40 are calibration data samples. Since there are 600 total detectors (or views), the accumulated data may be broken down as follows:

600 detectors × 552 data samples per detector = 331,200 total samples

600 detectors × 40 calibration data samples per detector = 24,000 calibration data samples

600 detectors × 512 image data samples per detector = 307,200 image data samples.

X-Ray Tube

Fourth generation units usually employ a continuously operating x-ray tube with a rotating anode. A typical tube current might be about 50–100 mA. This is only about a fifth of the tube current that the pulsed x-ray tubes of some third generation units use. However, since the pulsed tubes are generally operating with a duty cycle of 20%, the average current and resulting radiation from the two tubes may be comparable. For a pulsed tube:

$$500 \text{ mA} \times \tfrac{1}{5} \text{ (duty cycle)} \times 5 \text{ s} = 500 \text{ mAs}$$

For a continuous tube:

$$100 \text{ mA} \times 5 \text{ s} = 500 \text{ mAs}$$

The rotating anode tube permits the use of a relatively high anode current in combination with a small focal spot (e.g., .6–1.0 mm) for better resolution. Since a rotating anode tube is employed, the x-ray tube is oriented perpendicular to the scan plane, or parallel to the scan axis, to avoid the gyroscopic effect previously described (see Figure 3.5).

Collimation and Detector Spacing

Collimation is used at both the entrance and exit sides of the patient. The entrance collimators decrease unwanted radiation that would not pass through the tissue section in an appropriate path to the detector, resulting in useless patient irradiation and possible scatter radiation to the detectors. The primary purpose of the exit collimators in fourth generation units is to reduce the size of the detector aperture (the geometric aperture or slit through which x-rays pass); secondarily they decrease undesired scattered radiation that would result in increased noise. However, the exit collimators decrease the portion of the transmitted radiation that will be detected and recorded as a signal. The excluded radiation has traversed the patient uselessly and "wastes" the dose.

To maintain spatial resolution it is important to keep the individual detectors, or more correctly, the apertures of the detectors, as small as possible. Many of the typical scintillation crystal-photomultiplier tube combinations are relatively bulky and usually cannot be spaced more closely than 8–9 mm between centers. The collimation typically permits a reduction of the aperture size to about 4 mm, a relatively wide aperture. This is illustrated in Figure 3.13.

In the Technicare 2000 series, the crystal detector width and aperture size are both 4 mm. There is 4 mm of dead space between detectors, so that the spacing between crystal centers is 8 mm. In the Pfizer 0450 the physical width of the crystals is 5 mm, with 8 mm spacing between crystal centers (or 3 mm dead space between crystals). Collimators reduce the aperture size in the Pfizer 0450 to 4 mm. In the Picker Synerview 600 the physical width of the crystals is 8 mm, and the spacing between crystal centers is 8.9 mm, so there is only .9 mm dead space between crystals, but the typical aperture size between tungsten pin collimators is 4 mm. These units all employ bismuth germanate crystals.

The detector apertures thus occupy only a fraction (usually about half) of the area of the fan beam, the remainder of the fan beam being intercepted by the collimating elements. Only about half of the transmitted x-ray photons therefore enter the detectors. However, since nearly 100% of the photons entering the detectors are captured and converted into a signal, the wasted radiation dose associated with collimation is partly offset by the high photon conversion efficiency of the detectors.

Detectors

The most commonly used detector system to date consists of scintillation crystals with photomultiplier tubes. These are equally spaced in a large ring within the gantry, usually through 360°.

Different materials have been used for the scintillation crystals. The most frequently employed to date has been bismuth germanate, which has largely replaced the earlier sodium iodide and calcium fluoride crystals in currently manufactured translational-rotational units. Bismuth germanate crystals are used in the AS&E (600 crystals), the Pfizer/AS&E 0450 (600 crystals), the Picker Synerview 300, 600, and 1200 (360, 600, and 1200 crystals, respectively), the Technicare 2005 and 2010 (424 crystals), and the Technicare 2020 (720 crystals). The Technicare 2060 uses 720 crystals of bismuth germanate and cadmium tungstate.

An alternative detection system using 1,088 cesium iodide crystals interfaced to solid-state photodiodes was used by EMI in the CT 7070 (now the Omnimedical Quad I). These detectors are 1.8 mm in width, with a spacing between crystal centers of 2.3 mm, and .5-mm lead separators or collimators between the cesium iodide crystals. This gives a geometrical photon utilization efficiency of about 78%. Combining this with a photon absorption efficiency of 99% for cesium iodide (at the energy levels used in CT) results in a net photon utilization of about 77%. That is, 78% of the transmitted photons enter the detectors, and of these almost all (99%) are totally absorbed.

A total of 2,400 cadmium tungstate ($CdWO_4$) scintillation detectors were incorporated into the Pfizer PZ-2400. A photon collection rate of 84% was claimed for this unit, which was not produced commercially.

A complete scan can be performed in as rapidly as 1 or 2 s by some fourth generation units. A distinct

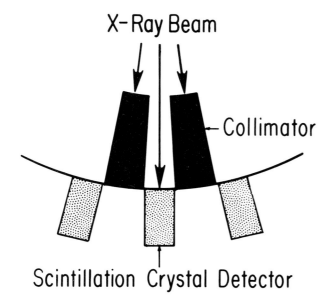

Figure 3.13. Approximately half of the x-ray beams may be intercepted by the relatively thick collimators between the individual scintillation detectors, thus decreasing the detected signal. In practice, round pins are usually employed for collimation, and the physical width of the detector may exceed the aperture width.

advantage of this system compared to the third generation rotating detection system is that during the course of the scan every detector in the system will sample a portion of the x-ray beam that has not travelled through the patient. This then allows a continuous calibration of the detectors and allows for some error in stability. However, this system of detectors is extremely costly because of the large number of scintillation detectors and photomultipliers that have been employed.

Variations in the Fourth Generation

One of the most significant limitations in the fourth generation of scanners is the necessity for having a large number (typically 600–720) of relatively expensive scintillation crystal and photomultipliers along the outer ring of detectors. One way of decreasing the required number of detectors is to place them only around part of the circumference, for example, 212° in the Technicare 2005 and 2010. This permits a decrease in the number of detectors involved as well as the photomultipliers, but scanning can be performed only through an angle smaller than 360°.

Another alternative is to use a smaller diameter ring of detectors, as introduced in the EMI 7070. The detectors may then still be placed around the entire 360° circumference and fewer scintillation crystal detectors would be needed. The x-ray tube is then placed in a larger diameter outer ring. This necessitates nutating or tilting the detector ring off its central axis to prevent the x-ray beam being intercepted by the back or outer portion of the inner detector ring. A small nutation or wobble of the detector ring off the main axis of the gantry permits the x-ray beam to traverse the gantry opening and strike the scintillation detectors on the opposite side of the ring (Figure 3.14).

A further variation that has been introduced with this latter system is the use of cesium iodide crystals in conjunction with photodiodes. The optical output of the cesium iodide crystals is coupled to solid-state silicon photodiodes. The output characteristics of the cesium iodide crystal match the input features of the photodiode, ensuring an optimal transfer of energy from the cesium iodide to the photodiode. The photodiode acts essentially as a solid-state photomultiplier tube, converting the optical energy from the cesium iodide scintillation crystals into electrical energy. Light from the cesium iodide scintillation crystals is transferred via a short light pipe to the silicon photodiode. The light striking the photosensitive surface of the photodiode generates a small current (of the order of 10^{-13} amperes). This current then enters

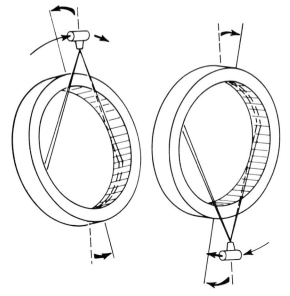

Figure 3.14. The slight tilting or nutation of the detector ring allows the x-ray beam to strike the crystals on the opposite side of the detector ring, without being intercepted by the back ends of the detection system in the proximal portion of the ring.

a low noise preamplifier immediately adjacent to the photodiode. The preamplifier is also a current-to-voltage converter. The preamplifier output ranges from 50 µV to 10 V.

A distinct advantage of the photodiode as compared to the photomultiplier tube is its lower cost, permitting a large number of these detectors (1,088 in the EMI 7070) to be used. The relatively small size of the cesium iodide scintillation crystals (1.8 mm wide) and the photodiodes allow them to be more closely spaced (less than ½ mm apart). The close spacing with a small detector aperture size may offer improved resolution. A small amount of exit collimation is used to reduce the amount of scatter entering the detectors.

The introduction of a system with 2,400 cadmium tungstate detectors, the Pfizer PZ-2400, had offered a further improvement in data collection and resolution. No collimators were used in this system, and the detector aperture size of 1.9 mm was virtually identical to the physical width of the crystal. There was very little dead space between detectors (about .1 mm), accounting for the claimed 93% geometric efficiency of this system. The overall capture efficiency (geometric and detector) was reputed to be 84%. In different operating modes (as determined by the computer programming or software) not only were different numbers of rays collected per view, but the quantity of data collected per ray, and the resulting statistical reliability of the measurement, could also be varied.

COMPARISON OF THIRD AND FOURTH GENERATION SCANNERS

The third and fourth generations both represent units with purely rotational geometries designed to gather the maximum amount of x-ray transmission data in the shortest possible time. The specific design features incorporated into each of these conceptually different approaches have been described. Each is an attempt to achieve the highest possible spatial and contrast resolution at the lowest radiation dose to the patient and with the fewest artifacts.

Factors determining spatial resolution include: 1) the aperture size of the detector, 2) the sampling rate, 3) the form of the algorithm used in reconstruction, and 4) the pixel size. The aperture size, or aperture function, determines the size of the x-ray beam each detector sees. This is related to the x-ray tube focal spot size and to the physical size of the detector aperture. As mentioned earlier, typical scintillation crystal/photomultiplier tube combinations employed in fourth generation units are relatively bulky, and commonly the individual detector centers cannot be spaced more closely than 8–9 mm (although this was reduced substantially in the EMI 7070 and the Pfizer PZ-2400). The actual detector aperture size is typically about 4 mm in the units employing bismuth germanate crystals and photomultiplier tubes. Even if physical limitations were not present, economic considerations might prevail, since close spacing would require more of these relatively expensive detectors. If the individual detector apertures were made smaller (by using physically smaller detectors and/or by greater collimation), a reduced portion of the radiation dose would be used for a signal. Thus, the fraction of wasted radiation would increase. Furthermore, for a fixed radiation dose to the patient the smaller aperture would detect less emerging radiation, and the greater spatial resolution would be offset by decreased contrast resolution secondary to increased quantum statistical noise related to the smaller signal. Increasing the total x-ray flux, either by raising tube output or by increasing scan time, into the narrow aperture detector in order to decrease quantum noise would result in increased patient dosage.

In the high pressure gas detection array used in most third generation units, the aperture of the different detector elements can be made smaller, typically 1.5 mm or less, without an associated decrease in utilization of patient radiation dose, since the individual detectors are separated only by the thin tungsten plates. Similarly, in modified third or fourth generation systems using physically smaller scintillation crystal-photodiode detectors, the aperture size may be reduced to 1.8 mm, as in the EMI 7070. For any system, however, the effective aperture size will be modified by the motion of the x-ray beam or the patient relative to the detector. In this regard it is interesting that in most translational-rotational units a wide aperture is required, because the x-ray flux, or number of photons, intercepted by a detector during one data sampling or measurement is limited by the low output of the stationary anode tube.

A wider aperture may be compensated for, at least in part, by a higher sampling rate. Faithful reproduction of a spatially varying object requires a spatial sampling frequency twice the highest spatial frequency or rate of change within the object (Nyquist theorem). For a scanning system with a sufficiently small detector aperture, the sampling need only be high enough to maintain the spatial resolution limit set by this aperture (aperture-limited frequency). In systems with a wide detector aperture (including most fourth generation units as well as the translational-rotational units of the first and second generations), the sampling frequency is much higher than twice the aperture-limited frequency. This permits the relatively broad detector aperture response function to be more accurately analyzed ("deconvolved") during reconstruction. This will then in part offset the larger aperture size. However, the high sampling rate increases noise in the reconstructed image. In other words, to compensate for a wide aperture, a high sampling rate is necessary, but this high sampling rate introduces noise.

Most commercially available units at this time use filtered back-projection (also called convolutional) algorithms. This and other reconstruction algorithms are described in detail in Chapter 5. Basically, however, the geometries in the third and fourth generations are seen from differing "points of view." This has consequences in both the physical gathering of data and the manner in which the algorithm instructs the computer to process the data.

In the third generation the point of view is taken from the x-ray tube. For a pulsed tube, each pulse forms a view (equivalent to a profile, projection, or view in translational-rotational systems). In a third generation system with a continuously operating tube, the view is formed over a single measuring time or signal integration period (Figure 3.15). During a single pulse or integration time, each detector intercepts a single ray and measures the ray-sum associated with that ray (Figure 3.16). The ray spacing is the

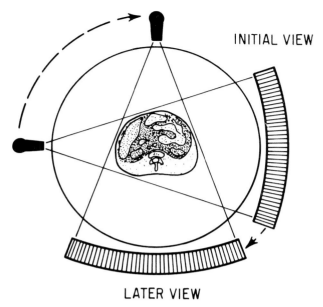

Figure 3.15. A view for a rotating x-ray tube and detector system is illustrated for two different positions during the rotation. The x-ray signals detected simultaneously by all the detectors during a single pulse constitute a single view in this geometric arrangement.

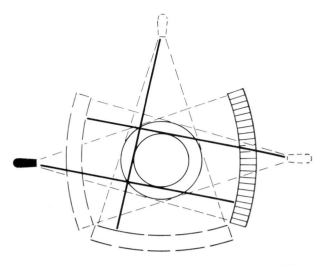

Figure 3.17. For a simultaneously rotating x-ray tube and detector array, a single detector sees a set of rays whose common paths form a circle within the object scanned.

physical spacing between detector elements. Each ray-sum constitutes a data sample or measurement. The sum total of all the rays for a single pulse or measurement time constitutes the view (Figure 3.15). Thus, all the detector elements participate in forming a view which results from one x-ray pulse. The number and spacing of the rays per view is fixed and is equal to the number of detectors in the array. The number of views is equal to the number of pulses or separate integration times per scan. The number of views can be varied in different units. Increasing the number of views increases the data and improves contrast resolution. There is, however, a concomitant increase in the scanning time and patient irradiation to acquire the additional views. Each detector records one ray in every view. The set of rays seen by a single detector during a scan describes a circle in the cross-section (Figure 3.17). That is, each detector effectively only sees or samples those volume elements that lie within a given circle within the slice. Thus, every voxel within the object slice is not seen by every detector. Detector failure or drift introduces an error which will be confined to volume elements on the circle seen by this detector. Thus, rather than averaging out all error over all the voxels in a tissue slice, the error is distributed over the elements on a circle, resulting in a localized circular artifact (Figure 3.18).

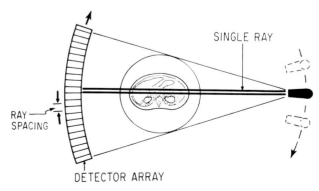

Figure 3.16. A ray is practically defined as that portion of the x-ray beam intercepted by a single detector.

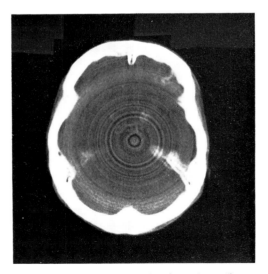

Figure 3.18. Clinical example of circular artifacts.

In a fourth generation system the point of view is an individual detector element. A view is formed over the time interval during which x-rays from the fan beam strike the detector (Figure 3.19). The number of views is equal to the number of detectors. Each view is composed of a number of rays, whose number and spacing are determined by the detector sampling rate, that is, the number of measurements made by each detector (Figure 3.19). This is determined by the computer programming or software. The sampling frequency can be varied as resolution requirements demand. During a scan, every detector in the fixed array surveys the entire cross-section; that is, every voxel in the cross-section is seen by the detector (Figure 3.20). Thus, the failure of any single detector will be averaged over all the voxels in the cross-section, rather than creating localized and easily noticed artifacts.

It is important that the pixel size be sufficiently small so that the spatial resolution achieved as a result of the aperture size, sampling rate, and algorithm is not lost because of an overly coarse matrix. However, it is also usually a waste of computer reconstruction time to demand a finer matrix than is justified by other factors determining the resolution. As a rule the matrix size should be chosen so that it is not a limiting factor in achieving the desired resolution. The display resolution or pixel size will be a function of the matrix size and the size of the field of view being reconstructed. A 512 matrix, for example, pro-

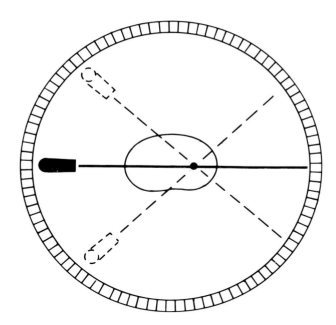

Figure 3.20. In the fixed detector geometry every voxel within the object scanned is seen by every detector.

vides pixel sizes of .5 mm, .8 mm, and 1.0 mm at field-of-view or scan circle diameters of 25, 40, and 50 cm, respectively. A 320 matrix will reconstruct a pixel of .8 mm in a 25-cm scan circle, and one of 1.3 mm when this field of view is increased to 42 cm.

Detection of low contrast objects (objects whose CT values differ only slightly from surrounding objects or organs) is usually limited by noise. The noise is related to statistical quantum fluctuations in the x-ray beam intensity, dose utilization, detector efficiency, sampling rate, detector noise, and associated electronic noise. The easiest way to decrease noise is to increase the number of x-ray photons detected, and hence, in general, the patient dose. It is thus also the least desirable way of reducing noise. Not infrequently, images of unusually high quality may be the result of the use of operating parameters (longer scanning time, high tube mA) that increase the patient's radiation dose. Crystal photomultiplier detectors and high pressure gas ionization detectors exhibit relatively low noise. The use of a narrow aperture detector decreases the need for high sampling rates with their increased noise level. It may also be helpful deliberately to use a coarser matrix. The larger voxels will individually contain more x-ray photons, with a concomitant decrease in the quantum statistical noise.

Scintillation detectors are inherently more efficient than high pressure xenon detectors, converting essentially 100% of the x-ray beam that strikes the detector into a signal as compared to about 50% for

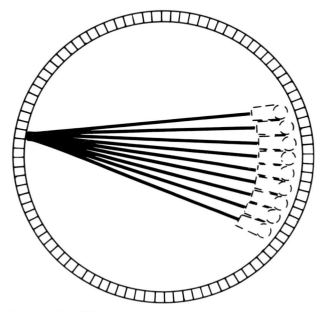

Figure 3.19. With a rotating x-ray tube and fixed circle of detectors, a view is the set of x-ray readings made by a single detector. These are consecutive (not simultaneous) readings made as the x-ray beam rotates into, through, and out of the view of that detector.

the xenon detectors. However, the virtual absence of collimators between the xenon gas cells allows nearly 100% of the transmitted x-ray beam to enter the xenon detectors. Because of the intervening collimators, the scintillation crystals see only about half of the transmitted beam that exits the patient. Thus, the overall efficiency for radiation capture and detection is about 50% for both detection systems. The close spacing and high absorption efficiency of cesium iodide crystals used with photodiodes, and of a system (PZ-2400) using 2,400 cadium tungstate crystals, have been promising developments in efficient utilization of the patient dose.

In fourth generation systems the patient does not completely fill the scanning field of view. Each detector thus intercepts the essentially unattenuated x-ray beam as it passes directly through air twice during a scan, before and after the patient interrupts rays passing from the tube to the detector (Figure 3.21). Therefore, each detector can be calibrated in air twice during a scan. Each detector's data profile through air can be normalized by the computer for the entire signal chain, including scintillation crystal, photomultiplier tube, and electronic circuitry. This normalization or correction after air calibration is performed for all detector signal chains during scanning. Hence, detector stability is only critical for the duration of that detector's view of the patient, and is usually very good over that very short period.

In a rotating detector system, however, each detector is fixed relative to the source. Some pe-

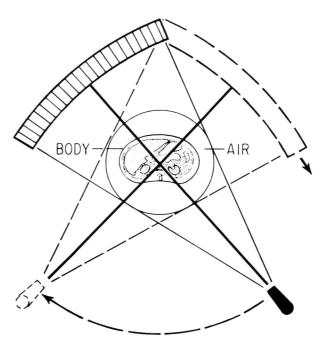

Figure 3.22. In a rotating tube and detector geometry, calibration of all the detectors through air cannot be done if the patient is in the gantry.

ripheral detectors will only see the x-ray source through air. Most of the detectors, and all of the centrally located ones, will only view the x-ray source through the patient, and hence cannot be calibrated through air so long as the patient is in the gantry (Figure 3.22). Thus, there is a much more stringent requirement for detector stability. During the scan, possible drifts in the output of the x-ray tube can be monitored and corrected by using the most peripheral detector elements as reference cells, typically up to 12 in number. In a pulsed tube system detector, electronic nulling (making sure that there is a zero electrical signal for zero x-ray intensity) can be performed between pulses. Further electronic corrections can be performed under computer control during scanning. Long-term stability and calibration can be tested periodically with phantoms.

Because in gas detector systems only one gas volume is present (the individual xenon cells are mechanically open to one another but electrically separate), the individual cells are more uniform than scintillation crystals, being identical in gas pressure and composition. Scintillation crystals will not possess the same uniformity from one to another, but individual detector calibration can eliminate this as a potential problem.

Ring artifacts have been prone to occur in rotating detector systems, as described earlier. These

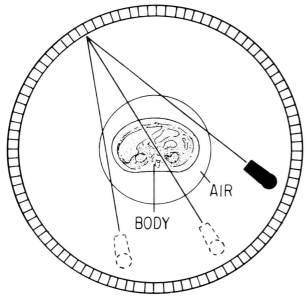

Figure 3.21. Calibration of the detectors through air is performed during each scan with a fixed detector geometry. This can be done even when the patient is in the gantry.

occur because failure of a single detector will result in an error that will not be averaged over all the voxels in the slice (since the detector will not see most of them) but will only be distributed among those voxels lying in the circle of points seen by the detector. Appropriate manufacturing design features, uniformity in detector linearity to changes in kVp, and periodic calibration based on phantom scanning have reduced this problem.

REFERENCES AND SUGGESTED READINGS

Adriaenssens, W., and Blumenfield, S. M. Dose utilization in the General Electric CT/T: Effects of narrow detector aperture sampling. *In* P. Gerhardt and G. van Kaick (eds.), Total Body Computerized Tomography. International Symposium, Heidelberg, 1977, pp. 284–290. Georg Thieme, Stuttgart, 1979.

Alfidi, R. J., MacIntyre, W. J., and Haaga, J. R. The effects of biological motion on CT resolution. American Journal of Roentgenology 127:11–15, 1976.

American Scientific and Engineering, Inc. AS&E CT scanner, 1976.

Brasch, R. C., Boyd, D. P., and Gooding, C. A. Computed tomographic scanning in children: Comparison of radiation dose and resolving power of commercial CT scanners. American Journal of Roentgenology 131:95–101, 1978.

Christensen, E. E., Curry, T. S., and Dowdey, J. E. Computed tomography. *In* An Introduction to the Physics of Diagnostic Radiology, Chap. 24, pp. 329–366. Lea & Febiger, Philadelphia, 1978.

Cohen, G. Contrast-detail-dose analysis of six different computed tomographic scanners. Journal of Computer Assisted Tomography 3:197–203, 1979.

General Electric Company. Introduction to computed tomography. General Electric Publication No. 4691, 1976.

General Electric Company. CT/T technology continuum: Technical performance of the CT/T system. General Electric Publication No. 4870.

General Electric Company. CT/T technology continuum update: The significance of dose and sensitivity profiles. General Electric Publication No. 4998, 1979.

Glover, G. H., and Eisner, R. L. Theoretical resolution of computed tomography systems. Journal of Computer Assisted Tomography 3:85–91, 1979.

Haque, P. Initial performance evaluation of the CT 7070 scanner. Presented at the 20th Annual Meeting of the American Association of Physicists in Medicine. San Francisco, July 30–August 3, 1978.

Haque, P. Scintillation crystal-photodiode array detectors. *In* T. H. Newton and D. G. Potts (eds.), Radiology of the Skull and Brain: Technical Aspects of Computed Tomography, Vol. 5, Chap. 118, Part XVII, Sect. IV, pp. 4127–4132. C. V. Mosby, St. Louis, 1981.

Harrel, G. S., Marshall, W. H., Breiman, R. S., and Seppi, E. J. Early experience with the Varian six-second body scanner in the diagnosis of hepatobiliary tract disease. Radiology 123:355–360, 1977.

Hounsfield, G. N. Picture quality of computed tomography. American Journal of Roentgenology 127:3–9, 1976.

Levitt, R. G., Stanley, R. J., Sagel, S. S., Lee, J. K. T., and Weyman, P. J. Computed tomography of the pancreas: Three-second versus 18-second scanning. Journal of Computer Assisted Tomography 6:259–267, 1982.

McCullough, E. C., and Payne, J. T. X-ray transmission computed tomography. Medical Physics 4:85–98, 1977.

McCullough, E. C., and Payne, J. T. Patient dosage in computed tomography. Radiology 129:457–463, 1978.

Margulis, A. R., Boyd, D. P., and Korobkin, M. T. Comparison of bimodal (translate-rotate) and pure rotary CT body scanners. *In* P. Gerhardt and G. van Kaick (eds.), Total Body Computerized Tomography. International Symposium, Heidelberg, 1977, pp. 10–15. Georg Thieme, Stuttgart, 1979.

Peschmann, K. R. Xenon gas ionization detectors. *In* T. H. Newton and D. G. Potts (eds., Radiology of the Skull and Brain: Technical Aspects of Computed Tomography, Vol. 5, Chap. 118, Part XVII, Sect. III, pp. 4112–4126. C. V. Mosby, St. Louis, 1981.

Peters, T. M., and Lewitt, R. M. Computed tomography with fan beam geometry. Journal of Computer Assisted Tomography 1:429–436, 1977.

Picker Corporation. Synerview 600 Computed Tomography: Performance Information.

Schwierz, G., and Ruhrnschopf, E. P. Characteristic properties of the fan beam technique. *In* P. Gerhardt and G. van Kaick (eds.), Total Body Computerized Tomography. International Symposium, Heidelberg, 1977, pp. 274–279. Georg Thieme, Stuttgart, 1979.

Technicare Corporation. Technical supplement: The Delta Scan 2000 series of computed tomography scanners, 1978.

Ter-Pogossian, M. M. Computerized cranial tomography: Equipment and physics. Seminars in Roentgenology 12:13–25, 1977.

Thompson, T. T. Computed tomography. *In* A Practical Approach to Modern X-Ray Equipment, Chap. 8, pp. 167–189. Little, Brown & Company, Boston, 1978.

Yaffe, M., Fenster, A., and Johns, H. E. Xenon ionization detectors for fan beam computed tomography scanners. Journal of Computer Assisted Tomography 1:419–428, 1977.

Zatz, L. M. General overview of computed tomography instrumentation. *In* T. H. Newton and D. G. Potts (eds.), Radiology of the Skull and Brain: Technical Aspects of Computed Tomography, Vol. 5, Chap. 116, Part XVII, pp. 4025–4057. C. V. Mosby, St. Louis, 1981.

Chapter 4
COMPUTER THEORY AND APPLICATIONS

Michael D. Miller, M.S., Ph.D., M.D.

COMPUTERS: BACKGROUND AND DEVELOPMENT

    Early Historical Background of Computer Development
    Analog and Digital Computers
    Number Systems
    Boolean Logic
    Early Electrical Representation of Binary States

HARDWARE

    Solid-State Devices
        Transistors
        Integrated Circuits
        Complex Integrated Circuits
        Large Scale Integrated Circuits
    Computer Organization
    Central Processor Unit
        Arithmetic Logic Unit
        Control Unit
    Memory
        Random Access Memory
        Auxiliary Memory
    Input and Output Devices
        Buffers
        Batch Devices
        Interactive Devices

SOFTWARE

    Machine Language
    Assembly Language
    Higher Languages
    Operating Systems and Applications Programs
        Operating Systems
        Applications Programs

COMPUTER APPLICATIONS IN COMPUTED
    TOMOGRAPHY

    General Description
    Hardware Installation

REFERENCES AND SUGGESTED READINGS

COMPUTERS: BACKGROUND AND DEVELOPMENT

Early Historical Background of Computer Development

The manual manipulation of numbers has always been slow, tedious, and of doubtful accuracy. Early mathematicians and accountants sought to increase computational speed by the use of tables and the abacus. These aids to computation remained in widespread use in Europe as late as the 17th century. The first working model of a mechanical adding machine was invented in 1642 by the 19-year-old Blaise Pascal (1623–1662). The primary innovation incorporated in this device was the automatic carryover, a function that had to be performed manually on an abacus.

Approximately 30 years later, Gottfried Wilhelm von Leibniz (1646–1716) proposed a design for a device that would multiply by successive additions. This machine incorporated the automatic carryover developed by Pascal as well as a new innovation, a moveable carriage, familiar to users of modern mechanical calculators. Fabrication of Leibniz's device required machine techniques beyond the state of the art at that time. The result was a calculator that was too unreliable for practical purposes.

No further significant progress was made in the development of the mechanical calculator until early in the 19th century when Charles Babbage (1792–1871) designed the difference engine. This mechanical device could generate complex tables for use in astronomy and navigation. The only mathematical function performed by the machine in generating these tables was addition. The success of this device led Babbage to design the analytical engine. This machine would have incorporated the major components of modern digital computers. Instructions were to be stored on punch cards, an idea earlier put into practice in the weaving industry by the French inventor Joseph Marie Jacquard (1752–1834) to control the operation of an automatic loom which wove complicated designs. Fabrication problems were compounded by the severe demands on the design imposed by Babbage, and a working model was never constructed.

By the end of the 19th century, improved technology finally allowed the construction of a reliable mechanical calculator. These machines could perform the four basic arithmetic functions by using concepts developed up to two centuries earlier. Other than the replacement of the hand crank by an electric motor, the mechanical calculator has changed little since that time.

Analog and Digital Computers

Two very different techniques are available for electronic or mechanical data processing. An approach using analog devices was most popular in the first half of this century. In the past two decades, this approach has been replaced almost completely by one using digital devices.

Analog computers depend on the amplitude of a signal to represent the numerical value of a variable. In a mechanical device, for example, this might be the number of degrees of rotation of a gear or wheel. Familiar analog devices still in common use are the conventional wristwatch and the electric, gas, and water meters in most homes. Electrical analog devices might use the voltage of a signal to represent the value of a variable. By using this representation, analog computers have been designed to represent complex mathematical functions, such as differential equations. The initial popularity of analog machines was primarily due to their relative ease of construction and simplicity. Accuracy of an analog device, however, is limited by the system capability for measuring, transmitting, and manipulating the signal amplitude. Any initial error in measurement is rapidly propagated and amplified within the machine, resulting in a progressive loss of accuracy. This problem of error propagation and amplification becomes particularly severe when a large number is to be combined with a smaller one, a situation that can result in complete loss of the smaller signal. The problem of "slide rule error" is a familiar example.

In contrast, in digital machines every instruction, variable, or logical element is represented as an array of elements, and each element in the array can assume only a limited number of discrete values. In modern computers, these values are 0 and 1, hence the use of the descriptive term, binary logic.

As binary switching elements became cheaper to produce, the advantages of versatility, precision, and stability available from digital computers began to outweigh the analog computer's advantage of relative simplicity of fabrication.

Number Systems

The number system in common daily use is a decimal system, based on the use of 10 different number elements or digits. To understand computer language, a familiarity with alternative number systems, in particular the binary number system using two digit elements, is required.

Number systems, such as the present-day Arabic (which actually originated in India) and the ancient

Roman systems, represent various quantities in an irregular fashion, much as our monetary system depends on the use of cents, nickles, and dimes as well as 5-, 10-, and 20-dollar bills. The place system allows combinations of a very limited number of distinct symbols to represent numbers of any desired magnitude to any degree of desired precision. In the place system, the numerical value of a symbol depends not only on the symbol itself, but also on the relative location of the symbol with respect to a reference. This reference may be with respect to another symbol as in the Roman system (e.g., IX = 9 and XI = 11) or with respect to an assigned point (the decimal point in a decimal system).

The base of a number system is the number of distinct symbols necessary to represent the value of a quantity in that system. For example, in the decimal system of everyday usage, 10 distinct symbols are used, 0 through 9. In the octal system, there are eight symbols, 0 through 7; and in a binary system there are only two symbols, 0 and 1. In situations where various number systems are intermixed, the base is indicated by a subscript following the number.

Table 4.1 summarizes these points and gives examples of the decimal number system and the number systems most commonly used in computer technology. The actual value represented by a symbol in the Nth place to the left of the reference point (called a decimal point when 10 different symbols are used) is the product of that symbol times the base of the particular number system in use raised to the $N - 1$ power. Thus, in the decimal system a 7 in the third place to the left of a decimal point represents 7 times 10 to the second power, that is, 7×10^2, or 700.

In the binary system, every number is represented by a string of 0s and 1s. This quickly becomes cumbersome. As can be seen from Table 4.1, representation of a number between 8 and 15 requires

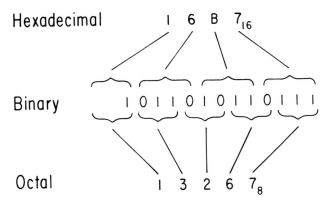

Figure 4.1. Equivalent expressions of a number in the hexadecimal, binary, and octal systems.

the use of four binary digits. By appropriately grouping binary numbers, a simple conversion can be made to a higher base number system (one with a base greater than 2), which is more familiar in appearance to an operator. If binary numbers are divided into groups of three digits, much as we divide decimal numbers into thousands, millions, and billions, each group of three binary digits can be represented by one of eight distinct symbols. This is an octal system. Similarly, it can be seen from Table 4.1 that four binary digits can represent 16 distinct values. This is a hexadecimal system. Because the decimal number system only associates numerical value with 10 different symbols, when the hexadecimal system is used, the first six letters of the alphabet, A through F, are recruited to represent the numbers 10 through 15, respectively. Table 4.1 illustrates this conversion. Figure 4.1 shows an example relating the binary, octal, and hexadecimal systems. Most computer systems use either the octal or hexadecimal system for ease of communication with the operator. The more complex conversion between binary and decimal is

Table 4.1. Commonly used number systems in computer technology.

System	Base	Digits	Decimal value of each unit in Nth place to left of decimal				
			1	2	3	4	5
Decimal	10	0, 1, 2, 3, 4, 5, 6, 7, 8, 9	1	10	100	1,000	10,000
Binary	2	0, 1	1	2	4	8	16
Octal	8	0, 1, 2, 3, 4, 5, 6, 7	1	8	64	512	4,096
Hexadecimal	16	0, 1, 2, 3, 4, 5, 6, 7, 8, 9, A, B, C, D, E, F	1	16	256	4,096	65,536
Exponential equivalent of each place to base n			10_n^0	10_n^1	10_n^2	10_n^3	10_n^4

made only when essential for communication with the user.

Because the conversion between the binary system and the decimal system is so clumsy, a variation of the binary system has been devised in situations requiring frequent conversions between these two systems. A common example of this situation is in devices where there is a high ratio of input and output to internal processing, for example, in calculators. Table 4.2 shows the conversion between decimal numbers and binary coded decimal, usually abbreviated BCD. A four-digit binary number is used to represent each decimal digit. A three-digit decimal number would therefore require use of twelve binary digits. Storage of a BCD variable is relatively inefficient, because a three-digit decimal number requires as much memory in this system as a three-digit hexadecimal number ordinarily would. In conventional binary notation, a three-digit decimal number would require only 10 binary digits. The trade-off is between expense of the additional memory locations versus the complexity of the processing circuits.

Boolean Logic

The rules for manipulation of binary variables are defined by a form of mathematics called Boolean logic or switching logic. A binary variable can take on only two values, 0 or 1. These two states can also

Table 4.2. Conversion between decimal and BCD numbers.

BCD[a]	Decimal equivalent
0000	0
0001	1
0010	2
0011	3
.	.
.	.
.	.
1001	9
0001 0000	10
0001 0001	11
0001 0010	12
0001 0011	13
.	.
.	.
.	.
0001 1001	19
0010 0000	20
.	.
.	.
0010 0011 1001	239

[a] BCD = binary coded decimal.

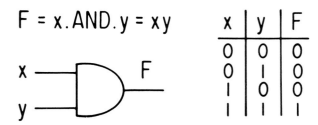

Figure 4.2. The mathematical representation, gate symbol, and truth table for the AND function.

be thought of as representation of the logic "true" and "false." Most commonly, logic true is represented by a binary state 1 and logic false by a binary state 0.

A logic function or operation defines the condition of a binary variable based on the states of one or more input variables. These operations are most clearly represented by a "truth table," a tabular representation of the output value for different values of the inputs. The customary mathematical representation, symbol, and truth table for each of the three basic operations or logic functions, AND, OR, and complement, are shown in Figures 4.2, 4.3, and 4.4, respectively. The complement function is also called the NOT or inverter function. The letters X and Y represent the independent input variables upon which the dependent output variable, or value of the function, depends. The AND and OR functions may have more than two inputs, but the additional independent variables would be handled in a fashion similar to the two shown. This is illustrated for each of these functions for three input variables in Figures 4.5 and 4.6. Other logic functions such as inverse functions of AND and OR, also called NAND and NOR functions, respectively (Figures 4.7 and 4.8), and the exclusive OR (Figure 4.9), can be defined in terms of these three basic functions.

A logic gate is a mechanical or electrical device that generates digital output, either 0 or 1, depending on the value of the input signals. The type of gate is determined by the relationship of the output to the input variables. For example, a dual input device

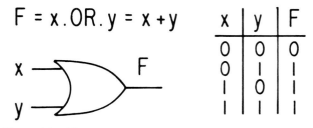

Figure 4.3. The mathematical representation, gate symbol, and truth table for the OR function.

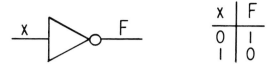

Figure 4.4. The mathematical representation, gate symbol, and truth table for the complement function.

which generates output as defined by the truth table shown in Figure 4.2 is called an AND gate. Figures 4.2–4.4 show the customary mathematical representations and the symbols commonly used in describing the gates within a complex electrical circuit as well as the truth tables. A combination of an AND gate followed by a complement (NOT or inverter) gate is called a NAND gate or AND inverse gate. This is illustrated in Figure 4.7. The NOR gate is similarly defined and is illustrated in Figure 4.8. The inverse or complement of a function or variable is indicated algebraically by an apostrophe following the name of the variables.

There are many similarities between the rules governing conventional algebra and the rules of the algebra involving logic circuits. The rules of manipulation of logic gates and the relationships between the various forms of logic gates are defined by the rules of Boolean algebra. The Boolean equivalents of addition and multiplication are the OR function and the AND function, respectively. Boolean variables obey the same distributive and associative laws of addition and multiplication as conventional algebra. The symbols 0 and 1 are also treated similarly in the equivalent operations of the algebras.

There are important differences, however. For example, logic functions do not always commute. That is, if the sequence in which functions are applied to input variables is altered, the output may be

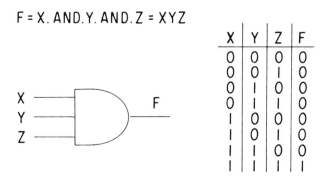

Figure 4.5. The mathematical representation, gate symbol, and truth table for the three-input AND function.

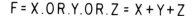

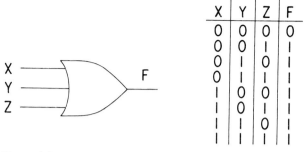

Figure 4.6. The mathematical representation, gate symbol, and truth table for the three-input OR function.

changed. Specifically, an AND gate followed by an inverter results in a truth table characteristic of the NAND function (Figure 4.7). In contrast, inverters preceding the input to an AND gate result in a truth table characteristic of the NOR function. This is shown in Figure 4.8.

Some of the other important relationships in Boolean algebra that differ from conventional algebra are described in Table 4.3. The noncommuting nature of the inverse operation with AND and OR functions is described in rules 3 and 4, commonly referred to as De Morgan's theorem. These are particularly useful in dealing with the relationships between NAND and NOR gates. The significance of these relationships is not apparent based on material presented to this point, but is based in part upon the relative ease of manufacture of NAND and NOR gates and the use of these gates in generating other logic functions.

Early Electrical Representation of Binary States

The logic circuits that manipulate binary data are called "gates." Examples of simple electrical gates representing the AND and OR functions are shown in Figures 4.10 and 4.11. Consider switches X and Y to be representations of the input data, in other words the independent variables, with an open switch representing logic state 0 and a closed switch representing logic state 1. The output, represented by a lamp, is in logic state 1 when lit and in logic state 0 when extinguished. The four possible combinations of states for the two switches in each circuit can then

Table 4.3. Selected relationships in Boolean algebra

1. $x + x = x$
2. $x * x = x$
3. $(x + y)' = x'y'$
4. $(xy)' = x' + y'$
5. $x + yz = (x + y)(x + z)$

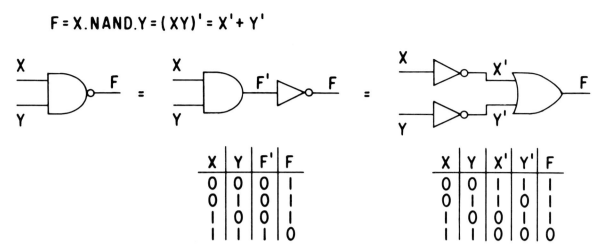

Figure 4.7. Two equivalent methods for generating the NAND function and the truth table for each.

be seen to reproduce the correct output previously defined for AND and OR gates in Figures 4.2 and 4.3.

Arrangements of mechanically activated switches are not practical for use as logic gates in computers. An electromagnetic relay consists of a switch that is activated by an electromagnet and returned to its resting position by a spring. If the input current through the electromagnet is sufficiently large, the relay circuits close for normally opened (NO) contacts and open for normally closed (NC) contacts. The current required to energize the electromagnet is called the lock-in current. When the current input to the electromagnet decreases below the drop-out value, the relay contact is returned to the resting state. Figure 4.12 shows a schematic diagram of a relay with both NO and NC contacts. The choice and number of contacts will determine the type of logic circuit represented by an individual relay. As with mechanical switches, closed contacts usually are defined as representing logic state 1 and open contacts as logic state 0. The normally closed contacts of a relay act as a logic inverter, whereas the normally opened contacts act as a buffer, that is, a gate for which the output equals the input.

Combinations of relays can replace similar combinations of manually operated switches to generate automatic logic switching circuits as shown in Figure 4.13 and 4.14. The input, X and Y, describes the state of the electromagnet in the relay as being energized (1) or idle (0). Figure 4.13 shows two relays connected to form a dual input AND gate. An OR gate is shown in Figure 4.14. These gates satisfy the truth tables of Figures 4.2 and 4.3, respectively.

Logic gates utilizing electromagnetic relays of

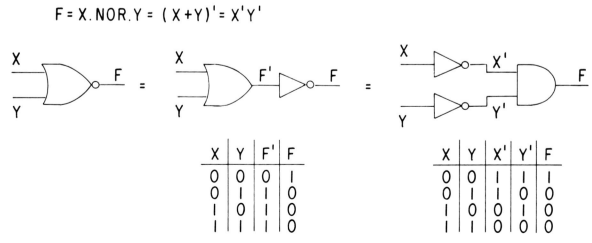

Figure 4.8. Two equivalent methods for generating the NOR function and the truth table for each.

Basic Principles of Computed Tomography

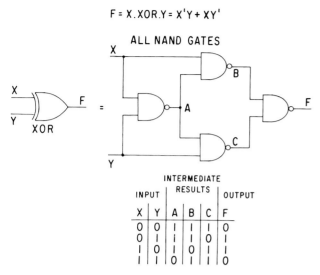

Figure 4.9. The use of four NAND gates to generate the exclusive OR function and the truth table showing the intermediate functions.

this type were employed in what is credited to be the first successful digital computer, the Mark I, which was used at Harvard from 1935 to 1944. It consisted essentially of a large number of IBM tabulating machines. Although they carried out their intended functions, these electromechanical devices are bulky and require large amounts of power to energize the electromagnets. This power is dissipated in the form of heat, which then must be removed from the computer room. Depending on size and design, the time taken for a relay to switch between one state and another is usually measured in tens of milliseconds. Finally, the moving parts, including the electrical contacts, are subject to wear, and reliability suffers. The

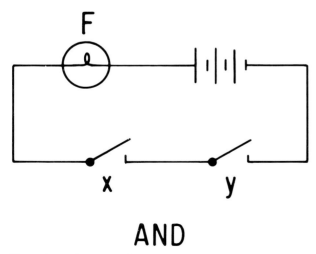

Figure 4.10. Example of a manual switching AND gate with two inputs.

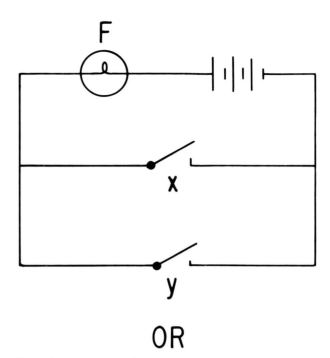

Figure 4.11. Example of a manual switching two-input OR gate.

Mark I required approximately .3 s for a single addition. A multiplication took 6 s, and a division approximately 16 s. The machine measured about 50 feet in length and weighed 5 tons.

Initially, these devices were replaced by electronic vacuum tubes, diodes and triodes, because of the more rapid switching times associated with the vacuum tubes. A vacuum tube diode, familiar to radiologists as the rectifier in x-ray tube high voltage power supplies, is illustrated in Figure 4.15. Electrons emitted by the hot cathode of the diode are attracted to the electrically positive anode or plate. The intensity of the electron flow or current between the cath-

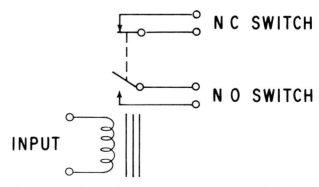

Figure 4.12. Relay with one set of normally open (NO) and one set of normally closed (NC) contacts shown in the idle state. When energized, the NO contacts close and the NC contacts open.

Computer Theory 75

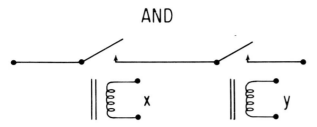

Figure 4.13. An electromagnetic AND gate equivalent to the switches used in Figure 4.10.

ode and anode of the diode is dependent on the temperature of the cathode and the potential difference between anode and cathode. The introduction of a third element, called a grid, between the cathode and anode converts the diode to a triode, illustrated in Figures 4.16 and 4.17. The current flowing between the cathode and anode of a triode is usually 10–100 times more sensitive to changes in grid voltage than to changes in plate voltage of an equivalent diode. When grid voltage becomes sufficiently negative with respect to the cathode, the current is reduced to zero. These characteristics of the triode allow it to be used as the active element in a switching circuit.

The first electronic digital computer, the ENIAC (Electronic Numerical Integrator and Calculator), was built at the University of Pennsylvania in 1946 by John Eckert and William Mauchley. It contained 18,000 electronic vacuum tubes wired together in appropriate logic circuits. The ENIAC could perform 300 multiplications per second, making it approximately 1,800 times faster than the Mark I. Like its electromechanical predecessor, the program or in-

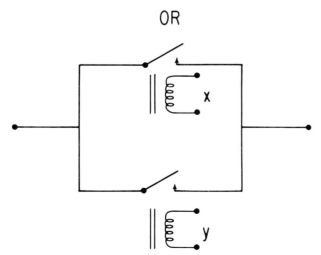

Figure 4.14. An electromagnetic OR gate equivalent to the switches used in Figure 4.11.

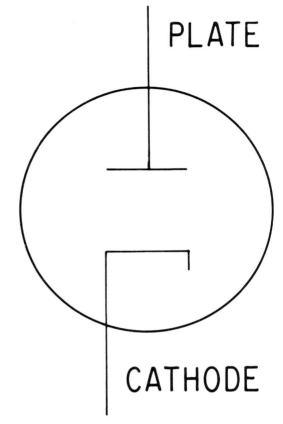

Figure 4.15. Vacuum tube diode.

structions determining the sequence of arithmetic and logic operations to be performed by the ENIAC were initially hardwired into the machine; that is, the program was incorporated into wired boards. A change in the program necessitated a change in one or more of these hardwired boards. In spite of its large size and number of components, only 20 10-digit numbers could be stored in this machine at one time. The ENIAC was used extensively to calculate ballistic tables for the U.S. Army.

About the time the ENIAC was constructed, the mathematician John von Neumann (1903–1957) proposed a method for storing the sequence of instructions in digital form in memory along with the data. Because of the ease of manipulation of these stored instructions, machines incorporating this feature can be used for many different purposes without extensive revision of the hardware for each function. This is probably the single most important innovation in the development of the modern computer. The ENIAC was successfully modified to incorporate this principle. The set of instructions stored in computer memory became known as software to distinguish it from the physical portion of the computer including

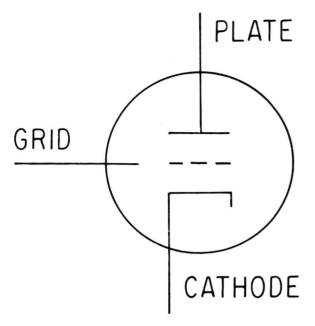

Figure 4.16. Schematic representation of a vacuum tube triode.

the hardwired plug-in boards that the numerical instructions replaced.

The first commercially available digital electronic computer, the UNIVAC, appeared about 1950. Electronic store-program digital computers, such as the ENIAC and UNIVAC, which are constructed with vacuum tubes, are referred to as the first generation of computers.

The relay functions in logic gates have now been completely taken over by solid-state devices (diodes, transistors, and integrated circuits), which are faster, cheaper to produce, more compact and reliable, and consume far less power per gate. The definition of logic gates is more complex for solid-state devices, which do not have distinct on and off conditions. Basically, the problem is solved by defining two ranges of input or output voltages without overlap such that input to a gate within either range will generate output, which will also fall unambiguously within one of these ranges. For example, an input or output voltage in the range 0–1 V might represent a logic state 0, and a voltage of 3–5 V might represent logic state 1. The design of the gate is such that input voltages in these ranges are never able to generate output voltages in the ambiguous 1- to 3-V range.

HARDWARE

Solid-State Devices

Transistors   The year 1948 marked the beginning of a revolution in electronics with the development of the transistor at Bell Telephone Laboratories by the physicists Walter Brattain, John Bardeen, and William Shockley. For this invention they were awarded the Nobel Prize in Physics in 1956. The earliest devices were generally made of germanium, a semiconductor with electrical properties between those of an insulator and metallic conductors. The majority of modern devices are now contructed from silicon, which is also a semiconductor but has superior thermal stability and can tolerate somewhat higher operating voltages.

The earliest transistors, and still the majority of transistors, are bipolar or junction-type transistors consisting of three elements: the base, the emitter, and the collector. This makes them analogous to the triode electron tube, although the latter is basically a voltage amplifier whereas bipolar transistors are current amplifiers.

The basic elements of a transistor circuit are illustrated in Figure 4.18. In the circuit illustrated here, a small current flowing in the base-emitter circuit results in a larger current flowing in the collector-emitter circuit. The ratio of the two currents, I_c/I_b, is the current gain, which depends not only on the

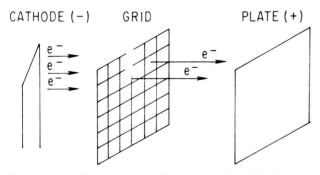

Figure 4.17. The elements of the vacuum tube triode showing the effect of the grid in attenuating the electron current.

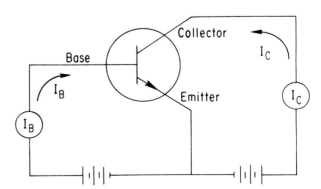

Figure 4.18. Basic circuit of a transistor current amplifier.

Computer Theory   77

design of the transistor itself but also on the particular operating conditions of the circuit. Gain, or amplification, and operating frequency are closely related factors in transistor circuits. Specifically, the gain of a transistor decreases as frequency increases. For each device, there is a frequency at which the amplitude of the output signal equals the amplitude of the input signal; that is, no amplification occurs. This characteristic sets an upper limit on the speed at which a transistor can function as a switching device. The earliest transistors were limited to audio frequencies, that is, switching times on the order of milliseconds. Modern transistors are capable of operation well into the ultrahigh frequency (UHF) range, with switching times on the order of nanoseconds (1 ns = 10^{-9} s).

The current requirements for power consumption of transistors are far less than those of similar circuits using electromagnetic relays or electron tubes. Nevertheless, as the complexity of the circuits increases, the total power consumption can still become appreciable. This takes on particular importance in computer circuits. As increasing numbers of current-dissipating devices, which include transistors as well as resistors, are packed into smaller volumes, the problem of dissipation of heat can again become significant. For this and other reasons it became necessary to develop devices with lower power requirements than the bipolar transistor. The prototype of a family of transistors with these desirable low power characteristics is the field effect transistor (FET). This device more nearly approximates a solid-state equivalent of the triode electron tube in that current flow through the input circuit is not necessary to control the amount of current flowing through the output circuit. The three basic elements of the FET are the gate, source, and drain (Figures 4.19 and 4.20). The gate performs the equivalent function of the grid in an electron tube. A voltage applied to the gate regulates the flow of current between source and drain without significant current flowing through the gate itself.

Most FETs manufactured today are of the metal-oxide-semiconductor (MOS) type, because of the ease of manufacturing large numbers of these devices in very small volumes, that is, at a high density. A further modification is the complementary metal-oxide-semiconductor (CMOS) device. These operate at even lower current levels then the MOS type of FET. CMOS devices are somewhat more complex to fabricate, however. Trade-offs have to be made between cost of manufacture and the actual need for their reduced power consumption. In spite of their relatively higher power requirements, the conventional bipolar transistors still have a speed advantage

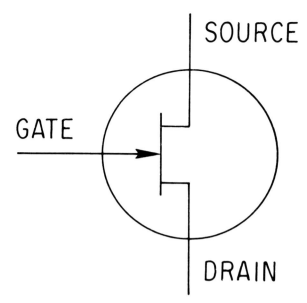

Figure 4.19. Schematic representation of the field effect transistor (FET).

over the MOS and CMOS devices. The trade-offs between power consumption, speed, and packing densities of the devices have to be made on the basis of the intended application.

Because of the tremendous improvement in power consumption, reliability, decrease in size, and increase in speed of operation, computers constructed of transistors instead of tubes have been referred to as second generation computers.

Integrated Circuits In spite of the dramatic improvements with the introduction of transistors into computer design, construction follows the same principles of forming logic gates from discrete electronic components. The next major breakthrough in the development of the computer came with the in-

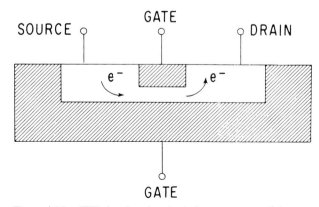

Figure 4.20. FET showing the physical arrangement of the semiconductors and the path of the electrons past the gate.

78 Basic Principles of Computed Tomography

troduction of integrated circuits in the early 1960s. Computers constructed using integrated circuits are called third generation computers.

Integrated circuits are devices composed of a semiconducting substrate upon which various layers of insulating, conducting, and semiconducting materials are deposited and etched into specific patterns. These then function as substitutes for assemblies of discrete transistors, resistors, capacitors, and diodes. The design and initial set-up for construction of these devices is more complex than for discrete components; however, once the manufacturing procedure has been established, large numbers of these integrated circuits can be manufactured at very low cost.

The earliest integrated circuits were attempts to reproduce faithfully on semiconductor chips the combinations of discrete components used in making similar gates by conventional techniques. It was soon found, however, that miniaturization of resistors was unreliable and that these components could be replaced more reliably and cheaply by additional transistors. The elimination of resistors from the coupling circuits between transistors also resulted in increased speed of operation of the circuits. The modern integrated circuit most commonly encountered is one using bipolar transistors directly coupled to each other and containing only a few resistors. Devices of this type are referred to as transistor-transistor-logic (TTL) circuits.

Typically, integrated circuits are assembled in packages measuring approximately 8 × 8 × 20 mm. The number of logic gates contained in one integrated circuit depends upon the complexity of the gate, usually measured in terms of the total number of inputs and outputs. Typically, six inverter gates might be included on one chip. The greater part of the volume of the integrated circuit is made up of the electrical leads and the inert plastic packaging material.

Although the AND and OR gates as well as the inverter were described as the three basic elements of Boolean or switching logic, the NAND and NOR gates are technically simpler to fabricate. Savings in cost of manufacture far outweigh the minor inconvenience of working with these inverse functions instead of their complements. All other gates are formed from combinations of these inverse functions. The versatility of the NAND gate is so great that the integrated circuit package containing four NAND gates is probably one of the most widely used. The construction of an exclusive OR gate from four NAND gates has been shown in Figure 4.9.

Digital integrated circuits of a single family such as the TTL type have the advantage of requiring a uniform supply voltage, in this case 5 V. In addition, the inputs and outputs are compatible, requiring no external matching devices. Thus, complex arrangements of logic gates can be assembled using only TTL integrated circuits with their inputs and outputs appropriately interconnected by jumper wires. This feature results in considerable simplification of design of complex circuits.

Other families of logic circuits have been created based on the MOS or CMOS devices. Gates of these types have particular advantages in high component density circuits or applications requiring very low power consumption. The TTL devices retain the advantage of highest operating speed.

Complex Integrated Circuits Although all logic operations can be performed by assembling inverters, NAND and NOR gates in the appropriate configurations, many combinations are encountered so frequently that it becomes more convenient to prepackage them into one integrated circuit.

Flip-Flops The flip-flop belongs to the family of devices known as sequential circuits. Its output depends not only upon the input, but also upon the state of the flip-flop at the time the input information is received. The flip-flop in its most basic form has one input and one output. The output cycles between 0 and 1 each time an appropriate pulse is received at the input. A circuit of this type can be constructed simply by the appropriate interconnection of a pair of NAND or a pair of NOR gates, as illustrated in Figures 4.21 and 4.22. The NAND gate flip-flops cycle on a 0 pulse. The NOR gate flip-flops cycle on a 1 pulse to the appropriate input. Even in its simplest form, there is provision for a reset input, which allows the flip-flop output to be started at a known value. This type of circuit is known as an asynchronous flip-flop or latch. Because it will maintain its output state indefinitely until instructed to change by a subsequent input pulse, a flip-flop is capable of storing a single unit of binary information, that is, one binary digit (1 bit). Flip-flops find widespread application within computers for storage of binary numbers.

The latch or asynchronous flip-flop can generate unpredictable output under certain input conditions and for this reason is rarely used. This problem can be resolved by allowing a change of state to occur only when the input pulse arrives coincidentally with a clock pulse. This modification is called a synchronous flip-flop. A device of this type can be constructed from four NAND gates appropriately interconnected. There are several types of synchronous flip-flops available, each defined by its own truth table. The basic function is the same, however.

The clock that generates the pulses that instruct

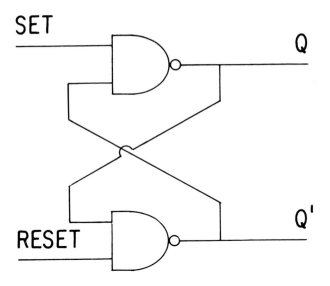

NAND GATE FLIP-FLOP   **NOR GATE FLIP-FLOP**

Figure 4.21. Pair of NAND gates connected to form an asynchronous flip-flop.

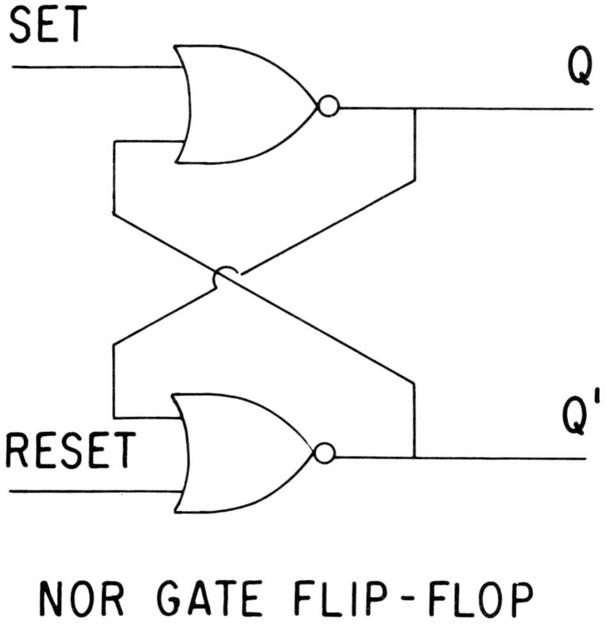

Figure 4.22. Pair of NOR gates connected to form an asynchronous flip-flop.

the synchronous flip-flops within the computer to respond to the input information provided them determines the overall speed of operation of the computer. The pulse interval must be sufficiently long to allow for the transit time between the input of data to any gate and the resultant change in output state. Short pulse intervals could result in incorrect transmission of information within a logic circuit. Unnecessarily long pulse intervals will still allow proper function but will result in unnecessarily slow operation of the computer. Typical propagation delays of signal within gates is on the order of 10 ns for the TTL family devices. For MOS integrated circuits, propagation delays are approximately 25 ns. A relatively newer family of devices, referred to as emitter coupled logic (ECL), has propagation delays as short as 2 ns.

Registers A group of flip-flops arranged to hold an entire binary word of information is called a register. The number of flip-flop elements in a register is determined by the intended organization of the computer. The smallest unit of binary information, the binary digit, is called a bit. A bit can have the value of 0 or 1, a rather limited range. For this reason, bits are usually organized in groups of 8, called bytes; this is the smallest unit of binary information usually transmitted within the computer. The largest number of bytes customarily manipulated within a computer is called a word. Depending on the computer design, a word usually consists of 1–4 bytes. The choice of word size is dependent upon the intended function of the computer. Where the computer is primarily required to manipulate alphanumeric data and perform simple calculations such as accounting procedures and formation of directories, word lengths of 8–16 bits usually suffice. In computers used for scientific or engineering applications, word lengths of 32 bits or more are generally chosen.

In addition to one flip-flop for each bit being stored, the register must have additional gates to control loading and unloading of information. There are two basic types of registers, the distinction between them being made on the basis of how data are loaded into and removed from the register. This distinction becomes important not only for data transmission within the computer but also for data transmission between the computer and peripheral devices that allow communication with the computer operator. The first type of register is called a parallel load register. The parallel load register has a separate input and output line for each flip-flop within the register. Thus, each bit can be loaded or transmitted to a new location simultaneously on receiving the appropriate instruction for this operation. In contrast, the shift register loads each bit sequentially into the register from a single input line. As each bit is loaded, the previously loaded bits are shifted sequentially one flip-flop at a time left or right to allow space for the incoming bit. Output from a shift register can either be in parallel mode, with all bits being transmitted simultaneously, or in serial mode along a single output line in the same manner in which the shift register was loaded.

The advantage of the parallel register is that transmission of data occurs much more rapidly. If speed is not a factor, the number of interconnecting wires can be reduced by using serial mode of transmission. Even in computers in which speed of execution is of primary importance, shift registers perform an important function. Multiplication and division operations are carried out by sequential additions or subtractions and shift operations. A computer that operates in the serial mode would require only shift registers for both data storage and manipulation.

Binary Counters An alternate configuration for grouping flip-flops is the binary counter. In devices of this type, the state of each flip-flop is determined by the number of input pulses received. As in registers, the size of the binary word or the maximum number of pulses that can be counted is determined by the number of flip-flops in the counter. Most commonly, 4- and 8-bit binary counters are assembled as integrated circuit packages. If a larger number of bits is required, these can be assembled from the smaller units. Decade counters are also available where counting in units of 10 is most convenient. In addition to keeping track of sequential operations or other data-gathering functions, binary and decade counters are convenient means for performing repeated divisions of input data by a fixed number.

Decoders A decoder is a device that converts binary information from one form to another. Common applications of decoders include the conversion of binary data into a form that can be displayed by digital readout devices. Examples of decoders are familiar to users of digital watches and calculators. Additionally, decoders provide a convenient means for locating information stored in memory, a topic that is discussed later.

Multiplexers A multiplexer is a device with multiple inputs, one of which is connected to the output when the appropriate binary signal is applied to the select line of this device. Control of 2^n input lines requires n select lines. Thus, the multiplexer shown in Figure 4.23 has three select lines. By applying a three-digit binary number to these lines, data from one of the eight input lines will be transmitted to the output line. The reverse function of connecting one input line to any one of 2^n output lines is performed by the demultiplexer. There is a strong similarity in design and operation between decoders and multiplexers. These devices are most commonly used in direction of transmission of data within the computer as well as in communication with peripheral devices.

Adders Another relatively simple but frequently encountered combination of the basic logic circuits is the adder. As the name implies, this circuit provides the function of addition of binary numbers. The most elementary form of this device is the half-adder which is composed of an AND gate and an exclusive OR gate. The half-adder generates only the sum of 2 binary bits and by itself is of limited usefulness. For practical addition of binary numbers, a full adder is required. This device not only can add 2 binary bits but can include in the addition a third bit that has been previously generated by a carryover from addition of the two adjacent bits of lesser significance within the two binary numbers. Although two binary numbers of any length can be added by

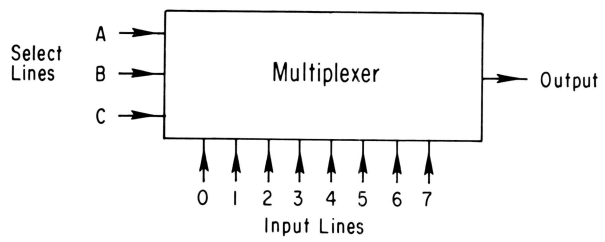

Figure 4.23. Control and data connections of the multiplexer.

sequentially shifting the numbers through a single bit full adder, more rapid processing can be achieved by using an array of full adders and loading the data in the parallel mode. Eight-bit adders are readily available in integrated circuits, and larger arrays can be constructed by combining several of these.

Large Scale Integrated Circuits The current state of the art in complexity of integrated circuits consists of devices containing in excess of 10,000 active elements. The original large scale integrated circuits (LSI) developed by Intel Corporation in the early 1970s included 1-kbit (kilobit) memories and 4-bit microprocessors, each entirely contained and fabricated as a unit on a single chip of silicon approximately 6 mm square. Within a few years, other companies joined Intel in producing increasingly complex LSIs. Current fourth generation computers are characterized by their use of LSIs as the basic building block, although smaller scale integrated circuits are still used extensively.

Although the transition from medium to large scale integrated circuits represents a tremendous jump in design and fabrication techniques, it was the logical progression from the technology that preceded it. Silicon crystals of increasing size and purity were being produced from which sufficiently large wafers could be cut to support the simultaneous production of approximately 100 LSIs. Because setup costs are relatively constant, it costs about the same to produce 100 chips simultaneously as it would to produce a single chip.

As the size of the individual chips increases, so does the probability that a chip will cross an imperfection in the silicon wafer. For chips 6 mm square, this probability is approximately 50%. Thus, only 40 to 50 of the LSIs produced on a single wafer will be usable. Increasing the complexity of circuits generally requires an increase in size, thereby reducing the yield per wafer and increasing the cost per unit significantly.

Because of the emphasis on high component density, most LSIs are produced using MOS transistors rather than the faster bipolar transistors usually incorporated in the TTL family of devices. A significant increase in packaging density has been accomplished simply from changes in layout of circuits to improve utilization of space. The components of the LSIs and their interconnections are produced by a sequence of deposition of conducting and insulating materials, etching, and oxidation. These processes are controlled by optical techniques, including the use of photo masks. The use of light in fabrication limits tolerances to measurements on the order of one wavelength of light, that is, a few ten-millionths of a meter. Because these tolerances are approaching the size of the conductors and other circuit elements, further reduction in component size to allow increased packaging density requires adoption of non-optical techniques such as electron or x-ray beam etching.

Random access memories (RAM) as large as 16K bits are now available on one chip, although cost considerations still favor the 4K- and 8K-bit memories in most applications. Sixteen-bit microprocessors are also readily available on one chip, as well as a wide selection of 8-bit microprocessors. Both microprocessors and memories can be combined with similar units to accommodate any desired word size, although this is easier to accomplish with memories than with microprocessors. In addition, memories can be combined to increase the total memory capacity of the computer to that allowed by the particular microprocessor used. For example, a small computer may consist of one 8-bit microprocessor and 32 4K-bit RAMs, the latter arranged with eight RAMs in parallel to accommodate the word size. The four rows of what now can be considered a 4K-byte (or, in this case, word) RAM provides a total memory of 16K bytes.

The availability of LSIs has had a dramatic impact on the computer industry from two viewpoints. The first of these is the market. Although size and cost had decreased dramatically and continuously through the third generation, computers were still large, expensive, and complicated to operate. This limited the market to large industry and business and research or teaching institutions. The development of the LSI reduced the size of a complete central processing unit (CPU) to a single chip, the power requirements to what could be supplied by a small battery, and the price initially below $100 and later below $10. Admittedly, a CPU having all of these characteristics would also have a more limited word size and a more limited set of basic operations than the CPU found in a larger computer. However, these limitations are readily acceptable in a variety of new applications. Typical of these are the hand or desk calculator, TV computer games, and, in small but otherwise traditional configuration, computers designed for use in the home or a small business.

These new applications brought about the introduction of new terminology to help distinguish these new computer systems from the larger machines. Two terms, minicomputer and microcomputer, are introduced here, although their meaning will probably become more apparent after reading the material presented in the next section. Three factors help distinguish full size computers from their smaller counterparts. First is the size of the word that the CPU is designed to manipulate. Microprocessors (a CPU contained on a single chip) capable of performing operations on 4- or 8-bit words are perfectly adequate to meet the requirements of a calculator or TV game computer. Operations requiring higher levels of precision, such as the addition or multiplication of a six-digit decimal number, are carried out by sequential operations on portions of the original operands. Although a 16- or 32-bit machine could carry out these operations much faster, the speed-limiting factor in calculators is usually the human operator.

The second distinguishing factor is the set of basic operations that the CPU is able to perform. It is important here to distinguish between those operations that are hardwired into the CPU and carried out on the basis of a single command and those operations that can only be performed by the proper sequence of commands initiating a corresponding sequence of less complex hardwired instructions. The machine with the more extensive instruction set will be able to perform a complex mathematical calculation more rapidly than a machine with a limited set of basic instructions.

The third feature that distinguishes the smaller from the larger machines is the amount of peripheral equipment utilized. Whereas the largest machines will include several of each of the types of input-output devices and peripheral memories described later in this chapter, the smallest may communicate with the operator through a keyboard having fewer than 20 buttons and a six- or eight-digit display output.

Although the exact boundaries are indistinct (and often blurred further by a sales pitch), the basic guidelines are as follows: A microcomputer is an LSI machine composed almost entirely of a microprocessor of 4- to 8- bit capacity and an extremely limited set of basic functions. There is usually no addressable memory or only one to four addressable registers. If any provision is made for connection to peripheral equipment, it is usually limited to one device such as a paper tape printer or television. Programming or software generation or modification is not usually available to the operator except through plug-in units.

A minicomputer is an LSI machine having one or more microprocessors, each with a capacity for direct manipulation of 8- to 16-bit words and a more extensive instruction set than the microcomputer. RAM capacity is usually between 4K and 64K bytes. Minimal peripheral support usually includes a cathode ray tube (CRT) display and typewriter keyboard but is readily extended to a printer and floppy disk or rigid disk drive. The larger minicomputers can support input and output devices but not to the extent that a full size computer can. Tape drives of the seven- or nine-track variety and card punches and readers are rarely available in minicomputer installations. Programming will be available in machine language and at least one higher language, often a simplified version or dialect of a conventional computer language.

The capabilities of full size computers are almost unlimited. The CPU may utilize LSI technology but will not be contained on a single chip. Word size is usually 32 or 64 bits for maximum speed. RAM size often exceeds one megabyte (Mbyte, or 1,000,000 bytes). The total number of peripheral devices in use can exceed 100, and some may be located many miles from the CPU.

The second change in computer technology brought about by LSI techniques is in the manner in which the CPU is used. As described above, a CPU on a single chip is called a microprocessor. In third generation and earlier computers, only one CPU was used. In fourth generation computers, microprocessors are often incorporated into peripheral devices to reduce the work load on the CPU, thereby increasing its efficiency and the speed of execution of a task. Even minicomputers often include more than one microprocessor.

Computer Organization

A computer is a complex system in which the discrete functional components illustrated in Figure 4.24 are closely integrated electronically. The CPU serves as the central nervous system of the computer. This unit not only performs the primary computer functions of carrying out rapid calculations but also directs the operations of the other major components. The input and output devices act as interpreters in their role of converting the digital electrical pulses understood by the CPU into forms of information useful to the

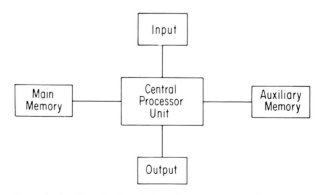

Figure 4.24. Organization of the major components of a computer.

operator. The computer memory provides a repository for data and instructions not in immediate use by the CPU.

Central Processor Unit

The two major components of the CPU are the control unit and the arithmetic logic unit, illustrated in Figure 4.25. Also vital to the function of the computer is the bus system. This system, which is under the direct control of the CPU, consists of a network of wires which allow communication among the various elements of the computer. One bus system is required to supply power to the components of the computer and is of relatively straightforward design. The remainder of the bus system is made up of two basic components. The control bus relays information regarding the basic operation of the computer between the CPU and the other sections. Data are transmitted between and within the sections of the computer along the data or address bus, as directed by the signals transmitted along the control bus.

In its simplest form, all of the logic elements of the computer could be connected directly to one another. Direct access between elements of the computer would provide the fastest execution time for programs. However, this rapidly becomes impractical for all but the simplest devices, and a less direct but more manageable system is used, as illustrated in Figure 4.26. This system is analogous to telephone or intercom communication via a switchboard using trunk lines. The blocks shown in Figure 4.26 could represent memory registers, registers in the arithmetic and logic unit, or output devices. Since not all of the elements connected to a bus line are to receive or respond to information being transmitted, the des-

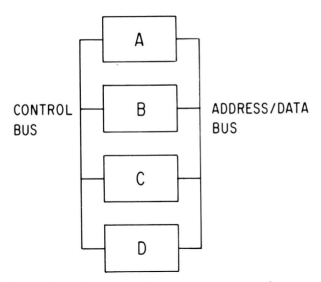

Figure 4.26. Use of a simplified bus circuit to couple four computer components.

tination device must be enabled (i.e., connected to the bus) by an appropriate binary control signal transmitted ahead of the data. The binary coded instructions applied to the control bus by the CPU determine which device is to be connected to the address/data bus as the transmitter of data and which other device is to receive the signal from the bus. The remaining devices are electrically isolated from the bus during the data transmission. The actual transmission of data takes place on arrival of the next clock pulse (a pulse that is transmitted at regular fixed intervals of time) along the control bus, after enabling of the origin and destination devices has occurred.

A simplified representation of the sequence of events described above is shown in Figure 4.27. In this particular case, enabling of the originating device is illustrated. The separate devices, labeled *1, 2,* and *3,* might represent a card reader, keyboard, and disk drive. In the top panel of Figure 4.27, all three devices are separated from the data bus, even though each is connected to the control bus and thus is able to receive signals along that line. In the middle panel, a binary representation of the signal to enable device *3* has been transmitted along the control bus. Devices *1* and *2* take no action on receipt of this signal; however, this same signal activates a gate on device *3* connecting it to the data bus. At this point, device *3* is able to transmit its data along the control bus where the data will be received by another device that has also been connected to the same line. To ensure that transmission of data does not occur until the receiving device is ready, transmission of data from device *3* does not occur until the next clock

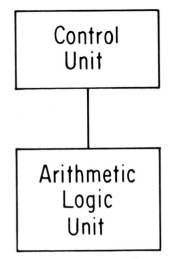

Figure 4.25. Organization of the CPU.

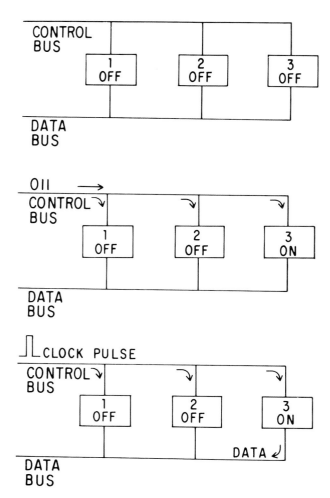

Figure 4.27. Operating sequence of a bus system.

pulse is received (bottom panel). In this illustration, the clock pulse is shown as arriving along the control bus, although in most installations a separate clock bus is provided for this purpose.

To ensure that data are not lost in the event that a receiving device has been accidentally turned off or otherwise disabled, an additional sequence of signals may take place along the control bus prior to transmission of data. When the enabled device is connected to the data bus, it sends a return signal along the control bus to the control unit, thereby informing the control unit that the activation signal has been received and interpreted appropriately. This sequence of operations is called a handshake.

Arithmetic Logic Unit The actual process of computation is carried out by the arithmetic logic unit (ALU). The fashion in which this unit is constructed, as well as the capabilities of the accompanying control unit, determine the nature of the operations that can ultimately be performed by the computer and the computer's speed and precision (measured in bits per word).

The basic operations of arithmetic are addition and shift operations. The binary adder has been previously described. Most common ALUs will include a 4-bit or 8-bit adder, which can be arranged in arrays to achieve higher precision if necessary. This device alone will handle addition as well as the complementary operation of subtraction on appropriately preprocessed data. To efficiently perform multiplication and its complementary operation, division, a shifter is included with the ALU. Each shift of input data to the left or right is equivalent to a multiplication or division, respectively, by the binary number 10 (which is equivalent to 2 in the decimal system).

The basic logic operation consists of comparing two pieces of data. This is accomplished by a series of gates, one for each bit, which compare the two words bit by bit. No numerical output based on the magnitude of either word is generated. Instead, the output might be assigned the value 1 if all bits are equal and 0 if they are not. The result of this calculation can be used to modify the instruction sequence most likely through the so-called JUMP instruction, described under "Software."

Complex logic and arithmetic functions can be carried out by sequential application of the basic arithmetic and logic operations. The ALU can be designed to carry out more complex functions as a one-step operation rather than as a succession of less complex steps under the direction of the control unit. By hardwiring in more complex functions, these operations can be carried out by the ALU with greater speed. However, the increased design complexity increases the cost of these units.

The complexity and expense of the ALU is also affected by the form of numerical data to be handled. The sequence of instructions, or algorithms, for handling floating point numbers, or numbers represented in scientific notation, are obviously more complex than required for manipulation of simple integers. The requirement to handle decimal or binary coded decimal (BCD) numbers rather than binary numbers also increases the complexity of arithmetic manipulation by the CPU.

In the earlier computers designed with discrete components as well as in later computers composed of small scale integrated circuitry, each ALU was tailored toward the intended application of the computer. With the availability of large scale integrated circuitry, there is greater incentive to reduce cost by tailoring the software of a readily available microprocessor unit.

Arithmetic and logic operations are not per-

Computer Theory 85

formed directly on data stored in either the peripheral or the core memory. Instead, data are transferred from these areas into specialized storage locations known as registers within the ALU. The number of these registers, usually two to eight, is determined again by the intended complexity of operations to be performed as well as the need for speed of operation. One of these registers, usually called the accumulator, will be designated as the location where results of the arithmetic operations will be stored prior to transmission back to core, peripheral memory, or a peripheral device.

Control Unit Ultimate responsibility for proper operation of each of the components of the computer lies within the control unit (CU). In its role as manager of operation of the computer, the CU must keep track of each step of the program as it is executed, locate and decode subsequent instructions, locate and direct recovery and transfer of data between the arithmetic units and peripheral devices, and control the operation of peripheral devices. Figure 4.28 summarizes the main components of the CU and provides a simplified representation of their interconnection internally as well as with the rest of the computer.

Control of instructions begins with the instruction counter, which keeps track of each step of the program as it is performed. The instruction counter is used to identify the location in memory of the next binary coded instruction, which is then transferred to the instruction register. The instruction is decoded by a read-only memory (ROM), which translates it into a sequence of instructions or micro-operations that can be performed by the ALU. A portion of the instruction word includes information regarding the location of the data to be used in this particular operation. As each step is completed, the instruction counter is incremented and the cycle is repeated.

Also included in the CU are timing circuits, which regulate synchronization of operation of the components of the computer; bus control circuits, which control intracomputer communications; and interrupt circuits, which allow communication between the operator and the CU when necessary for smooth functioning of the machine. Examples of this form of intervention that are outside the normal programming routine include requests by the computer for a change in a disk pack or magnetic tape or to alert the operator that a printer needed for output has not yet been turned on.

A single large scale integrated circuit consisting of an ALU as well as a CU, and including timing circuits, bus control circuits, and several registers of memory, is referred to as a microprocessor and requires only the addition of memory and appropriate input and output devices to form a complete computer.

Memory

There is a wide variety of devices available for storage of digital information. There are several characteristics of the various forms of memory that determine their specific application. Probably the most important of these is the method by which information is retrieved from memory. There are two basic forms of access: random and sequential. In a random access memory, each word can be immediately retrieved for processing by specifying its location in the memory unit. In sequential storage, in contrast, the memory must be examined word by word until the required piece of information is located. An analogy might be drawn to locating a phone number in a directory by looking up the name of the subscriber, as opposed to locating a subscriber's name by sequentially reading down the phone numbers until the specified number is identified. The advantage of RAM is speed of retrieval; however, it is more expensive to construct

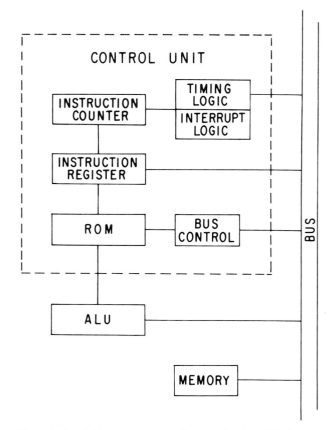

Figure 4.28. Major components of a control unit (within broken line) and their interconnection with the bus, ALU, and memory. Coupling to the input-output devices also takes place via the bus system.

and requires establishment of an index or directory for location of stored information.

Memories can also be characterized by whether or not energy is required (volatile) or is not required (nonvolatile) for maintenance of stored information. Permanent storage of data or program instructions obviously should be in a form that does not depend on whether power to the computer is accidentally or deliberately removed. The characteristics of the various forms of memory are discussed in more detail in subsequent paragraphs.

From the standpoint of operation of the computer, an alternate classification of memory has been previously indicated in Figure 4.24. Main memory refers to storage locations, invariably of the random access type, which are used by the CPU exclusively during the execution of program. Auxiliary memory relies on nonvolatile, sequential storage of data. Generally, the information is loaded into or retrieved from auxiliary memory in the form of blocks rather than individual words. Transfer takes place to and from the main memory under the control of the CPU, with any required manipulation of the data taking place between the CPU and the main memory.

Random Access Memory There are two basic forms of RAM currently available. The oldest, and until recently the cheapest and most widely used, is magnetic core memory. This form of memory is constructed by assembling large numbers of small toroidal cores made of ferrite material on a matrix of wires. The basic construction is shown in Figure 4.29. Each ferrite core is capable of two distinct magnetization states. Transitions between these two states can be induced by passing a sufficiently large current through the opening in the core in the appropriate direction. The core will maintain its state of magnetization in either direction indefinitely in the absence of an externally applied magnetic field of sufficient intensity to cause a transition. It is the ability of the ferrite cores to retain these two discrete states of magnetization that gives them their usefulness for storage of binary numbers, either 0 or 1, depending upon the state or direction of magnetization. Because no power is required to retain the information, this form of memory is nonvolatile.

The magnetic cores are arranged in two-dimensional arrays, which are then stacked one upon the other. A word or address is located in memory by specifying its X and Y coordinates. This information is applied to each layer simultaneously, with 1 bit being retrieved from each of the two-dimensional arrays. These bits are then assembled into 1 byte of information, the length of which is determined by the depth to which the two-dimensional arrays are

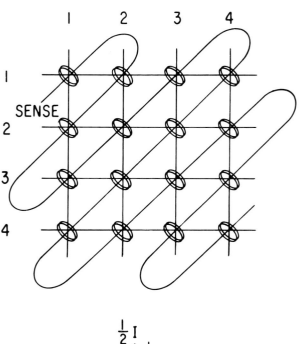

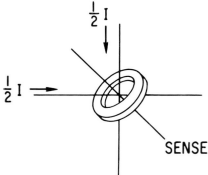

Figure 4.29. A 4 × 4 × 1 ferrite core memory with one element (bit) shown in more detail.

stacked. The word retrieved from core is assembled and temporarily stored in either a series or parallel register called a buffer, from which it can then be transmitted to other parts of the computer.

Reading and loading (writing) information into core memory are performed in similar fashions. Two of the wires passing through each toroid perform the function of locating the desired element. A pulse equal in amplitude to one-half of the current required to cause a transition to the desired form of magnetization is passed through the appropriate wire along the X axis. A similar signal is passed simultaneously through the appropriate Y coordinate wire. Only ferrite cores lying along one of these two wires will receive any magnetic field pulse at all, and only the core at the intersection of these two wires will experience a pulse of sufficient magnitude to cause a transition in magnetic state. The selection of the appropriate X and Y coordinate wires is carried out by demultiplexers, as previously described. When information is to be loaded or written into memory, a current of sufficient magnitude and appropriate polarity with respect to the appropriate X and Y coordinate wires is necessary to achieve the required state of magnetization. If the core element is in the correct state, its sense of magnetization will be maintained. If the sense of magnetization is incorrect initially, it will be changed by the current.

Reading from memory utilizes the same localization procedure as writing, but additional steps are required following localization of the desired address. Each time a core changes its state of magnetization, the changing magnetic field will induce a pulse of current in a wire passing through the center of the core. This is illustrated in Figure 4.29 as the "sense" wire. This is a continuous wire passing through each element in the two-dimensional core array. A current pulse detected in the sense wire indicates a magnetic transition in one of the elements. Because a transition can occur only in the presence of a sufficiently large inducing current, the presence of this pulse in the sense wire indicates that the current in the X and Y wires has induced a change in the state of magnetization of the core at their intersection. Conversely, the absence of a current pulse in the sense wire indicates that the state of magnetization of the core element at the intersection of the X and Y wires was already in the appropriate direction and therefore not changed by the write signal. A particular element can therefore be interrogated by sending an instruction corresponding to the loading of binary 0. If no signal is detected in the sense wire, then that element already is in the state of magnetization corresponding to binary 0. A signal in the sense wire indicates the presence of binary 1 in the address in question, which has subsequently been changed to a binary 0.

From the above discussion, it can be seen that although information stored in core memory can be retained indefinitely in the absence of power, the operation of reading information from core memory can result in a change in the information stored. Therefore, each request to read information from core memory must be followed by an instruction to reload the originally contained information back in the original location. Although the process sounds complex, it actually takes place very rapidly and automatically under the control of the memory unit.

In the early days, core memory was assembled manually by stringing beads of ferrite material measuring only about 1 mm in diameter on very fine wires. Because moderate to large computing systems required memories using millions of these cores, the manual assembly process was eventually replaced with automatic devices.

The second form of RAM currently available consists of solid-state devices. Basically, these consist of an assembly of registers, described earlier in this chapter. Most forms of solid-state memory require the continuous application of power for preservation of the stored information. Exceptions to this are discussed later. An instruction to read information stored in solid-state RAM does not change that information as it does in core memory. Thus, the "refresh" instruction required following a read from core memory is not necessary in solid-state RAM. Solid-state memory is produced by the same technology used to produce other integrated circuit components of the digital computer. For this reason, the cost and size of solid-state RAM have continued to decrease rapidly with time. In contrast, the cost and size of core memory have remained relatively stable. In the past few years, the crossover in cost advantage has shifted toward solid-state memory, which eventually will probably replace core memory except in those applications where nonvolatile RAM is essential.

There are certain situations in which the advantage of rapid access of information is vital but the ability to change the stored information is not required. For these situations, two specialized forms of solid-state memory are available. The first of these is read-only memory. Reading information stored in ROM is performed with the same ease and speed as in RAM; however, the option of changing the information is not available. The information stored in ROM is determined at the time of manufacture and cannot be changed by the user, nor is energy required to retain this information. A closely related family of devices known as programmable read-only memory (PROM) is also available. As manufactured, PROM contains fusible links in each storage location. By passing an appropriate current through the appropriate leads in these devices, some of these links can be destroyed, resulting in an open circuit in those locations. The manner in which links are either destroyed or left intact determines the binary value of each bit in PROM at the time a read instruction is received. This allows users the flexibility of generating specialized ROM in small quantities. Once PROM has been programmed, it functions in the same manner as ROM and, except under limited circumstances, cannot be modified for a different purpose. Application of these devices is discussed later under "Software." It should be understood that RAM, ROM, and PROM are all random access devices in that information may be retrieved from any location within any of these forms of memory merely or the sheet film to allow multiple images to be recorded on one piece of film.

It is frequently useful to enter the location of a particular element of an output image as input. Rather than typing in the coordinates of the particular point or points of interest, the information can be conveyed by either of two separate devices. The first of these utilizes a joystick or a trackball, either of which allows the operator to describe motion in two dimensions. These devices control the motion of a cursor on the CRT, which simultaneously displays the output image. The input data is generated by the movement of the joystick or trackball. The cursor provides feedback from the computer, indicating to the operator the information that has already been entered. The second form of image location input is the light pen. When held over the CRT by the operator, the light pen detects the arrival of the bright spot formed by the electron beam sweeping the face of the CRT at a fixed rate. The input location is calculated by the computer based on the time interval between the synchronization pulse which indicates the beginning of a new frame on the CRT, and the arrival of the next light pulse at the light pen.

As in the case of the cursor, the light pen is most commonly used in conjunction with output previously generated by the computer and displayed on the CRT. Both of these are labor-saving devices in that they reduce significantly the time it would otherwise take the computer operator to input additional information. Common uses of the light pen and joystick in CT include marking areas of interest for enlargement of the image, making densitometer readings, and measuring the size of structures.

The choice between the use of the light pen or the joystick is based primarily on personal preference. The light pen is probably easier to use in drawing irregular areas of interest or for operations requiring rapid motions across large areas of the CRT. The joystick probably is better suited for smooth, controlled motion of the cursor or an existing rectangular area of interest. Function of the light pen can be affected by ambient lighting as well as adjustment of CRT brightness and contrast, whereas the joystick is independent of these factors.

SOFTWARE

The set of instructions that controls the operation of a computer is referred to as software. Whereas the hardware is almost invariably purchased in complete form from a computer manufacturer, the software may be generated in whole or in part by the user, depending on the intended application of the computer and the sophistication of the user. As recently as a decade ago, the majority of computer installations were dependent on at least some user-generated software. Now, with the proliferation of computer applications, most computer installations consist of complete hardware and software packages, which the user operates as he or she would any other electrical or electronic device. This situation is usually referred to as a "turnkey" operation. The hardware and software may be purchased from separate sources or even assembled from a variety of sources. Additional software may be added later, as new applications are found, in the same manner that additional hardware, in the form of additional memory or input and output devices, may be added. The application of computers in CT is an example of a turnkey operation.

In the previous section on hardware, the computer was shown to be an assembly of components, each of which could be further broken down into successive levels of subcomponents characterized by an increasing number of elements and a decreasing complexity for each element. In this section, software, or the programming of computers, is discussed at four levels. Most programming done today is accomplished using so-called higher languages. An example of one of the oldest of these languages and one which is familiar by name to many people with little background in computers is **FORTRAN**. This language as well as several other commonly used higher languages are discussed briefly below. The higher languages provide a convenient means of communication between the user and a machine that ultimately is only able to respond to an appropriate series of electrical pulses.

The relationship between the four levels of programming is illustrated in Figure 4.30. The lowest level accessible to the user is machine language. Each instruction of machine language consists of a binary number that is converted by the ROM within the CPU into a more detailed set of instructions that is actually executed by the CPU. This lowest level of instruction is referred to as a microinstruction, discussion of which is beyond the scope of this chapter. The translation of a higher language into machine language takes place through the use of a compiler, which is itself a piece of software. Similarly, assembly language, discussed below, is translated into machine language by the use of a specialized form of compiler called an assembler.

Machine Language

Each type of CPU is characterized not only by the specific set of basic operations it is able to perform, but also by the binary number that causes the CPU

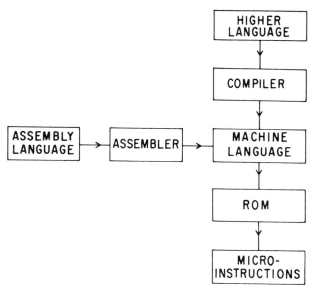

Figure 4.30. The four levels of programming and the software that couples them.

to carry out each instruction. Because of these different characteristics of CPUs, a machine language program written for a computer utilizing, for example, a Z80 microprocessor would not work on another computer utilizing an LSI-11 microprocessor. Machine language, therefore, is said to be machine-dependent.

An exception to the rule of machine dependence of machine language instructions is found in the concept of the virtual computer. The most basic set of hardwired instructions that an ALU can carry out defines the basic operational properties of that microprocessor. In earlier computer design, these operations were accessed directly by the machine language instructions without any intervening software. The introduction of microprogramming, illustrated in Figure 4.30, between machine language programming and the computer hardware increases the flexibility of CPU design. Consider, for example, two ALUs labeled A and B. Unit A includes only the most basic set of arithmetic and shift operations required for number manipulation. In contrast, unit B includes in its design the hardwired capability for performing more advanced arithmetic manipulation, including perhaps manipulation of floating point numbers. The hardwired features of both machines can be implemented by a single machine language instruction. All the operations performed by the more complex unit B can be performed by unit A, although more steps would be involved. This is accomplished by connecting unit A behind an ROM designed so that the input of a type B machine language instruction into the ROM will result in output from the ROM of the sequence of type A instructions required to perform the same mathematical manipulations.

From the standpoint of the machine language programmer, the operation of these two units is identical, although the execution time would be much faster for unit B than for unit A. In many applications, however, this time difference will not be noticeable to the operator. The combination of the type A microprocessor coupled with the appropriate ROM can be considered a virtual computer which simulates the operation of a CPU incorporating type B hardware.

Manufacturers of microprocessors use this concept of the virtual computer extensively in designing a single general purpose microprocessor that can fill a variety of roles when coupled with the appropriate ROM. The concept of the virtual computer can be applied at other levels of programming as well, although the machine language simulation is the most important one.

A single instruction in machine language is divided into two parts. The first part includes the instruction itself, or operation. The second part consists of the address or operand, which may represent a number or address at which a number can be found. In the process known as indirect addressing, the operand may represent the address in memory at which the address of a particular piece of data has previously been stored. The structure of the entire machine language instruction is as rigidly machine-dependent as the instruction set itself. A general example is shown in Figure 4.31. This might represent a complete machine language instruction for an 8-bit word CPU. In this particular case, the 3 leftmost binary bits have been reserved for identification of the operation. The remaining 5 specify the address associated with the instruction. This particular CPU is assumed to have two registers labeled R_0 and R_1. The register involved in this operation is designated by the left-most bit within the address field. In this case, the 0 specifies R_0 or the accumulator. In this hypothetical CPU, the operations characterized by the binary representation of the number 3, or 011, is an instruction to store the contents of the specified register in the specified address in memory. Figure 4.31 therefore represents an instruction to store the contents of the accumulator in location 1110_2, that is, the 14th location in memory. The machine language instruction that carries out the complementary operation to the STORE instruction of Figure 4.31 is shown in Figure 4.32. In this case, the contents of memory address 1001_2, or location 9_{10}, are transferred into register 1 of the microprocessor.

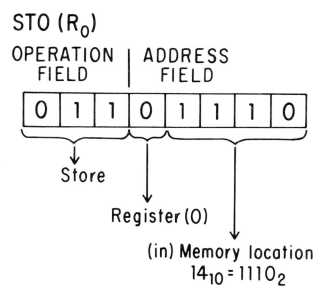

Figure 4.31. The structure of the machine language instruction to store the contents of the accumulator in memory.

Some of the variations in the forms taken by the instructions are shown in Figure 4.33. The HALT instruction, which terminates execution of the program, requires no further information for execution. Consequently, no address need be given with this instruction, and the 5-bit address field is ignored in the execution of this instruction. No register need be identified in the HALT instruction. The JUMP instruction utilizes the entire 5-bit address field to spec-

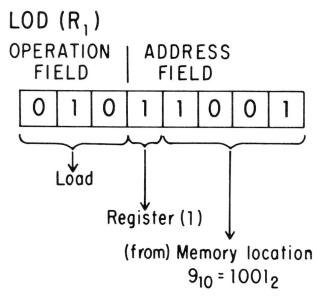

Figure 4.32. The structure of the machine language instruction to load the contents of a particular address in memory into register 1 in the ALU.

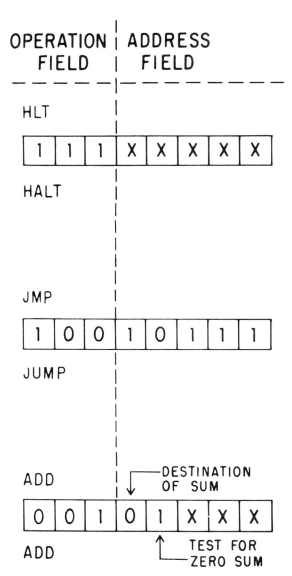

Figure 4.33. Machine language instructions illustrating three different methods of using the address field.

ify the location of the next instruction to be executed. Like the HALT instruction, identification of the register is unnecessary; however, the address field is critical. This is an extremely powerful instruction in that it permits the execution of nonlinear programs. A linear program is one in which each instruction is carried out sequentially with the program counter incremented by 1 as each step is executed. In all but the most elementary programs, it quickly becomes apparent that certain sequences of operations are being carried out repeatedly. Utilizing the JUMP instruction, the programmer can save large amounts of memory by writing these sequences of instructions only once. Where execution of these common sub-

Computer Theory 95

programs is required, appropriate JUMP instructions are inserted which cause the program counter to jump ahead or backward to the beginning of that particular subprogram and, following execution, return to what otherwise would have been the next step. This is illustrated in Figure 4.34, where five steps of the program, steps *3* through *7*, would otherwise recur three times. In this case, instructions *9* and *13* instruct the program counter to jump back to instruction *3*. Instruction *7* is also a JUMP operation. It initially instructs the program counter to jump to instruction *8*. On the second and third passes through this subprogram, the jump is to instructions *10* and *14*, respectively.

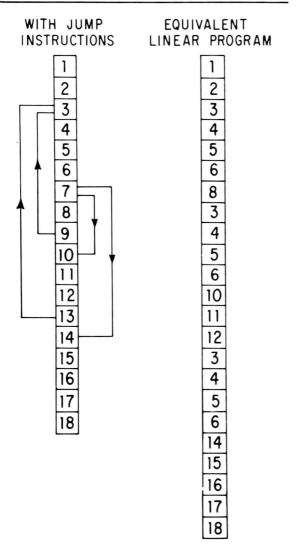

Figure 4.34. Comparison of linear programming with a program using JUMP instructions.

The third type of instruction format illustrated in Figure 4.33 is the ADD instruction. In this hypothetical CPU, the addition takes place between two numbers that have previously been stored in registers R_0 and R_1. Only the identity of the register that will store the sum needs to be specified. Customarily this is the accumulator, R_0, and it is specified by placing a 0 in the leftmost bit of the address portion of the instruction. This leaves 4 bits of the address unused. Another powerful programming tool provided in most CPUs is called the conditional jump. For example, if the address bit adjacent to the register bit contains the value 0, then following the addition directed by that instruction, the program counter will increment by 1 and execution of the program will continue in a linear fashion. If, however, that address bit contains a 1, the microprocessor will execute a subprogram that tests the value of the number stored in the accumulator. If the value of the contents of the accumulator is equal to 0, then execution will still proceed in a linear fashion. If the contents of the accumulator are not equal to 0, however, the program counter will be incremented by 2, bypassing the next instruction in the program. In most cases, this process would only be a useful technique if the bypassed instruction were a JUMP instruction.

These examples illustrate some of the alternative uses of the address field in an instruction. The HALT instruction ignores the address field. The JUMP instruction utilizes the entire field as an address in memory. Several instructions in this hypothetical computer utilize 1 bit of the address to designate a register. The ADD instruction uses portions of the address field not only to designate registers but also to instruct the computer to modify the instruction sequence based on the result of an arithmetic process. Although primitive in its machine language form, it is this form of instruction that gives the illusion that the computer is making decisions based on intermediate results of complex calculations in the absence of human intervention.

The limitations of this hypothetical machine are obvious. With only 3 bits available in the operation field of machine language instruction, only 2^3 or 8 separate operations can be coded. Furthermore, the address field is limited to using only 2^5 or 32 distinct locations in memory, and then only if a register specification is unnecessary. This limits the size of the program that can be executed by this machine. The obvious solution is to increase the number of bits per word, although this would increase the cost of the machine. An alternative is to allow the use of two or more words per instruction when needed. As previously mentioned, the address field of an instruction could identify the address of the location in memory where the 8-bit address of the operand is stored. This is referred to as indirect addressing and can be expanded to multiple levels. For example, Figure 4.35 illustrates an instruction to load the contents of a location in memory into the accumulator. The address field of the instruction, 1001_2, identifies a location in memory containing an 8-bit binary number. In this particular case, that number is not the datum but rather its location in memory, specifically 01101101_2. The content of this memory location is identified in the last line of the figure and contains the binary equivalent of 127_8. This illustration ignored the fact that in order to distinguish direct from indirect addressing one further bit of the address portion of the instruction word must be used; however, the concept remains valid.

An example of the set of instructions necessary to add two numbers in memory and store the result in memory is shown in Figure 4.36. The first step of the instruction loads the contents of address 5 in memory into register R_1. Step 2 then loads the contents of memory location 6 into register R_0, the accumulator. Step 3 adds the contents of the two registers and stores the results back in the accumulator. The final step of this sequence of instructions stores the contents of the accumulator back in memory address number 5, destroying the previously stored contents of that register.

The complexity of writing even a simple program in machine language is obvious from the preceding paragraphs even in this hypothetical situation. The programmer must not only correctly associate a binary number with each instruction, but must keep track of the precise location of each piece of data in memory throughout execution of the program. This is difficult enough in an 8-bit computer but becomes

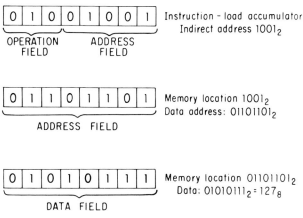

Figure 4.35. An example of indirect addressing.

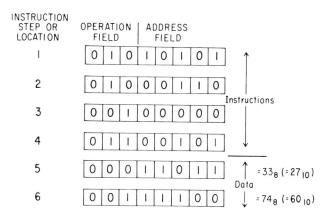

Figure 4.36. The set of machine language instructions required to add two data in memory.

totally unmanageable in 16-, 32-, and 64-bit computers with larger instruction sets and generally more complex programs. Knowledge of machine language is primarily of value in understanding the operation of the computer, design of hardware and compilers, and occasionally in debugging or improving more complex programs.

Assembly Language

An immediate improvement in the ease of manipulation of machine language would be provided if the binary coded instructions could be instead represented by a mnemonic. This is illustrated in Figures 4.31–4.33 where a three-letter mnemonic has been included along with the binary representation of the instruction. Using these mnemonics, the instruction to add registers R_0 and R_1 and store the contents in register R_0 would now be encoded as ADD rather than 0010. The ability to use a symbolic address in assembly language is at least as important as the use of a mnemonic rather than a binary instruction code. In machine language, the programmer is required to specify the exact location in memory of each fixed or variable number, a difficult task in a lengthy program whose size would be difficult to determine in the early stages of programming and which might change many times during the evolution of the program. A symbolic address is simply the association of an alphanumeric mnemonic with each datum. As it translates each instruction from assembly language to machine language, the assembler not only converts the mnemonic operation code into the binary operation code but also assigns to each symbol associated with the datum a specific address in memory. Table 4.5 shows the assembly language equivalent of the machine language program illustrated in Figure 4.36. The shorter alphanumeric strings make it easier for

Table 4.5. Assembly language equivalent of program in Figure 4.36.

Instruction step or location	Symbolic address	Instruction	
1		LOD 1	X
2		LOD 0	Y
3		ADD 0	
4		STO 0	X
5	X,	OCT	33
6	Y,	OCT	74

the programmer later to identify specific sections of the program. The major improvement, however, is that as the load and store instructions are written, only a symbol, in this case X or Y, needs to be written by the programmer. The assembler automatically assigns symbol X location 5 and symbol Y location 6 and, as directed by the programmer, stores the binary equivalent of the octal numbers 33 and 74 (equivalent to the numbers 27 and 60, respectively, in the decimal system) to these two locations, respectively. Both the machine language and assembly language version of this program are incomplete and are intended only to illustrate a machine language and assembly language version of a portion of a more extensive program.

Higher Languages

Although assembly language simplifies some of the bookkeeping chores for the programmer, it does little else to facilitate writing of involved programs. The assembler is basically a translator in that it converts the assembly language version of the program line for line into the machine language program that is directly usable by the CPU. There are many commonly utilized sequences of machine language instructions. One example of these has already been illustrated in both its machine and assembly language versions in Figure 4.36. In the FORTRAN language, the four instructions required in machine language to carry out the addition are replaced by one statement, X = X + Y. As it stands, the statement is not algebraically correct except in the circumstance Y equals 0, and should not be thought of as an algebraic expression. The correct interpretation of that statement is for the computer to add the contents of memory location X to the contents of memory location Y and store the result in memory location X, destroying the original contents at that location. As these instructions are received by the computer, they are converted by the compiler back into the four steps of machine language previously illustrated. Other examples of FORTRAN instructions are shown in Table 4.6. The first of these FORTRAN statements will be translated by the compiler into a series of machine language statements that calculates the square root of the datum stored in the location identified by the symbol X and stores the result in the location of memory associated with symbol Y. The second instruction will make extensive use of the JUMP and conditional JUMP instructions described in the section on machine language. The value of the data stored in locations X and Y will be compared. If X is greater than or equal to Y, an unconditional jump will be made to statement number 31, ignoring all intervening instructions. If X is less than Y, then the program will proceed in linear fashion. There are many variations of this general form of IF statement, the most obvious being the replacement of "greater than or equal to" by "less than," "less than or equal to," or "equal to." More complex conditional jumps can be constructed using the logical AND, OR, or complement instructions within the parentheses to link arithmetic conditions.

A third class of FORTRAN instruction used extensively in most programs is the "do loop." This instruction causes all subsequent instructions up to and including statement 29 to be executed repeatedly, initially with the value of the variable I equal to 2. Each time the series of statements is executed, the value of the variable I is incremented by 1 until it reaches the value 25, at which point control is transferred back out of the loop.

The three examples in Table 4.6 serve to illustrate the tremendous power of higher languages in simplifying programming. A long complex sequence of machine language instructions is reduced to a one-line instruction which has the appearance of an abbreviation of the English instruction. In contrast to machine or assembly language programming, a beginner can learn to write useful programs using the higher languages in a matter of days or weeks.

The compiler, in contrast to the assembler, not only has the job of translating the symbolic instructions into an appropriate series of machine language instructions and assigning specific locations in memory to symbolic addresses but also takes further steps to improve the efficiency of the resulting machine language program. This optimization step has a significant effect on the efficiency with which a program is executed. The compiler also informs the programmer of some forms of errors in the program.

Table 4.6. Examples of FORTRAN statements

Y = SQRT (X)
IF (X.GE.Y) GO TO 31
DO 29 I = 2, 25

FORTRAN is one of the oldest of the higher languages and is still in widespread use. It is designed for, and optimally suited for, scientific and engineering applications, as its name (FORmula TRANslation) implies. Although virtually any computer task can be coded using FORTRAN, the FORTRAN language lacks many features required for efficient manipulation of long strings of alphanumeric characters. An example of this type of operation might be in compiling a telephone directory. Languages particularly suited to this task include LISP and SNOBOL 4. Business applications frequently require the ability to manipulate lists as well as the ability to manipulate numbers. Number manipulating ability is never as extensive as in the engineering and scientific applications, however, making many of the features of FORTRAN unnecessary in these applications. An example of a specialized business-oriented language that has achieved widespread popularity is COBOL (Common Business Oriented Language). Programs written in this language are characterized by their easy readability, as they consist almost entirely of familiar English words. A drawback of this language, however, is that even short programs tend to become rather cumbersome. More recently, relatively simple, general purpose languages have been developed which are gaining increasing popularity. Among the most familiar of these are BASIC and PL/1 (Programming Language 1). These two languages are the ones most commonly taught to beginning general purpose programmers. From there, a transition to FORTRAN for scientific applications is relatively easy.

Operating Systems and Applications Programs

The highest level of complexity in software is found in operating systems and applications programs. Both of these consist of the complete set of instructions necessary to carry out a particular task, expressed in machine language, a higher language, or some combination. The distinction between these two types of software is based on their utilization. The operating system defines the complete set of software that is available to the user as part of the initial computer system. It is the software that comes with the computer. The operating system together with the hardware represents the complete computer system. The perception of the hardware to a user who has access to an entire operating system is usually quite different from that of an individual who deals with the hardware alone, without benefit of the complete operating system. The modified image of the hardware as generated by the operating system is sometimes referred to as the virtual computer. Application programs are software packages generated by the user to perform a particular task. They represent additional software to what was supplied with the computer system initially.

Operating Systems Operating systems can be divided into two categories. The first of these, control programs or control systems, consists of the set of housekeeping instructions necessary for practical operation of the computer. These software packages can become quite extensive, particularly in cases where one computer may be utilized by a number of different users simultaneously. In these situations, the control system must determine which user has priority in access to the hardware, allow him access to enough memory to carry out his operation, and keep track of his utilization of the CPU, memory, and peripheral devices for accounting purposes.

In addition to the time-shared functions described above, the control system is responsible for communications with the operator, particularly for those situations that cannot be controlled by the computer. These include requests to activate portions of the machine or to change a tape or a disk pack. Some of these functions have been previously mentioned in the discussion of the control unit portion of the CPU. The control system is also involved in the instruction of the control unit in operation of the input and output units as well as the peripheral memory devices. The control system also restricts access to certain areas of the hardware and software of the computer. Specifically, the user will be unable to generate any applications program that is able to alter any portion of the operating system. In most cases, this is for the user's own protection, since inadvertent modification of the operating system could render the system unusable. Of comparable importance in time-shared systems is preventing users from modifying the accounting functions as well as ensuring that one user is not able to access portions of another user's data or instruction field.

The second portion of the operating system consists of the processing system. In contrast to the control program, which is responsible for the basic operation of the hardware, the processing system provides a number of software packages which simplify the task of generating applications programs. Processing systems can be divided into two broad areas, compilers and utility programs. Compilers have been described previously. They provide the function of translation of higher languages into machine languages as well as provide some error detection features. The higher language application program is initially reviewed by the compiler, where it is screened for errors. These errors consist of incorrect use of the programming language, equivalent to spelling or grammatical errors in English. Once these errors have been corrected by the programmer, the set of instructions is referred to as a source program. This is translated and optimized by the compiler into a set of machine language instructions referred to as the object program. This object program can be stored on disks or tape or in the form of Hollerith cards for subsequent use without the need for a repeated pass of the source program through the compiler. The operating system of a large computer will probably contain several compilers. This allows the user to generate the program in the language with which he is most familiar or which is best suited for the intended application. In some cases, one program may be generated by using more than one language. When a portion of an extremely large program must be modified, it is possible to utilize a previously generated object program and only recompile the small portion of the instruction set that needs modification.

Utility programs not only carry out routine functions such as linking the components of an object program with programs or data already stored in an auxiliary memory, but also provide many software functions which would otherwise be a part of many applications programs. These include instructions for sorting and updating data files, and involved statistical and mathematical functions. The distinction between some utility programs and applications programs is often only on the basis of whether or not they have been generated by the user rather than their exact application. Occasionally a user-generated application program will achieve sufficient popularity that it will be incorporated into subsequent editions of a computer-operating system as a utility program.

Applications Programs In the past fifteen years, there has been a dramatic expansion in the generation of applications programs. These applications can be broken down into four major areas: scientific, information, control systems, and personal use.

The oldest of these four applications is the scientific. This includes the generation of mathematical functions and ballistic tables, which were among the earliest applications of the stored program computer. From this early start, the application software expanded, no longer simply replacing a human in the performance of tedious arithmetic calculations but now making possible solutions to problems too complex to allow practical solution by the unaided human mind. Meteorology is one field that has benefited tremendously from the rapid development of computer hardware and software. Rather than dealing with weather primarily on a local level, the modern meteorologist now has available a few charts, graphs, and numbers summarizing the results of a tremendous amount of data collected on a worldwide basis only a short time earlier.

The engineer concerned with design of a particular piece of machinery can generate a program that computes the operating characteristics of the machine based on the variable design parameters. This allows the engineer to tailor those design parameters to the necessary constraints of intended application and cost. Applications programs utilizing the ability of the computer to generate a visual image are extremely helpful to the design engineer in controlling cosmetic features of a product such as an automobile or a building. Prior to the construction of a solid model, information on the appearance of the structure in three standard projections can be entered. A computer-simulated three-dimensional image of the model can then be generated on the CRT. The image may be rotated along any arbitrary axis on the CRT, allowing the viewer to visualize it from any projection. The combination of this visual simulation of a solid object with the concept of the virtual computer allows the user to program the computer so that it may behave like many mechanical or even biological devices. One example of this application is the simulation of a ship or airplane control system by a computer, allowing personnel to be instructed safely and repetitively in the management of emergency conditions.

The second principal application of modern computers is information processing. This comprises two sometimes overlapping areas: non-numerical and numerical. The non-numerical area includes language translation and generation of data reference files such as telephone directories, library file systems, and storage of records. Numerical information processing includes business applications such as accounting. The U.S. Census Bureau was one of the earliest users of computers in information processing, although their earliest machines were entirely hardwired and therefore did not contain applications programs in the true sense. Overlapping areas in information processing include the use of a computer in maintaining an inventory in a large business or the application of a computer system by airlines in making reservations.

The third category of applications programs is control systems. This is to be distinguished from the control systems described earlier under "Operating Systems." In this application, the operation of a machine is simplified for the operator by two features of computer interfacing. The first is preprocessing of information from the device to be controlled and the display of this information in a form more easily utilized by the operator. The second is the use of the computer to perform routine chores previously performed by the human operator. Operators can thus be allowed to concentrate their efforts on avoiding dangerous or critical situations. Control system applications include air traffic control, complex communications networks, missile guidance systems including spacecraft, and control of industrial machinery such as steel mills, nuclear power plants, and the machinery involved in the design and manufacture of computers.

The most recent area of computer application is in personal use. An increasing number of small, inexpensive computers are now being sold to individuals for other than business applications. Although some of these do find their way into limited practical use, such as management of home finances and education, the majority are intended for hobby use, including the popular computer games. Hobbyists may generate a variety of applications programs on their own, but most home computers probably are utilized by people having no training in computer programming. In this sense, it could be argued that the software containing the instructions for the game or other application is not an application program in the strict sense, but for that user just an extension of the operating system.

COMPUTER APPLICATIONS IN COMPUTED TOMOGRAPHY

The computer used in CT scanning is a specialized assembly of hardware and software components. The discussion of the CT computer architecture in this chapter is based on the American Science and Engineering (AS&E)/Pfizer models. Typical hardware organization is illustrated in Figure 4.37. The central hardware component is a large disk drive system typically with a capacity of 80 Mbytes. The large capacity of this disk drive allows storage of over 100 reconstructed images. Each replaceable disk pack allows fairly rapid access to another 100 or more images for review on the CRT. In addition to providing a nonvolatile, rapid access storage medium for the reconstructed images, a portion of the space available on this disk drive is allocated to storage of the computer-operating system, from which it may be loaded into the computer RAM. The operating system may include specialized utility programs, including features for radiation therapy treatment planning or maintenance of teaching files, if required by the user.

General Description

The computer system used in CT provides four basic functions: control of the scanning operation, acquisition and storage of the raw data, reconstruction of the image, and display of the reconstructed image. These tasks may be divided between two separate computers as shown in Figure 4.37. In this diagram, one computer is devoted entirely to display of the reconstructed image and transfer of the image to long-term storage. The computer that carries out this function is called the display computer. The remaining three functions are carried out by the scan/reconstruction computer. This segregation of tasks allows physicians to review the reconstructed images

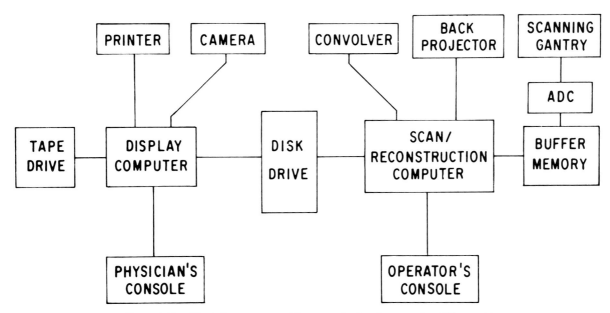

Figure 4.37. Typical computer architecture of a fourth generation CT scanner.

obtained on one patient while another patient is being scanned. Both computers share one disk drive; thus, the two tasks are not entirely independent. Because the process of scanning and initial storage of data prior to reconstruction cannot be interrupted without loss of data, this process generally takes priority over other functions, with the result that the scan-reconstruction computer gets a higher priority in access to the disk drive during scanning. Consequently, during the scanning process, the user of the display computer may notice a delayed response to a request for new or modified images, in comparison to when scanning is not underway. This time-shared use of the disk drive is directed by the control unit of the scan/reconstruction computer.

The CPUs of the scan/reconstruction and display computers are 16-bit word devices, each word consisting of two 8-bit bytes. Each of these computers will typically have approximately 32 kbytes of core memory. A computer of this configuration is adequate to process a reconstructed image and to direct the scanning process and initial acquisition and storage of data, but it cannot efficiently reconstruct the large amount of data into the final image within a practical time frame. For this reason, the scan/reconstruction computer performs primarily a control function in directing the flow of data into two highly specialized processor units called the convolver and the back projector. Both of these units have much more extensive RAMs. For example, the memory in the AS&E back projector provides storage for 256,000 words, each of 27 bits. This computer within a computer initially performs rebinning (a data reorganizing process) and data correction operations on the scan data under the control of the main scan/reconstruction computer. After these initial data correction and preliminary processing operations have been performed, the data are transferred to the memory of the convolver, where the Fourier transforms are calculated as required by the reconstruction algorithm. The convolver ALU includes a much more extensive set of instructions for arithmetic operations than the other CPUs in the CT scanner's collection of computers, thereby allowing these involved mathematical functions to be calculated efficiently and accurately. Following convolution, the data are again transferred to the back projector where the actual back-projecttions or reconstruction of the image from the processed data takes place. As the images are reconstructed, they are stored on disk under the direction of the scan/reconstruction computer.

Positioning of the patient, quality and intensity of the x-ray beam, and initiation of scanning are controlled by the scan-reconstruction computer through instructions generated at the operator console. The operator console consists of one or two CRTs, a teletype keyboard which includes additional specialized sets of switches that allow the operator to input instructions to the computer, and meters to monitor the operation of the x-ray unit. The reconstructed image is viewed at the operator console to confirm positioning.

At the direction of the operator, a scan cycle is initiated. This causes the x-ray tube to swing in a complete circle around the patient, emitting radiation that is attenuated by the patient before reaching the detectors. In fourth generation machines, the signal received by a detector during the scanning cycle consists of a number of separate pulses, each representing the amplitude of the x-ray beam received by the detector at the moment when each sampling instruction is received. The actual number of pulses and the number of pulses per angle of view depends on the scanner manufacturer and model. In spite of the fact that the signal from each detector is in the form of a series of pulses, it does not represent digital information because the signal amplitude is a continuous variable, depending upon the intensity of the beam produced by the x-ray tube and attenuated by the intervening air, patient, and portions of the CT scanning table before being received by the detector. Before digital data processing techniques can be applied to the signal, it must therefore be converted into a binary digital signal by an analog-to-digital converter. The first digital operation performed on the converted data is storage in buffer memory before further transmission. Consequently, analog-to-digital conversion must be accomplished rapidly, that is, immediately after the generation of the x-ray attenuation signal. The initial buffer is sufficiently large to store the complete set of raw data generated by one scan cycle. In some CT scanners, a second scanning cycle can begin before reconstruction of the first scanning cycle has been completed, in which case raw data from subsequent scanning cycles will be transferred to the disk while awaiting reconstruction.

Although Figure 4.37 shows a separate display computer, this is a desirable but not a necessary feature for a CT scanning installation. The functions carried out by the display computer could be carried out by the scan/reconstruction computer after scanning has been completed. The advantage of the display computer in allowing simultaneous processing of two patient files resident on the disk drive has been previously mentioned. An additional advantage is that the display computer can be located at a site remote to the CT scanning suite. The tasks performed by the display computer are much less extensive than those of the scan/reconstruction computer. The display computer is only required to retrieve already reconstructed images from the disk drive and to perform limited image enhancement operations and other restricted forms of data manipulation. Generally, facilities for long-term storage of the digital information onto magnetic tape are also controlled via the display computer.

The display computer also allows later retrieval of information from magnetic tape. Although coupling of a camera to provide hard copies of the images on sheet film could be made either to the scan or display computers, the display computer is a more convenient location, as images are generally represented on this computer in a form in which they are most useful for diagnostic purposes. A line printer may also be coupled to the display computer to allow permanent recording of x-ray attenuation data for research purposes or to allow more extensive diagnostic testing to be performed on a malfunctioning computer.

In some installations, a papertape reader is provided in conjunction with the scan/reconstruction computer for the purpose of booting the system when it is first turned on or recovering from a fault condition. In other installations, the sequence of boot instructions will be permanently stored in nonvolatile memory and can be accessed merely by flipping one of two switches on the operator's console.

In most installations, software details will be of no concern to the operator. For special research projects, however, there is no reason why the CT computer cannot be used in other applications within its hardware limitations. For these situations, it is often possible to obtain **BASIC** or **FORTRAN** compilers as software accessories. Many applications programs generated by earlier users of CT installations are currently available within the operating systems of subsequent machines. Examples of these include teaching file packages, radiation therapy treatment planning packages, and routines for multiplanar reconstruction.

A particularly interesting example of the versatility of the computer hardware package is the scan localizer application (computed radiography or digital computed radiography). In this application, not only is the computer used to reconstruct a nontomographic radiographic image, but the data for the radiographic image itself are obtained by a modified operating mode of the x-ray tube and detectors in the gantry. In this case, the x-ray tube irradiates the detectors (a fixed set in a fourth generation unit, and all of the detectors in a third generation unit), and the patient is slowly moved through the gantry as data are collected. In some installations, the CT computer is used, after scanning hours, for scheduling, accounting, and report-generating purposes.

Hardware Installation

Performance of even the best CT scanner can be severely degraded if careful attention is not given to the manufacturers' recommendations regarding installation. As with all radiographic equipment, sufficient power must be provided for operation of the x-ray tube, and the floor must be able to withstand the load of the heavy equipment without allowing even small amounts of motion which could degrade performance. There must be sufficient space around the gantry and table to allow easy access for patients and patient support devices as well as for personnel to assist in moving the patients and supporting them while they are being examined.

There are additional factors to be considered that are peculiar to computer installations. Although the electrical power requirements of a computer installation are not unusually large, particularly by radiographic standards, the computer is much more sensitive to fluctuations in the wave pattern of the supply voltage than are other radiographic devices. These fluctuations can not only result in loss of data, but in some circumstances can cause actual damage to the computer. Noise in the power line, often characterized by an unusually large voltage spike of very short duration, may propagate through the power supply to the solid-state devices, which are easily damaged by an overvoltage even of very short duration. Even if the overvoltage is of insufficient amplitude to damage a device, it can under certain circumstances be misinterpreted as a legitimate data bit and result in an incorrect result in the calculation or transmission of an incorrect instruction. These noise pulses may come either from natural phenomena such as lightning, even though fairly remote, or from man-made noise. The best protection against man-made noise is obtained by providing a separate power line from the circuit breaker panel to the computer installation. Adequate grounding is extremely important. Further reduction of both man-made and natural noise can be provided by filters on the power lines. Many of these are already built into the computer installation.

Lower frequency fluctuations in voltage levels, particularly those lasting from a few tenths of a second to hours, require different forms of protection. An overvoltage condition can, as previously described for pulses, result in damage to solid-state devices. Electrical motors generally are fairly resistant to moderate overvoltage. In contrast, motors are more sensitive to burnout from lowering of voltage such as occurs during a brownout, whereas solid-state devices are more resistant to failure from this condition. If the voltage drops too low, the solid-state devices may not be operating within their permissible envelope, and errors in processing may occur. One method of protection from over- and undervoltage conditions is turning off the CT scanner when they occur, although this is obviously not a desirable situation. Alternatively, the installation may be protected with a constant voltage transformer. This device supplies a virtually constant output voltage in spite of input voltages that may range 20% or more above or below the optimal level.

The ultimate low voltage condition, of course, is total power failure. The disk drive is particularly sensitive to this power abnormality, and irreparable damage can result to the drive as well as to the disk if adequate protection is not provided. The problem arises in that the recording/playback heads of the disk drive are supported under normal operating conditions by a thin layer of air just above the rapidly turning disk. Under normal shutdown procedures, the heads retract before the disk stops spinning. In an uncontrolled shutdown, the disk can lose speed while the heads are still in their extended position, with the result that the heads "crash" onto the disk surface. The resulting abrasion can irreparably damage the recording heads as well as the disk, with irretrievable loss of data stored on the disk. Modern disk drives incorporate devices intended to prevent this type of accident from occurring; however, if the power cycles off and on rapidly several times, as often occurs during a major power outage, damage can still occur. Whenever significant abnormalities in powerline voltage are noted, particularly when there is evidence suggestive of an impending power outage, the operator should be prepared to effect a prompt, controlled shutdown of the computer system until proper operating conditions can be reestablished. A transition from conventional power to a hospital emergency standby system can result in particularly dangerous voltage fluctuations. Whenever possible, the computer system should be turned off or put in a safe standby mode during this transition.

Portions of the computer are also more sensitive to extremes of temperature and humidity than conventional x-ray equipment. For this reason, manufacturers' recommendations regarding air conditioner installations should be closely adhered to. Whenever possible, a backup air-conditioning system should be provided. When the computer system is installed in a separate room, this backup system may be as simple as a moderate-sized window air-conditioning unit and may mean the difference between shutdown and continued operation of the CT unit. The low temperature limits below which solid-state devices can operate will probably never be encountered in a hospital installation. On the other hand, the high temperature limits can easily be reached in a confined space. Some portions of the computer system, particularly the disk drive, generate moderate amounts of heat, which can rapidly raise temperatures of adjacent components. Failure usually does not occur in the form of a spectacular cloud of smoke. Instead, failure from moderately increased temperature, as well as humidity, will frequently take the form of unexplained malfunctions of the computer, including increasing numbers of artifacts and inappropriate responses to instructions. Prolonged operation under these circumstances can result in a shortened lifetime of the components as well as in failures that can rapidly spread to involve multiple boards of the computer installation, making diagnostic testing prior to repair difficult. The magnetic core memory is the component of the computer most sensitive to high humidity. Although the humidity range of operation is rather limited, excursions outside the normal operating envelope rarely result in permanent damage, and reduction of the humidity to the normal operating range usually restores function. Unusually dry conditions interfere with operation, most commonly by increased generation of static electricity and consequently of noise. Continuously recording thermometers and hygrometers are particularly helpful in monitoring the performance of the air-conditioning system and in avoiding computer problems due to improper environment.

One final aspect of the computer environment that must be considered is dust particle size. Although the solid-state devices themselves can operate under thick layers of dust, this is undesirable for two reasons. First, accumulation of dust can interfere with heat transfer and, therefore, with maintaining proper temperature. More important than this, however, is that the disks and recording playback heads in the disk drive can be damaged by even very small dust particles in the air. This occurs because of the support of the flying head above the moving disk on a layer of air that usually measures only about .0001 inch thick. Common airborne contaminants including normal dust particles are usually much larger than this. Cigarette smoke, a frequent source of dust contamination, is particularly hazardous. The particle size of cigarette smoke is only slightly larger than the size of the air gap between the head and disk. In addition, its relatively small size makes it particularly difficult to filter from the atmosphere. For this reason, smoking within the computer room should be strictly forbidden.

Adequate lighting and space should be provided around the computer equipment to allow easy access and good working conditions for necessary repairs and routine maintenance.

REFERENCES AND SUGGESTED READINGS

Bell, C. G., Mudge, J. C., and McNamara, J. E. Computer Engineering, Digital Equipment Corp., Bedford, Mass., 1978.

Gear C. W. Computers and Systems. Science Research Associates, Chicago, 1978.

Greenberg, D. P. Computer graphics in architecture. Scientific American 230:98–106, May 1974.

Mano, M. M. Computer System Architecture. Prentice-Hall, Inc., Englewood Cliffs, NJ, 1976.

Matisoo, J. The superconducting computer. Scientific American 242:50–65, May 1980.

McWhorter, E. W. The small electronic calculator. Scientific American 234:88–98, March 1976.

Pratt, T. W. Programming Languages: Design and Implementation. Prentice-Hall, Inc., Englewood Cliffs, N.J., 1975.

Scientific American. Issue on microelectronics, September 1977.

Vacroux, A. G. Microcomputers. Scientific American 232:32–40, May 1975.

White, R. Disk-storage technology. Scientific American 243:138–148, August 1980.

Chapter 5
THEORY AND TECHNIQUES OF RECONSTRUCTION

RECONSTRUCTION TECHNIQUES

BACK-PROJECTION
    General Description
    Advantages and Limitations of Back-Projection

ITERATION
    Simultaneous Correction
    Ray-by-Ray Correction
    Point-by-Point Correction
    Further Variations and Constraints
    Advantages and Limitations of Iterative Techniques

ANALYTICAL METHODS
    Fourier Analysis
    Filtered Back-Projection
    Advantages and Limitations of Analytical Methods

COMPARISON BETWEEN ITERATIVE
    AND ANALYTICAL TECHNIQUES

RECONSTRUCTION TECHNIQUES
    FOR DIVERGENT BEAMS

REFERENCES AND SUGGESTED READINGS

RECONSTRUCTION TECHNIQUES

Computed tomography is the technique of computer-assisted image reconstruction of anatomical cross-sections. The reconstructed or synthesized image is composed of multiple voxels. Associated with each voxel is a linear x-ray attenuation coefficient, expressed as a CT number. The value of the CT number for each voxel is calculated from the numerous measurements of x-ray beam attenuation performed during scanning. The storage and manipulation of the large quantity of data compiled during scanning require the use of a computer that is programmed to follow a specific set of instructions, as described in Chapter 4.

Several conceptually distinct methods of image reconstruction have been developed, characterized by different mathematical theories and computational techniques. Each different approach is referred to as an algorithm, which may be regarded as a mathematical recipe for image reconstruction. Several algorithms have been devised for the analysis of the projection data and synthesis of the reconstructed image. The principal methods involve 1) back-projection or summation, 2) iteration, a technique used in the first EMI Mark I head scanner, and 3) analytic methods, which include two-dimensional Fourier analysis and filtered back-projection, the latter being the reconstruction technique currently used in CT units. These different reconstruction techniques are listed in Table 5.1. These algorithms are described in this chapter, using a conceptual rather than a mathematical approach, and their relative merits and lim-

Table 5.1. Reconstruction techniques

Back-projection (simple back-projection, summation method, method of linear superposition)
Iterative reconstruction
   Simultaneous correction (iterative least squares technique, ILST)
   Ray-by-ray correction (algebraic reconstruction technique, ART)
   Point-by-point correction (simultaneous iterative reconstruction technique, SIRT)
Analytical reconstruction
   Two-dimensional Fourier reconstruction
   Filtered back-projection (convolution method, convolutional integral, integral equation)
     Fourier filtering
     Radon filtering
     Convolution filtering

itations are analyzed. The mathematics of reconstruction are described in Appendix II.

BACK-PROJECTION

General Description

Back-projection, also referred to as the summation method, is the oldest form of image reconstruction and probably the simplest to understand. Although it is not used in any commercial models, the concepts underlying this technique serve as a good introductory model for understanding the general principles of reconstruction. Kuhl and Edwards (1963) originally used this technique in reconstructing radioisotope emission tomograms as described in Chapter 1.

The principle of this reconstruction technique is as follows: For a single ray (the x-ray beam traversing a core of tissue, or the bundle of paths from the x-ray source to a detector through the core of tissue), the resulting ray-sum (the detector signal or experimentally measured total attenuation of the ray after it has passed through the tissue core) is assumed to result from equal attenuation of the ray by all elements (the voxels from a three-dimensional viewpoint, or the pixels from a two-dimensional viewpoint) in the path of the ray. In other words, the core of tissue through which a ray has passed is assumed to be homogeneous in its x-ray attenuation. The ray-sum is then projected back into the core of tissue through which the ray has passed, where it is equally distributed throughout all elements in the path of the

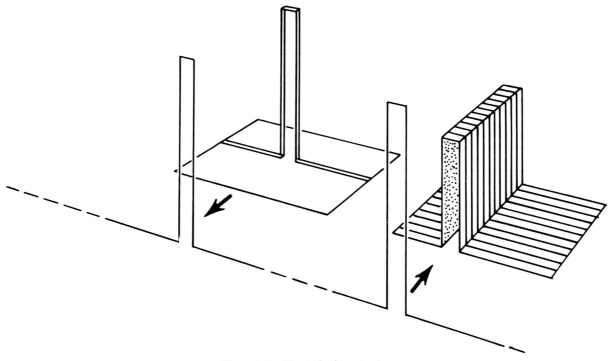

Figure 5.1. Simple back-projection.

ray. That is, the total x-ray attenuation (ray-sum) is divided equally among all the elements through which the ray passed (Figure 5.1).

This is illustrated schematically in Figure 5.2. A single dense point (e.g., an iron nail or a piece of calcium) is taken as the only object in the field of view to be reconstructed. Everything else in this field is assumed to be air. The x-ray beam is attenuated nowhere in the field of view except for those rays that pass through the high density point. After a single linear scan, the only ray-sum that shows a nonzero attenuation or signal is that associated with the ray-path or the strip in which the dense point lies. All other rays contribute nothing (zero attenuation) to the elements in their path after back-projection. The ray passing through the dense point will have its nonzero ray-sum (attenuation) distributed equally or homogeneously among all the elements through which it passed. Hence, the dense point appears to be located within a strip within the slice, or, in a three-dimensional view (considering the thickness of the slice), within a core (Figure 5.2A). It cannot be localized more precisely than this. The assumption is then made that the ray was equally attenuated by all elements within the strip or core.

Following an angular rotation, a second linear scan is performed and again a nonzero signal corresponding to attenuation is seen only in that path of the x-ray beam for the ray that passes through the strip containing the dense point. Thus, the ray-sum again differs from zero only in a single strip; its value will be distributed equally throughout this new strip containing the dense point. This is done for multiple projections (Figure 5.2B). Each time, a new back-projection is formed.

Finally, the back-projections are summed, giving rise to a starlike image (Figure 5.2C). The region of highest density corresponds to the location of the dense point. However, spokes appear to radiate from the region of highest density to the periphery (Figure 5.2C). This represents a point-spread function produced by the back projection and summation process; that is, a highly localized object has been spread out in space as a result of the reconstruction. A point has

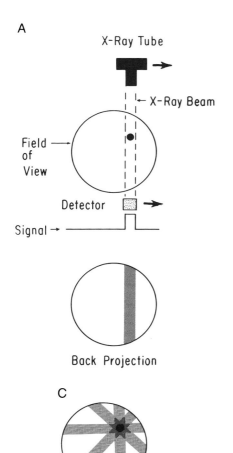

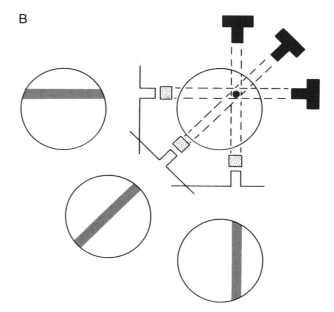

Figure 5.2. Simple back-projection. *A*, The ray-sum or total x-ray attentuation resulting from a single dense object is back-projected so that is is distributed homogeneously throughout the core of tissue in which the measurement of the ray-sum was made. The well-localized object is thus smeared out within the core. *B*, As different projections are performed, the dense object is identified within differently oriented tissue cores. *C*, The individual back-projections are summated. The resulting spoke pattern represents blurring of the object in space by the back-projection technique. Because of the basic assumption used in the back-projection method (the dense object is equally likely to be anywhere within a core of tissue), the final distribution may be thought of as a probability distribution for the likelihood of the object being at any position within the field.

been imaged as a star. An exact reconstruction should reproduce a point as a point, not as a star. Figure 5.3 illustrates further the concept of back-projection.

Any structure can be taken as a collection of points of varying density. The process of back-projection and summation leads to each individual point being reconstructed as a starlike image or as an ill defined central density with peripherally radiating spokes. The presence of these unwanted spokes associated with each reconstructed image point results in blurring of the composite synthesized image. Thus, there is a background density which exists as noise.

Conventional tomographic techniques involving coordinated movements of the x-ray tube and film are three-dimensional versions of the back-projection or summation method. Early work by Kuhl and Edwards (1963, 1968) in isotope emission tomography and by Oldendorf (1961) in radiographic transmission tomography used back-projection techniques.

Advantages and Limitations of Back-Projection

The advantage of back-projection is that the technique is relatively easy to conceptualize and to implement. Kuhl and Edwards (1968) performed back projection in a nonmathematical manner utilizing an oscilloscope whose light trace was coupled to and modulated by the gamma detector and later computerized.

However, the significant disadvantage is that the resulting image is only a crude approximation of the original object and is of very limited accuracy. There is a great deal of background noise or fogging. The most striking artifact is the well known star pattern, in which a highly localized object or spike, as illustrated in Figure 5.2C, is converted into a series of spokes. These limitations result from the fact that each ray-sum is back-projected not only to points of high density but to all points along the ray; that is, points outside the localized object are assigned some of the back projection density. This effect is additive, so that if there are multiple localized points of non-zero x-ray attenuation (as is the case for any realistic image), each point contributes to the back-projection intensity or x-ray attenuation of every other point. This reduces contrast. Thus, unlike conventional tomography, blurring in back-projection occurs within the plane of interest and not from the overlying planes.

Although the technique is presently only of historical interest, it is an approach whose ready conceptualization may help to understand the basic principles of image reconstruction. In particular, a modified form of this technique, filtered back-projection, is presently the most widely used algorithm in commercial units. An understanding of simple back-projection serves as an intellectual stepping stone to a discussion of filtered back-projection. This is taken up later in this chapter.

ITERATION

The iterative techniques are based on the principle of successive approximations, using the calculating capabilities of the computer to derive successively better approximations to the value of the attenuation coefficient in each voxel. An arbitrary set of values for these attenuation coefficients or an initial image is assumed for a first approximation, and serial corrections are made until the calculated ray-sums or projections from the reconstructed image are in agreement with the measured values. Iteration has been commonly used by mathematicians in solving complex matrix equations. Iterative methods were first introduced for image reconstruction by Bracewell (1956) in radio astronomy and by Gordon et al. (1970) in electron microscopy. Hounsfield (1972, 1973) developed an iteration algorithm for the orig-

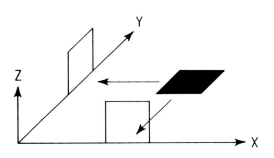

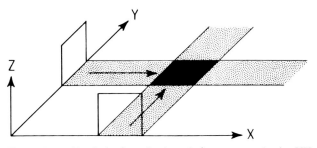

Figure 5.3. Simple back-projection. A dense square in the *XY* plane is projected onto the *X* and the *Y* axes (two independent projections). When the vertical projections are back-projected onto the *XY* plane, a cross-pattern is obtained. The intersection of the two back-projections corresponds to the original high density square.

inal EMI Mark I head CT scanner. As a rule, iterative techniques are tedious and time-consuming.

There are three variations of iterative reconstruction currently employed: simultaneous correction (iterative least-squares technique, or ILST), ray-by-ray correction (algebraic reconstruction technique, or ART), and point-by-point correction (simultaneous iterative reconstruction technique, or SIRT). Their differences are based on whether the sequence in which successive corrections are made involve the whole matrix simultaneously, a ray at a time, or point by point.

Simultaneous Correction

The simplest variation is simultaneous correction. This technique was first attempted in radio astronomy in the reconstruction of a map of solar microwave emissions (Bracewell, 1956). Since the microwave antennas could not focus on points, the total radiation from ribbon-like strips was measured. The solar microwave map was then reconstructed using a series of these "strip-sums" from different directions. Unfortunately, the simultaneous correction did not converge because of a vast overcorrection (Brooks and Di Chiro, 1976).

In simultaneous correction, all the projections for the entire matrix are calculated at the beginning of each iteration, and corrections are made simultaneously for each element or pixel in the matrix at the end of the iteration (Figure 5.4). No further correction or updating is performed for any element or pixel until the end of the next iteration; that is, each element is corrected once and only once during each iteration. This approach unfortunately leads to overcorrection, since each element in the matrix is re-corrected for every ray passing through it, so that the successive iterations actually oscillate about the correct solution. Thus, there is a lack of convergence to a final solution. This may be alleviated by applying a damping factor to all corrections (Goitein, 1972). This variation of simultaneous correction is referred to as the iterative least-squares technique because the original damping factor was selected for the best least-squares fit after each iteration. It appears that the exact form of the damping factor is not critical, however.

Ray-by-Ray Correction

In the ray-by-ray correction, a ray-sum is calculated at the beginning of each iteration and corrections are made for each element or point in that ray (Figure 5.5). This is done sequentially for each ray in each

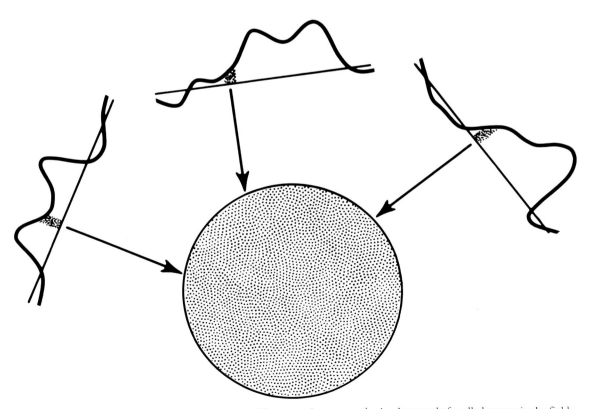

Figure 5.4. Iteration with simultaneous correction. The corrections are made simultaneously for all elements in the field.

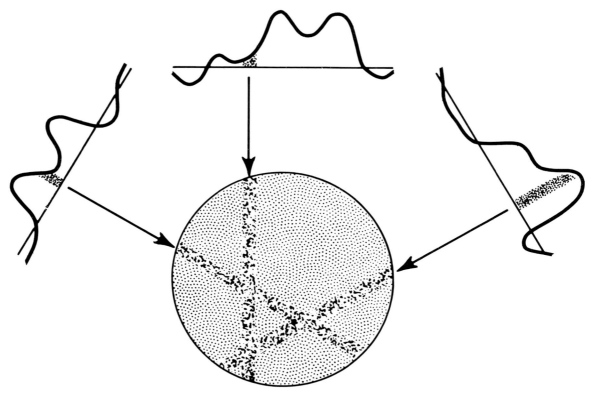

Figure 5.5. Iteration with ray-by-ray correction. All the elements and only those elements in a ray are corrected. This is repeated sequentially one ray at a time. Three successive ray-by-ray corrections are shown.

projection, always incorporating corrections made in previous rays into each new calculation. After this has been done for all rays in all projections in that iteration, a new iteration is begun. This approach was used by Hounsfield (1972, 1973) in the original EMI Mark I CT scanner and by Gordon et al. (1970).

A numerical example of a ray-by-ray correction is illustrated in Figure 5.6. Ray-sums first measured for horizontal (Figure 5.6A), vertical (Figure 5.6B), and oblique (Figure 5.6, C and D) rays. These ray-sums are the experimentally obtained data; that is, each ray-sum corresponds to the measured value of the x-ray attenuation for corresponding horizontal, vertical, and oblique rays. The individual elements in the matrix corresponding to the attenuation coefficients in each pixel are not known initially; they are to be found by iteration.

In the first step (Figure 5.6E), the value of each measured horizontal ray-sum is divided equally (as in back-projection) among the elements in its ray (11 ÷ 2 and 9 ÷ 2). In this example, there are two elements in each horizontal ray. An initial starting matrix is thus formed at the beginning of the iteration.

In the next step (Figure 5.6F), vertical ray-sums are calculated from the starting matrix of Figure 5.6E. These calculated ray-sums are compared to the true or measured vertical ray-sums (from Figure 5.6B). The difference for each vertical ray-sum (12 − 10 and 8 − 10) is divided by the number of elements in each ray (two in this example), and this correction is made for each element in the ray. A new working matrix is thus formed. Note the similarity in either of these two steps to back-projection.

The ray-sums from the new working matrix are now calculated for a set of oblique rays (Figure 5.6, G and H) and compared to the measured values (from Figure 5.6, C and D). In Figure 5.6G, there are three such oblique rays, two containing only one element and the third containing two elements. The difference for each oblique ray-sum (7 − 4.5, 5 − 10, and 8 − 5.5) is then divided equally among the elements in that ray. This gives a new working matrix. In this example, this last correction within the first iteration gives a matrix whose ray-sums in all directions correspond to the measured values (this also occurs if the other set of oblique rays from Figure 5.6H is used). Therefore, no more corrections are required. If this had not been the case, corrections for other oblique ray-sums would have been necessary and would have ended the first iteration. A new iteration, starting with the horizontal ray-sums, would have been performed if the first iteration were not successful. The process would be repeated until the calculated and measured ray-sums for all rays were equal, or until the computer was instructed that the differences were sufficiently small that no further calculations were needed.

The ray-by-ray correction is most effective if successive corrections within a particular iteration sequence are made one projection at a time, for example, all the horizontal ray-sums at once or all the

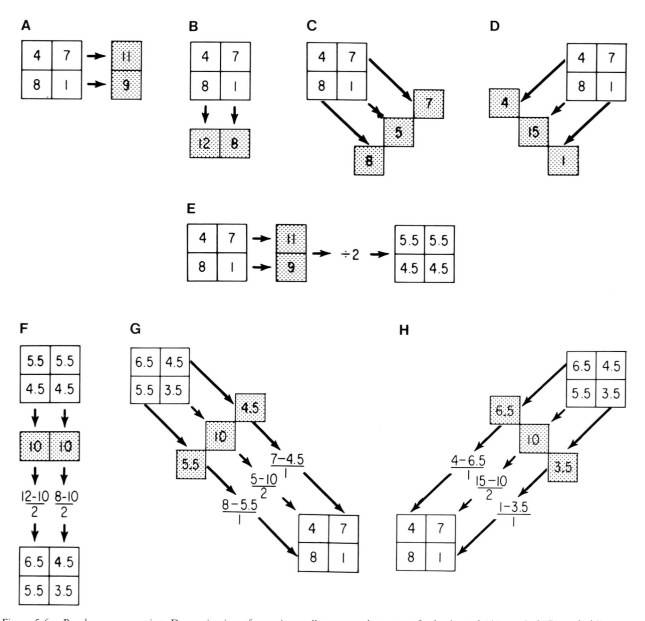

Figure 5.6. Ray-by-ray correction. Determination of experimentally measured ray-sums for horizontal (A), vertical (B), and oblique rays (C and D). E, Equal distribution of the ray-sum for horizontal rays among the elements in the ray. This is equivalent to back-projection. F, Vertical ray-sums are calculated from the matrix in E and compared to the true or measured values of the ray-sums from B. The difference between the calculated value and the measured value is distributed equally among the elements in each vertical ray. A new working matrix is obtained. G, Ray-sums from the new working matrix are calculated for oblique rays. These ray-sums are then compared to the true or measured ray-sums for these oblique rays from C. The difference is then distributed equally among each element in the ray. The original or true matrix has now been obtained. H, The ray-sums from the working matrix in F are calculated for a different set of oblique rays. These ray-sums are compared to the true or measured ray-sums for these oblique rays from D. The difference is then distributed equally among each element in the ray. The original or true matrix has now been obtained.

Reconstruction   113

vertical ray-sums at once. Also, it should be done with large angles between consecutive projections, that is, first the horizontal ray-sums and then the vertical ray-sums, rather than consecutive projections separated by only 1° or 2° (this refers to the calculation sequence for reconstructing the image, not the measurement sequence for obtaining the data). If the angles between successive corrections in a single iteration are large, then the corrections are relatively independent of one another; that is, the maximum difference for a correction will be obtained. If, on the other hand, they are close together (small angular difference), each successive correction will be nearly the same as the previous one and errors may accumulate. Hounsfield (1972) recognized this and used 40° increments in the first head scanner, the EMI Mark I. Kuhl et al. (1973) used projections that were orthogonal, that is, at 90° to each other.

Point-by-Point Correction

In point-by-point correction each iteration initially corrects a single pixel or element for all rays passing through it (Figure 5.7). The process is repeated sequentially for all pixels or elements in the matrix, but with the incorporation of the successive corrections made during the iteration. Gilbert (1972) introduced this variation in electron microscopy, calling it the simultaneous iterative reconstruction technique (SIRT). Bracewell (1956) used a similar method in radio astronomy (Brooks and Di Chiro, 1975).

Further Variations and Constraints

In each of these variations, two correction mechanisms are available: additive and multiplicative. The additive mechanism divides the correction among the different pixels or elements in a ray in proportion to their weighting factors. The most accurate weighting function has been thought to be the actual area of intersection of the pixel and ray (the fraction of the pixel that lies within the ray under consideration; Figure 5.8). Other weighting factors have been used. In a multiplicative method, each pixel is corrected in proportion to its most current density or attenuation; that is, the brightest elements get the largest corrections. The additive method is more commonly used (Brooks and Di Chiro, 1975, 1976).

Finally, constraints are introduced to increase the speed and accuracy of iteration. These include: 1) no attenuation value can be less than zero, 2) no attenuation value can exceed a specific maximum, and 3) pixels within rays whose ray-sum is zero are assigned attenuation values of zero (Brooks and Di Chiro, 1976).

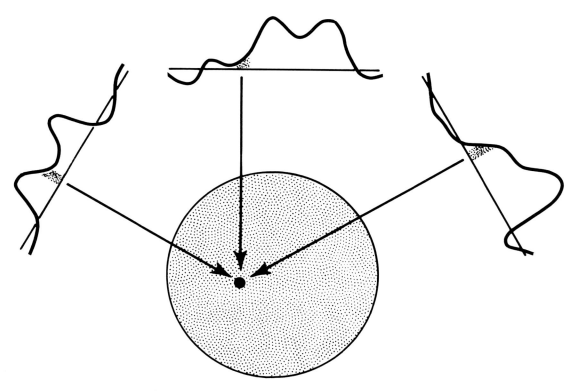

Figure 5.7. Point-by-point correction. The correction is performed for a single point at a time.

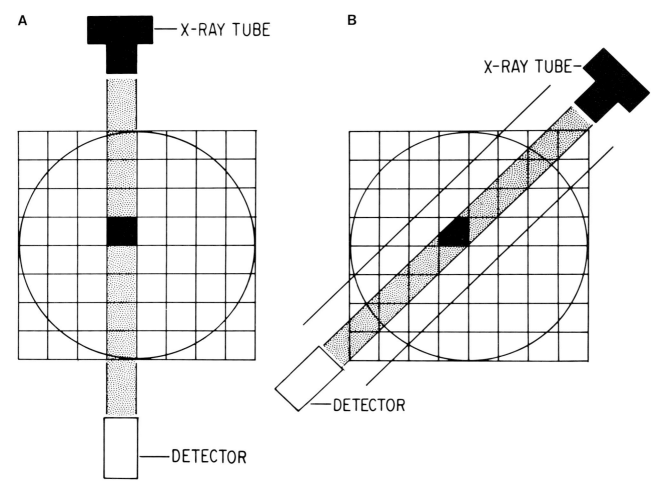

Figure 5.8. Additive correction mechanism. *A*, The entire area of a pixel lies within the ray. Its weighting factor is 1. *B*, Only a portion of the pixel lies within the ray. Its weighting factor is the ratio of the area of the portion of the pixel contained within the ray to the entire area of the pixel. The amount of a correction applied to each pixel in a ray is proportional to its weighting factor for that ray.

Advantages and Limitations of Iterative Techniques

Iterative techniques are well established in the solution of multiple simultaneous equations. The approach is relatively easy to conceptualize. The details of programming computers to solve simultaneous equations by iteration are not difficult. Finally, quite adequate images can frequently be obtained with this approach.

Iterative methods are beset by two significant limitations: the relatively long time required to perform the iteration (finite iteration time) and the possible lack of convergence of the calculated results to the true values of the attenuation coefficients (Brooks and Di Chiro, 1975).

The method of successive approximations or iterative techniques requires the gathering of all the data before calculations can be performed. Furthermore, multiple successive approximations may be required until the correct values of attenuation coefficients are obtained. The time delay is a significant limitation. Of the different methods, the ray-by-ray correction is the most efficient of the iterative techniques because it incorporates corrections during the iteration without a significant increase in computation time. Between the point-by-point and simultaneous correction methods, the simultaneous correction method is the faster of the two (Brooks and Di Chiro, 1976).

Balanced against the greater efficiency of the ray-by-ray technique is its increased susceptibility to noise compared to the simultaneous and point-by-point methods. The presence of noise results in inconsistencies within the various projection data. Thus, it really may not be possible to solve the equations. In this instance, values of the attenuation coefficients are obtained which satisfy the best least-

Reconstruction 115

squares fit to the projection data. The simultaneous and point-by-point corrections are better able to produce a satisfactory least-squares fit than the ray-by-ray correction. With a ray-by-ray technique, each element is corrected one ray at a time. This process results in the value of the element being weighted more heavily by the rays in the last projection than by rays in earlier projections in that iteration. This is not really a true averaging process. Noisy data will cause a ray-by-ray reconstruction to oscillate and possibly even to diverge during later iterations in trying to follow the successively calculated ray-sums. As mentioned earlier, this can be partially offset by a damping factor (Brooks and Di Chiro, 1976).

If the data are not noisy, the simultaneous correction and point-by-point techniques do not converge as rapidly as the ray-by-ray technique. All of these methods, however, may fail to converge or may not converge rapidly enough toward the appropriate values of the linear attenuation coefficients.

Clinically, the long reconstruction time with iteration often resulted in the patient being removed from the gantry and another patient being examined before the data on the first patient were available for display. Because the computer is often not capable of simultaneously performing scans, taking new data, and calculating the old data from the previous scan, it was often necessary to scan patients earlier in the day and then allow the computer to perform the reconstruction on all the scans for these patients later in the day. This can be extremely cumbersome in an active clinical setting. Because of these often unacceptable time delays in reconstructing the data, most units now utilize one of the analytical methods for reconstruction.

ANALYTICAL METHODS

Analytical reconstruction is characterized by a direct solution of the basic equation for reconstruction. Precise mathematical formulae are used to achieve an analytical reconstruction. The first analytical reconstruction of an x-ray image was performed by Cormack in 1963. Analytical reconstruction is currently the exclusive reconstruction technique in the commercially available CT units. The two most common forms of analytical reconstruction are Fourier analysis and filtered back projection.

Fourier Analysis

The basic concept of Fourier analysis is that any function or variation of a quantity in time or space can be expressed as a sum of sine and cosine waves, each of different frequencies with appropriate amplitudes assigned to each frequency component (Figure 5.9). Each frequency component is also referred to as a harmonic, analogous to the different frequency components associated with a musical note. The amplitude associated with each frequency component is referred to as the Fourier coefficient.

Initially, Fourier analysis for image reconstruction was first used by Bracewell (1956) in radioastronomy. The calculational difficulties of two-dimensional Fourier integrals were prohibitive, forcing Bracewell to use an iterative approach (Brooks and Di Chiro, 1975). The technique was introduced independently into electron microscopy by DeRosier and Klug (1968).

In a two-dimensional tomographic slice, there are spatial variations in the x-ray attenuation coefficient. By the Fourier theorem, this spatially varying x-ray attenuation coefficient can be expressed as a sum of spatially oriented sine and cosine waves. Each of these spatial harmonics is characterized by its frequency, the direction in space in which it is propagating, and its amplitude, which expresses its relative contribution. The mathematical basis of Fourier reconstruction is that the Fourier coefficients of the image can be expressed in terms of the Fourier coefficients of the projections. The amplitudes of spatial waves at any given angle are actually equal to the Fourier coefficients of the projection at that same angle. This allows the Fourier coefficients of the image to be derived from those of the projections. The picture image is then synthesized from its Fourier coefficients (Brooks and Di Chiro, 1975). This is illustrated in Figure 5.10 for a homogeneous rectangle in two projections.

Although the technique of Fourier analysis is frequently hard to conceptualize for an individual not trained in mathematics, it is a familiar mathematical approach to scientists and engineers. Conceptually and practically, it is has a wide range of ramifications in many different fields. Finally, the technique is not difficult to implement with a computer.

Filtered Back-Projection

In filtered back-projection, the profiles obtained in simple back-projection are modified or filtered prior to being back-projected. This is done to correct for the background density that occurs in simple back-projection. Because the problem can be reduced to the solution of a one-dimensional integral equation, this technique is sometimes referred to as an integral equation method.

The convolution method is a type of integral equation approach with proven accuracy and speed. The basic problem is to find a mathematical function,

Table 5.2. Comparison of iterative and analytical methods

	Iterative method	Analytical method
Speed	Considerably slower unless the data are incomplete	Significantly faster; also can be performed during scanning
Accuracy	Limited by finite iteration time and lack of convergence	Problems with band limiting and interpolation
Incomplete data	Assumed that the final image should be as smooth as possible; time for reconstruction is decreased; performs even with asymmetry	Assumed that missing projections are similar to measured projections; time for reconstruction is increased; works best when there is symmetry
Noise	Equivalent when data are complete; less affected by noise when data are incomplete	Equivalent when data are complete, generally more affected by noise when data are incomplete
Constraints	Allows introduction of additional information or constraints into algorithm	Constraints not allowed

The time to perform a reconstruction is also dependent upon the number of projections measured, the size of the reconstructed matrix, particular features of the algorithm, and the speed and capability of the computer and ancillary data-processing equipment. This ancillary equipment may include hardwiring (fixed hardwired circuit boards), which can perform specific calculations or data-processing techniques for a particular algorithm. The data are essentially taken out of the computer and put into the hardwired circuits, where the data are processed and then reentered into the computer. This permits much faster data processing than with the computer alone. However, it introduces a certain amount of inflexibility into the system. Any alteration in the algorithm now requires physical replacement of circuit boards rather than just a relatively simpler and less expensive software change or reprogramming of the computer.

As described earlier, the principal limitations to the accuracy of analytical techniques are band limiting and interpolation; the accuracy of iteration is limited by the finite iteration time and the possible lack of convergence to an appropriate set of attenuation coefficients.

The lack of convergence in iteration may result in wandering of the best guess for the attenuation coefficients among nearly equivalent reconstructions. It is affected by the details of implementation of the algorithm (e.g., the sequence in which production data are processed, what damping factors are applied to the data) and by constraints placed on allowable values of the attenuation coefficients.

Finally, a criterion must be adopted to end the iteration scheme. This stopping criterion affects the accuracy of the reconstruction as well. Analytical techniques do not require any such arbitrary criterion.

When the number of projections is less than that required for the necessary image reconstruction, the data are incomplete. To solve the large number of simultaneous equations, as illustrated by Equation 2.12, so that each unknown (the value of an attenuation coefficient for a particular voxel) has a specific fixed value, it is necessary to have more equations than unknowns. Having incomplete data, or an insufficient number of projections, results in having fewer equations than unknowns. The requirement for the necessary number of projections for the complete specification of a circularly bounded image is illustrated in Figure 5.13. The number of cells (specifically, the number of voxels or pixels) in a diameter of the field of view to be reconstructed is n. There are thus $n/2$ cells in a radius of the field of view and $\pi(n/2)^2 = \pi n^2/4$ cells in the entire area encompassed within the circular field of view. In a typical first generation translation-rotation system, measure-

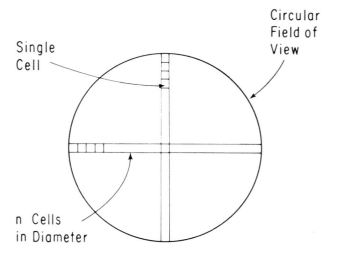

Figure 5.13. Illustration of a circular field of view (area of reconstruction) containing n cells in a diameter. The total number of cells in the circle is equal to $\pi(\text{diameter})^2/4$ or $\pi n^2/4$. This represents the number of independent variables or quantities to be determined in the reconstruction. The number of independent data measurements, or equations, must equal or exceed this number.

ments might be taken n times during a single translation corresponding to a particular projection. Each measurement corresponds to a single equation of the form of Equation 2.10. A single projection would thus typically give n equations. The total number of equations, which is equal to the total number of measurements, will then be n times the number of projections. This total number of equations must be equal to or greater than the number of unknowns, which is $\pi n^2/4$.

$$n \times \text{number of projections} = \pi n^2/4 \qquad (5.1)$$
$$\therefore \text{number of projections} = \pi n/4$$

For other than first generation translational-rotational systems, the number of measurements taken for a single projection may be the same, greater than, or less than n (depending upon how a projection is defined). If fewer measurements are made for each projection, more projections will be required, and vice versa. The required number of projections, or more precisely the total number of measurements, may be modified if the sampling theorem is rigorously followed. This would require taking more data for greater statistical reliability. That is, the sampling rate, or frequency of taking data, is increased over the requirements summarized in Equation 5.1. Although the earliest versions of the first translation-rotation system, the EMI Mark I, did eventually make 160 measurements during a single linear translation or projection for their 160 × 160 matrix, this was later modified so that 240 measurements were performed, thus adhering to the sampling theory. Similarly, in the original ACTA scanner, 160 measurements were performed in a single linear translation for a 160 × 160 matrix. This also has been changed with successive modifications of the unit to adapt to the sampling theorem.

When the data are incomplete, assumptions must be made in order to derive the attenuation coefficients. In analytical techniques, the assumption is made that the missing projections are similar to those that have been measured, and a time-consuming interpolation process is used to fill in the missing projection data. This assumption of similarity is most effective when there is circular symmetry in the object being reconstructed. Iteration assumes that the final image should be as smooth as possible, that is, without abrupt changes. Unlike the analytical techniques in which the additional interpolation requires longer reconstruction time, the iterative method is actually reduced. With incomplete data, iterative approaches may become as fast as analytical techniques. Furthermore, iteration performs better when there is asymmetry in the image. It may in fact use projection data that do not span a complete semicircular arc, unlike the analytical techniques.

Noise refers to statistical fluctuations in the projection data. At its most fundamental level, noise arises from the statistical variations in x-ray measurement occurring because of the limited number of x-ray photons.

When the projection data are complete and an accurate reconstruction technique is used, the noise is generally independent of the specific algorithm used. However, when the projection data are incomplete, the assumptions made about the incomplete data become very important. Iterative methods will generally produce the smoothest possible picture. Analytical techniques will usually maintain the full noise spectrum, unless additional filtering is introduced. Among the iterative methods, both the simultaneous (ILST) and point-by-point (SIRT) corrections perform better with noisy data than the ray-by-ray correction (ART).

As described earlier, the various iterative techniques also permit the use of additional information or conditions referred to as constraints. This introduces an added degree of flexibility, allowing modification of the basic algorithm.

RECONSTRUCTION TECHNIQUES FOR DIVERGENT BEAMS

With the development of CT units that can scan in 5 s or less, compared to the 4.5-min scanning time of the earliest machines, the geometry of data collection has undergone significant alteration. The use of a single circular motion has led to the discarding of the parallel beam technique in favor of a fan beam of divergent x-rays from a single source for each projection.

This change to a divergent or fan beam geometry necessitates modification of the algorithm. The algorithm must have the capability for extremely rapid data processing without sacrificing any accuracy. Because of these requirements for speed as well as accuracy in data processing, an analytical method, generally convolution, is used.

Convolution methods for processing data collected by parallel beams are well developed. One approach involves reordering the data obtained from divergent beams into a form based on collection from parallel (or nearly parallel) rays coming from different projections. Convolution methods for parallel beam geometry may then be used. This approach thus requires two separate steps in data processing: conversion of the data collected by divergent beams into a parallel beam format, and application of a parallel beam convolution algorithm.

Another approach involves the use of a diverging beam convolution method that does not require reordering of the data into parallel beam form (Herman et al., 1976; Edelheit et al., 1977). This technique permits both rapid data collection and rapid and accurate reconstruction. The final results are still expressed in rectilinear or Cartesian coordinates; that is, the attenuation coefficients are derived for voxels arranged in a square matrix format.

The latter approach is the most commonly used method for data processing in divergent beam geometry. It is utilized, for example, in the GE CT/T 8800 and the Pfizer 0450. Although the convolution method is generally the form currently used for divergent beam geometry reconstruction, an alternative analytical approach using a Fourier transform may be feasible if there is a sufficiently large quantity of data.

REFERENCES AND SUGGESTED READINGS

Bracewell, R. N. Strip integration in radio astronomy. Australian Journal of Physics 9:198–217, 1956.

Bracewell, R. N., and Riddle, A. C. Inversion of fan-beam scans in radio astronomy. Astrophysical Journal 150:427–434, 1967.

Brooks, R. A., and Di Chiro, G. Theory of image reconstruction in computed tomography. Radiology 117:561–572, 1975.

Brooks, R. A., and Di Chiro, G. Principles of computer assisted tomography (CAT) in radiographic and radioisotopic imaging. Physics in Medicine and Biology 21:689–732, 1976.

Cormack, A. M. Representation of a function by its line integrals, with some radiological applications. Journal of Applied Physics 34:2722–2727, 1963.

Cormack, A. M. Representation of a function by its line integrals, with some radiological applications. Journal of Applied Physics 34:2908–2913, 1964.

Cormack, A. M. Reconstruction of densities from their projections, with applications in radiological physics. Physics in Medicine and Biology 18:195–207, 1973.

Cormack, A. M. Early two-dimensional reconstruction (CT scanning) and recent topics stemming from it. Nobel Lecture, December 8, 1979. Journal of Computer Assisted Tomography 4:658–664, 1980.

DeRosier, D. J., and Klug, A. Reconstruction of three-dimensional structures from electron micrographs. Nature 217:130–134, 1968.

Edelheit, L. S., Herman, G. T., and Lakshminarayanan, A. V. Reconstruction of objects from diverging x-rays. Medical Physics 4:226–231, 1977.

Gilbert, P. Iterative methods for the three-dimensional reconstruction of an object from projections. Journal of Theoretical Biology 36:105–117, 1972.

Gilbert, P. F. C. The reconstruction of a three-dimensional structure from projections and its application to electron microscopy. II. Direct methods. Proceedings of the Royal Society of London, B. 182:89–102, 1972.

Goitein, M. Three-dimensional density reconstruction from a series of two-dimensional projections. Nuclear Instruments and Methods 101:509–518, 1972.

Gordon, R., Bender, R., and Herman, G. T. Algebraic reconstruction techniques (ART) for three-dimensional electron microscopy and x-ray photography. Theoretical Biology 29:471–481, 1970.

Gordon, R., and Herman, G. T. Three-dimensional reconstruction from projections: A review of algorithms. International Review of Cytology 38:111–151, 1974.

Gordon, R., Herman, G. T., and Johnson, S. A. Image reconstruction from projections. Scientific American 233:56–68, October 1975.

Herman, G. T. Advanced principles of reconstruction algorithms. *In* T. H. Newton and D. G. Potts (eds.), Radiology of the Skull and Brain: Technical Aspects of Computed Tomography, Vol. 5, Chap. 110, Part XVI, Sect. II, pp. 3888–3903. C. V. Mosby, St. Louis, 1981.

Herman, G. T., Lakshminarayanan, A. V., and Naparstek, A. Convolution reconstruction techniques for divergent beams. Computers in Biology and Medicine 6:259–271, 1976.

Herman, G. T., and Rowland, S. W. Three methods for reconstructing objects from x-rays: A comparative study. Computer Graphics and Image Processing 2:151–178, 1973.

Hounsfield, G. N. A method of and apparatus for examination of a body by radiation such as x- or gamma-radiation. British patent No. 1283915, London, 1972. Issued to EMI Ltd. Application filed August 1968.

Hounsfield, G. N. Computerized transverse axial scanning (tomography): I. Description of system. British Journal of Radiology 46:1016–1022, 1973.

Katz, M. Principles and technique of image reconstruction with CT. *In* Leon Weisberg (ed.), Cerebral Computed Tomography: A Text-Atlas, Chap. 2. W. B. Saunders Co., Philadelphia, 1978.

Kuhl, D. E., and Edwards, R. Q. Image separation radioisotope scanning. Radiology 80:653–661, 1963.

Kuhl, D. E., and Edwards, R. Q. Reorganizing data from transverse section scans of the brain using digital processing. Radiology 91:975–983, 1968.

Kuhl, D. E., Edwards, R. Q., Ricci, A. R., et al. Quantitative section scanning using orthogonal tangent correction. Journal of Nuclear Medicine 14:196–200, 1973.

McCullough, E. C., and Payne, J. T. X-ray transmission computed tomography. Medical Physics 4:85–98, 1977.

Macovski, A. Basic concepts of reconstruction algorithms. *In* T. H. Newton and D. G. Potts (eds.), Radiology of the Skull and Brain: Technical Aspects of Computed Tomography, Vol. 5, Chap. 110, Part XVI, Sect. I, pp. 3877–3887. C. V. Mosby, St. Louis, 1981.

Oldendorf, W. H. Isolated flying spot detection of radiodensity discontinuities—displaying the internal structural pattern of a complex object. I.E.E.E. Transactions on Biomedical Electronics, Vol. BMW 8:68–72, 1961.

Payne, J. T., and McCullough, E. C. Basic principles of computer-assisted tomography. Applied Radiology 5:March/April, 53–60, 1976.

Radon, J. On the determination of functions from their integrals along certain manifolds. Berichte über die Verhandlungen der königlichen Sächsischen Gesellschaft der Wissenschaften zu Leipzig. Mathematisch-Physische Klasse 69:262–277, 1917.

Ramachandran, G. N., and Lakshminarayanan, A. V. Three-dimensional reconstruction from radiographs and electron micrographs: Application of convolutions instead of Fourier transforms. Proceedings of the National Academy of Science 68:2236–2240, 1971.

Shepp, L. A., and Logan, B. F. The Fourier reconstruction of a head section. I.E.E.E. Transactions on Nuclear Science NS-21 (3):21–43, 1974.

Smith, K. T., Solomon, D. C., and Wagner, S. L. Practical and mathematical aspects of the problem of reconstructing objects from radiographs. Bulletin of the American Mathematical Society 83:1227–1270, 1977.

Smith, P. R., Peters, T. M., and Bates, R. H. T. Image reconstruction from finite numbers of projections. Journal of Physics A. Mathematical, Nuclear, and General 6:361–382, 1973.

CHAPTER 6
THE IMAGE DISPLAY

THE SYNTHESIZED IMAGE

DISPLAY MONITOR: THE CATHODE RAY TUBE

BASIC IMAGE PRESENTATION AND MANIPULATION

CT Number Scale
Window Settings
  Window Level
  Window Width
  Optimization of Window Settings
  Multiple Windows
  Extended CT Number Scale
Image Reversals
  Image Polarity
  Image Position
Magnification
Multi-Image Display
Color Display

COMPUTER GRAPHICS AND MEASUREMENTS

Computer Graphics
  Cursor
  Interactive Devices
  Line
  Trace
  Annotation
  Grid
Measurements
  CT Numbers
  Spatial Measurements

CONTRAST ENHANCEMENT

Oral Contrast
Intravenous Contrast
Intrathecal Contrast
Biliary Contrast
Other Contrast Studies

FILTERING

Smoothing
Edge Enhancement

HARD COPY

Positive Print Film (Polaroid)
Transilluminated Film with a Multiformat Camera

Film Size and Format
Multiformat Camera Design
Photography and Film Requirements

REFERENCES AND SUGGESTED READINGS

THE SYNTHESIZED IMAGE

All the information available from a conventional radiographic examination is on the film itself. The composite of shadows comprising the conventional radiograph is fixed on the film and may not be varied after the film is exposed and processed. The image is determined by a multitude of factors including the x-ray tube voltage (usually expressed as the maximum x-ray tube kilovoltage, kVp) and current (in milliamperes), the time of exposure (in seconds), the size of the patient, and the x-ray film (or, more correctly, the film-screen combination). The radiographic end product, an image of a three-dimensional object displayed on a hard copy, two-dimensional film, cannot be altered or varied in appearance, aside perhaps from brightlighting an overexposed film to better illuminate the darker shades of gray.

If better or additional detail of a particular region or tissue is required, then a new radiograph must be made; the examination must be repeated and the patient again exposed to x-rays. Usually, at least two different projections, at 90° to each other, are required for an adequate examination of a body region. Generally, if a radiograph is performed with technique optimized for one type of tissue detail (e.g., bone), then it is not optimal for another tissue (e.g., soft tissues). Different radiographs may be needed to obtain the requested detail for different tissues. For example, if a radiograph of the chest does not display sufficient detail of the thoracic spine, then another radiograph must be performed with different techniques (e.g., different kVp and mAs), optimized for the bone detail of the thoracic spine.

In computed tomography, the end product is not really an image but a matrix of x-ray attenuation coefficients expressed as CT numbers. These numbers are obtained by computer calculations using the input data from the x-ray intensity recording devices (e.g., scintillation crystals and photomultiplier tubes, high pressure gas ionization chambers, scintillation crystals with photodiodes). This matrix of numbers forms the primary image information basis in CT. The actual visualized image, usually displayed on Polaroid or x-ray film, is derived from the matrix by assignment of a shade of gray in the visual scale to each range of CT numbers.

The usual convention is to assign progressively lighter shades of gray to groups of CT numbers with progressively higher values. The total range of CT numbers spanned in passing from black (the darkest gray) to white (the lightest gray) is the CT window width. The CT number at the midpoint of the gray scale (the central gray value) is the window level. Both the window width and the window level may be freely varied by arbitrarily altering the manner in which shades of gray are assigned to ranges of CT numbers; that is, a single shade of gray may be made to encompass a larger or smaller range of CT numbers. Also, the central gray shade may be shifted from a higher to a lower CT value.

The polarity of the image itself may be readily altered between white-on-black or black-on-white display modes. The usual convention is that higher CT numbers (associated with denser tissues such as bone) are assigned lighter shades of gray, and lower CT numbers (associated with less dense tissues such as lung parenchyma) are assigned darker shades of gray. This is similar to a conventional radiograph or x-ray negative (called a negative since the exposed film is viewed directly, rather than making a positive print). The CT image following this convention is also referred to as a negative. Reversing the polarity results in a positive CT image. For example, the bones at the higher end of the density scale are displayed in darker shades of gray, and the lungs at the lower end of the density scale are shown in lighter shades of gray. Although the negative image polarity is by far the more widely accepted convention, the positive image mode has found support for bone display.

In addition to alterations in the window settings and polarity reversal, numerous other manipulations can be performed on the computer-synthesized CT image. These manipulations may accentuate certain features or structures within the image; they may also quantify the information within the image. Computer storage of the image data facilitates measurements of contrast (CT numbers) and spatial (distances and areas) parameters. Modification of both the raw data (the actual x-ray intensity measurements) and the processed CT numbers can be done. The appropriate use of various contrast agents can significantly enhance natural differences in tissue contrast and hence increase the information available in the CT image. The results of this image manipulation can be viewed on a display monitor (a television monitor) from which hard copy (film) pictures can be obtained.

DISPLAY MONITOR: THE CATHODE RAY TUBE

The monitor on which the visual image is displayed is a cathode ray tube (CRT) used in a television monitor format. In a CRT a maneuverable electron beam strikes a phosphorescent screen, causing emission of light. The electron beam arises from a heated wire element (electron gun) and is focused by electrodes, which function as an electric lens, or by an electrical coil functioning as a magnetic lens. The concept of an electric or a magnetic lens is borrowed from conventional optics and refers to devices whose only common feature with optical lenses is the capability of focusing or concentrating rays. In the case of a CRT, the rays are electron rays. The electron beam is accelerated across the vacuum within the monitor or picture tube by a high electrical voltage applied to the tube anode. This anode is plated on the inside surface of the picture tube by the phosphorescent screen.

In traveling across the tube from the electron gun to the screen, the electron beam can be deflected in two directions, horizontal and vertical. This deflection is accomplished by either of two pairs of mutually perpendicular electrical plates (electrodes) or by a magnetic deflecting coil. The advantage of a magnetic deflection compared to an electrical one is that a larger deflection angle can be achieved at a lower voltage. This enables the CRT to be made shorter and its face flatter. By application of the appropriate voltage to these deflecting electrodes or coils, the focused electron beam is directed to a specific point or dot on the phosphorescent screen. The amount of light emitted from a particular dot on the screen depends upon the number of electrons in the electron beam as well as on the efficiency of the phosphorescent screen. An electrical control grid is used to regulate the number of electrons in the beam.

When a CRT is used as a television monitor, the electron beam sequentially scans a series of horizontal lines across the phosphorescent screen. This is often referred to as the television raster. In the United States the standard television raster consists of 525 horizontal lines scanned in $1/30$ s. In Europe the raster contains 625 lines scanned in $1/25$ s.

The electron beam scans each line from left to right, illuminating each dot in the scan line by an amount determined by the number of electrons in the beam at the instant it strikes the dot. Display information is fed into the control grid and synchronized with the scanning beam. After scanning a line, the electron beam quickly returns to the left side of the monitor to begin scanning the next line. During its return the beam is blanked out. This process is continued until the last line at the bottom of the screen has been generated. The beam is then again blanked out while it returns rapidly to the top left-hand corner of the screen to begin scanning again.

In American television an interlaced scanning format is used. In this format $262\frac{1}{2}$ alternate lines are scanned initially in $1/60$ s ($16\frac{2}{3}$ ms). Each of these alternate scanning sequences is referred to as a field. The interlaced fields comprise a single frame generated in $1/30$ s. The frame rate of 30 per s is sufficiently fast to give the appearance to the eye of a continuous motion, thus avoiding any bothersome motion flicker. One field consists of the odd-numbered lines; the second field consists of the even-numbered lines. The purpose of interlacing two separate scans or fields of $262\frac{1}{2}$ lines each into a single frame of 525 lines, rather than simply scanning all 525 lines consecutively from top to bottom in a single scan, is to prevent brightness flicker. The eye can detect individual light flashes at a rate of up to 50 per s. Each time the electron beam scans through the entire area of the monitor, a light flash occurs. At a frame rate of 30 per s without interlacing, there would be a perceptible flicker of light on the monitor as the electron beam passed over the entire screen during each $1/30$ s. With interlacing, the electron beam scans the entire monitor screen each $1/60$ s. The light flashes are therefore sufficiently close together in time to avoid brightness flicker.

In some CT display systems a noninterlaced format is used; all the lines comprising a single image frame are scanned sequentially. This format is called repeat field scanning. However, to avoid flicker, the CT image frame in the noninterlaced format must still be repeated every $1/60$ s, the same time as a single field in television. Thus, if the same number of lines is used for displaying the CT image as for a television image (525 lines), the CT system must have a line rate (rate of scanning lines) twice that of a television system. The time during which an individual element within a line is exposed to the scanning electron beam is correspondingly reduced to half that for television. Some CT display systems may, however, use the more conventional interlaced format. An example is the General Electric CT/T system, in which each field is scanned in $1/60$ s and the entire frame in $1/30$ s.

A CT system may also use display monitors employing raster scan formats with more than 525 lines, permitting increased monitor resolution. The General Electric CT/T system, for example, has a display monitor with about 680 lines per frame. Increasing the number of lines in a frame also necessitates an increase in the line rate, and a further decrease in the time one element in a line is scanned.

As a consequence of increasing the line rate, either by the use of a repeat field scanning format or by employing a monitor with a higher number of lines per frame, a larger electronic bandwidth is required than for an interlaced television image with 525 lines. This involves added cost for electronics and monitors.

The CT numbers that form the basis of the CT image must be stored in some type of memory that can be read at a very rapid rate to provide the appropriate modulation of the electron beam, and hence the appropriate light output (gray scale) on the monitor. Since the CT numbers are digital in form, it is appropriate to use a digital (as opposed to an analog) memory to modulate the intensity of the electron beam. A memory of this type is referred to as a refresh memory, since it is read repeatedly at a high rate to refresh the image on the CRT display monitors. There is a specific location or address in the refresh memory for every element or position on the face of the CRT. The values in the refresh memory are read sequentially in synchronization with the scanning of the electron beam. In this way the refresh memory determines the electron beam intensity and resulting light output or gray scale for every element on the face of the CRT.

BASIC IMAGE PRESENTATION AND MANIPULATION

CT Number Scale

The display of the CT image and its manipulation are generally done at a display terminal (display or viewer's console). This display terminal includes an image monitor; appropriate controls for adjustments of the window settings; an alphanumeric and multiple function keyboard for communication with the computer in order to perform image manipulation, analysis and annotation; and, usually, a second monitor for displaying commands and receiving information or prompts (instruction on how to proceed) from the computer.

A CT image with the routine or conventional annotation and window settings is shown in Figure 6.1. This is the standard format in the General Electric CT/T 8800. Other units incorporate basically the

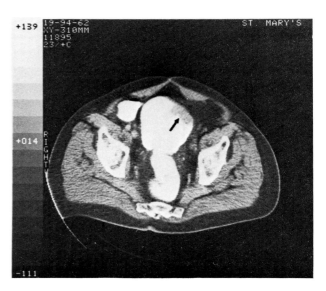

Figure 6.1. Conventional annotation and window settings. The four rows of annotation in the upper left indicate the patient's identification number (19-94-62), the slice location (310 mm below the anatomical reference, the xyphoid (XY)), the CT run number (11895), the slice number (23), and the use of intravenous contrast (+C). In the upper righthand corner the hospital is indicated, the patient's name and date below having been deleted. The right side of the patient is indicated. Other routine information that may be annotated includes the slice thickness, the time, kVp, and mA. The gray scale bar on the left illustrates 16 shades of gray for a window width of 250 that extends from −111 to +139 with a level (center) or +014. A bladder tumor (arrow) is present in this patient.

same and perhaps additional information in their formats.

Of particular importance is the scale for the window settings on the left side of the image. Sixteen shades of gray are displayed, from white at the top through successively darker shades of gray to black at the bottom. The CT number scale is shown for a system using a scale factor of 500 (−500 to +500). As discussed in Chapter 2, the scale factor is the constant K in the formula

$$\text{CT number} = \frac{\mu_{\text{substance}} - \mu_{H_2O}}{\mu_{H_2O}} \times K, \quad (6.1)$$

where $\mu_{\text{substance}}$ and μ_{H_2O} are the linear attenuation coefficients of a particular tissue and of water, respectively. The CT number is a linear function of the attenuation coefficient $\mu_{\text{substance}}$. The window selected in Figure 6.1 displays the range of CT numbers from −111 to +139.

The widest CT window would correspond to one extending over the entire range of CT numbers (from −500 to +500). In this window the darkest shade of gray (black) is assigned to those regions having a CT number of -500, the value of air.

Actually, a rigorous application of Equation 6.1 shows that a CT number of -500 corresponds to a value for $\mu_{substance}$, or linear attenuation coefficient, of zero, that is, a total vacuum. For practical purposes the linear attenuation coefficient μ for air is so small compared to water and body tissues that it approximates the zero value of a vacuum.

Any part of the reconstructed image having a CT number of $+500$ or greater (e.g. metal), as in a prosthesis or dense bone, will be given the value $+500$ and will appear white (the lightest shade of gray). Therefore, white corresponds to CT numbers in the range from $+500$ to $+\infty$.

A block of CT numbers is assigned to each intermediate shade of gray. The range or size of the block of CT numbers in this shade of gray depends on the window width (the total range of CT numbers displayed) and the number of shades of gray available. The darker the shade of gray, the lower the values of the particular range of CT numbers depicted in that shade of gray.

The center of the total range of CT numbers depicted throughout the entire gray scale is the window level. It is the arithmetic average of the highest and lowest CT numbers depicted and is assigned the center shade of gray. In Figure 6.1 its value is $+14$. Since 16 shades of gray are illustrated in the scale in Figure 6.1, the window level of $+14$ is the lowest CT number in the range of CT values depicted in the upper center (i.e., ninth from the bottom or seventh from the top) gray shade.

Increasing the CT scale factor from 500 (EMI or old Hounsfield units) to 1,000 (new Hounsfield units) does not imply an extension of the range of x-ray attenuation values (linear attenuation coefficients) over which individual CT numbers are assigned. Rather, it implies that a smaller change in the x-ray attenuation is needed to change the CT number by 1. General Electric CT/T 8800 units are available with both 500- and 1,000-scale factors (the units with a 500-scale factor are generally units updated from a CT/T 7800 to a CT/T 8800 model). The same range of linear x-ray attenuation coefficients is covered in both scales, but this range uses twice as many numbers in the 1,000-scale factor compared to the 500-scale factor. An alternative way of understanding this difference is that an incrementation of the CT number by 1 in a system with a 1,000-scale factor corresponds to only half the change in the x-ray attenuation coefficient that must occur to increment the CT number by 1 in a 500-scale factor system.

In old Hounsfield units, air has a value of -500 and dense bone $+500$; in new Hounsfield units the corresponding values are $-1,000$ and $+1,000$. In both systems water has the value of zero.

Particularly in the early history of CT there was a great deal more variation and confusion in the value of a CT number. Different units might use not only different scale factors but also assign different values to the CT number of water. In the ACTA scanner the range of CT numbers extended from zero (air) to $+400$ (bone), with water having a value of 200.

Also adding to the confusion have been the different names assigned to each scale and the numbers in that scale. The 500-scale factor system and its CT units have been described as EMI, old Hounsfield, and old EMI. The 1,000-scale factor system and its corresponding CT units have been designated as Hounsfield, Delta (from its initial use in the Delta scanner), and new EMI. The ACTA scale and its CT units have usually been referred to simply by the term ACTA. Zatz (1981) has suggested the following convenient notation: ES for the EMI scale (scale factor of 500), HS for the New Hounsfield scale (scale factor of 1,000), and AS for the ACTA scale.

Fortunately, standardization has removed most of this confusion except for the differences in scale factors. Since the common scale factors are either 500 (EMI or old Hounsfield units) or 1,000 (new Hounsfield units), transposition between these two scales is accomplished by multiplying or dividing by 2. The illustrations shown in this chapter (and throughout most of this text) are seen to have a scale factor of 500, since this was the scale factor on the unit previously used by the author.

Window Settings

Window Level The effect of varying the window level for a fixed window width is illustrated in Figure 6.2. When the window level is low, all the bony structures are completely white, the medullary as well as the cortical bone. The soft tissues are shown in white or lighter shades of gray. Even fat appears portrayed in a lighter shade of gray. Only air or air-containing structures appear black or in darker shades of gray.

When the window level is raised, the nonfatty soft tissues and organs are displayed in the mid-gray range. Fat is seen in the darker gray range, and air and air-filled bowel lumen appear as black. The cortical bone appears white, medullary bone as a lighter gray.

Raising the window level further results in a dark appearing image. All soft tissues, fatty and nonfatty,

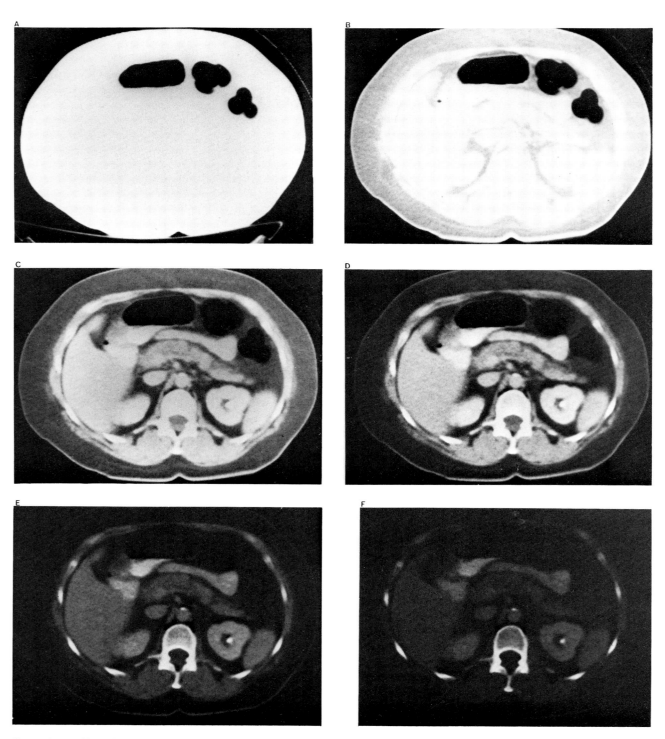

Figure 6.2. Effect of variations in the window level. With the window width held constant at 250, the image is displayed for window levels of (A) −200, (B) −100, (C) −50, (D) 0, (E) +50, and (F) +100.

130 Basic Principles of Computed Tomography

fall in the dark range of grays. Even the medullary bone appears in the mid-gray range. Only cortical bone appears lighter.

For lower window levels, aerated structures such as lung parenchyma are seen in better detail. Successively higher window levels optimize visualization of less dense soft tissues (e.g., fat) and water, denser soft tissues (e.g., liver), contrast-enhanced structures (e.g., enhanced renal parenchyma), and bone.

Window Width The change in the image display as the window width is varied is shown in Figure 6.3.

A narrow window with the window level centered at +20 results in a high contrast image. Fat appears black; both medullary and cortical bone are white. Small variations in density are readily perceived. Statistical variations in the x-ray attenuation and subtle artifacts may become more apparent.

A wider window leads to less contrast; a wider range of tissue densities is included within the gray scale. Fat is seen as a darker gray; some medullary and cortical bone differentiation is noted.

A very wide range yields a low contrast scale. There is minimal differentiation between soft tissues, even between fatty and nonfatty soft tissues. Smaller variations in x-ray attenuation may not be seen, or at least not be obvious with this type of display.

Narrowing the window width effectively increases the image contrast. The image tends to appear more black and white with less intervening gray. This is equivalent to a short-scale contrast in radiography. Increasing the window width effectively decreases the image contrast. There is less black and white and more intervening gray shades. This is equivalent to a long-scale contrast in radiography.

Optimization of Window Settings One of the most significant advantages of CT is the capability of altering the image display to optimize the features and details of particular organs or tissues. Theoretically, each organ or tissue might be visualized independently, with its own optimum CT window. Exactly what is optional, of course, will show some variation from one viewer to another. Practically, several organs and tissues (e.g., liver, kidneys, fat) may be satisfactorily viewed at the same window settings. Tissues that are widely disparate in their CT levels (bone, soft tissues, lung) need to be viewed separately at the appropriate window for each. Generally, bone needs a high window level (e.g., +150 to +300 in a 500 CT scale) and broad window width (e.g., 250–500). These parameters will vary with the particular bone and the degree of calcification. Soft tissues can usually be optimized with a window level of zero to +20 and a relatively narrow width of 150–250. Lung requires a low level (e.g., −200 to −300) and a greater width (e.g., 250–500).

This optimization of window settings is illustrated in Figures 6.4 through 6.6. Figure 6.4 shows how a metastatic lesion in the liver barely if at all perceptible at greater window widths becomes more and more readily apparent as the window width is narrowed, that is, as the image contrast is increased. Figure 6.5 shows that a window setting optimized for mediastinal detail fails entirely in demonstrating the lung parenchyma. In particular, a pulmonary nodule in this patient with testicular cancer can only be seen by adjusting the window settings for lung detail. Figure 6.6 shows the difference in detail between the brain and the skull at two different window settings in a head scan.

Multiple Windows Some CT units offer the option of multiple windows, typically either two or three separate windows. The center or level of each window and its width can be optimized for a specific tissue or group of tissues. In the abdomen, two windows might be used, one for the soft tissues and one for bone. In the chest, three windows could be used, one for lung, one for the mediastinum and superficial soft tissues, and one for bone. Each window would be assigned a certain number or fraction of the gray scale levels. The level and width can be varied for each window to optimize the display of the tissues lying within that window with the gray scale shades assigned to the window. The range or number of CT values assigned to a shade of gray is the same for each level of gray in a particular window; however, it is usually different for different windows.

For example, in the abdomen the gray levels in the darker half of the gray scale range would be assigned to the soft tissues, and the remaining, lighter half of the gray scale would have its gray levels assigned to the bone. The level for the soft tissue window might be centered at 0 to +20 (for a CT scale factor of 500); the level of the bone window might be centered somewhere from +150 to +350. The width of the soft tissue window might be about 50–100, and the width for the bone window 200–400. If there were 16 gray levels, the eight darker shades would be assigned to the soft tissues and the eight lighter shades to the bones.

In a chest image with three windows, the darkest gray shades would be assigned to the lung, the middle gray shades to the soft tissues other than lung, and the light gray shades to the bones. Each window level and width could be adjusted for optimal display of the tissues within that window.

The advantage of multiple window displays is that tissues with greatly different ranges of CT num-

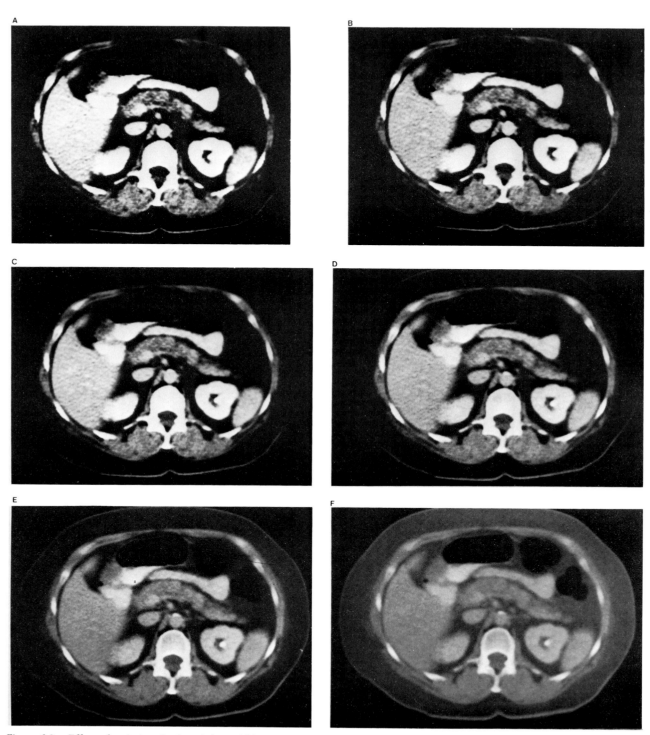

Figure 6.3. Effect of variations in the window width. With the window level held constant at +20, the image is displayed for window widths of (A) 50, (B) 75, (C) 100, (D) 150, (E) 250, and (F) 500.

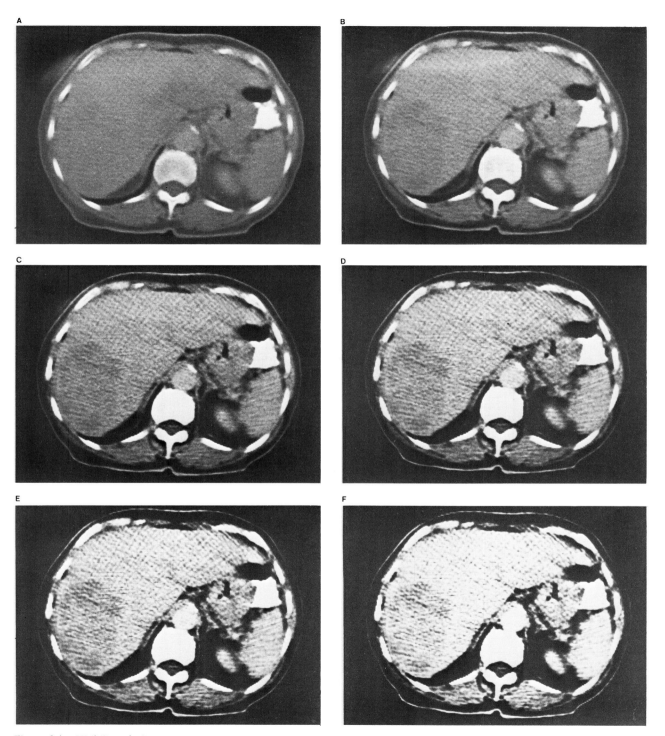

Figure 6.4. Visibility of a liver metastasis with variation in the window width. With the window level held constant at +025 the window width is progressively narrowed: (A) 500, (B) 250, (C) 150, (D) 100, (E) 75, (F) 50. The lesion, which can barely be seen at a window width of 500, becomes more perceptible as the window is narrowed.

Extended CT Number Scale It is useful to have the capability of extending the CT scale for certain examinations, usually those involving bony structures. The lower end of the normal scale corresponds to the CT number of air, this being equal to −500 in EMI or old Hounsfield units and −1,000 in new Hounsfield units (HU). However, the range of potential bone densities is very wide, with significant portions of bony structures having CT values considerably in excess of +500 EMI units (+1,000 HU). Thus it would be useful to be able to retain the information acquired from scanning and reconstruction to permit display of an extended CT range to

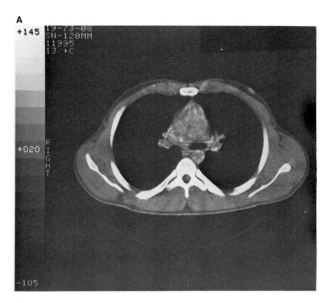

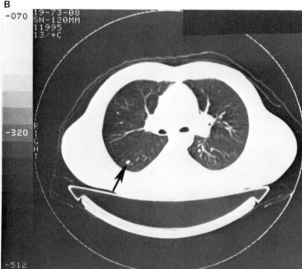

Figure 6.5. Chest images should be examined at window settings optimized for mediastinal/soft tissue detail (*A*) and for pulmonary detail (*B*). The pulmonary nodule (arrow) in this patient with testicular cancer is only seen with lung detail settings.

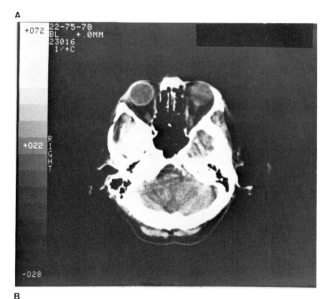

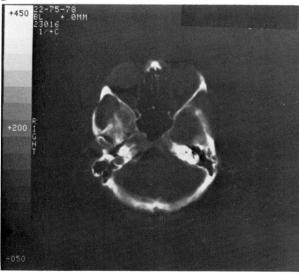

Figure 6.6. *A*, Detail of the brain and eyes is optimized with a window level of +022 and a width of 100; *B*, Bone detail is optimized with a window level of +200 and a width of 500.

bers can be simultaneously displayed on one image. One disadvantage is that the number of gray levels assigned to each window for different tissues is only a fraction of the total number of levels available. Alternatively, individual images, each optimized to a tissue with a particular range of CT numbers, can be displayed. This permits the full gray scale range to be used for each set of tissues, so that small or subtle variations in the distribution of CT numbers are more apparent. Another disadvantage of multiple windows is the time involved in estimating and assigning optimal levels and widths for each window.

include values greater than +500 EMI units (+1,000 HU). In the extended scale, pixels whose CT values are greater than +500 EMI units but less than the new upper limit of the extended scale will be assigned their measured CT value, not the value +500 as before. Pixels with measured CT values greater than the new upper limit of the extended scale will be assigned the value of this upper limit.

As an example, in the General Electric CT/T system the following extended CT scale may be displayed:

	Normal Scale	Extended Scale
EMI units	−500 to +500	−500 to +1,500
New HU	−1,000 to +1,000	−1,000 to +3,000

Actually, the ranges are slightly wider than the above at the lower and upper ends of both the normal and extended scales. This is a consequence of the binary nature of the memory in the display memory (Ramtek). Thus, rather than −500 EMI units (−1,000

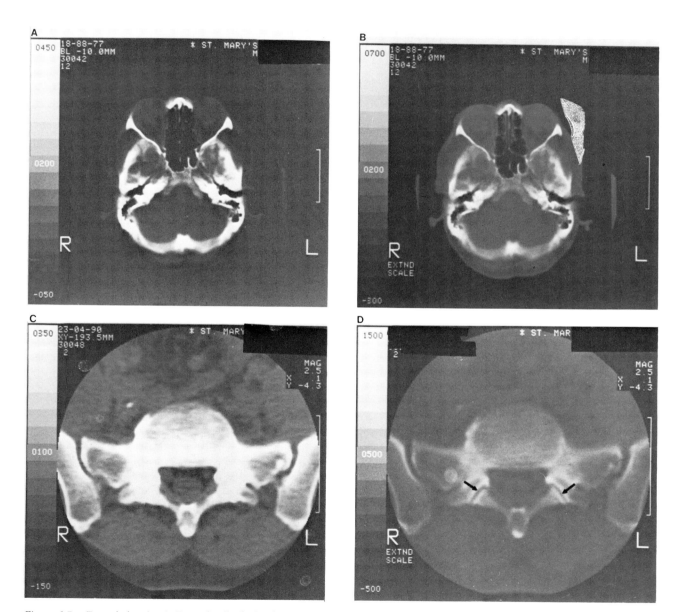

Figure 6.7. Extended scale. A, Bone detail of a head scan is shown on the conventional scale with a window level of +200 and a width of 500. The effect of the extended scale is shown in B, where the level is kept at +200 but the width is increased to 1,000. C, A scan of the sacrum is displayed on a nonextended scale with a level of +100 and a width of 500. D, the window width is extended to 2,000 (−500 to +1,500) at a level of +500. There is virtually no soft tissue detail in D, but note the better definition of the posteriorly located apophyseal joints (arrows).

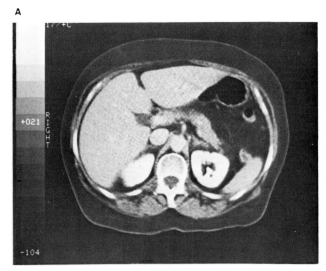

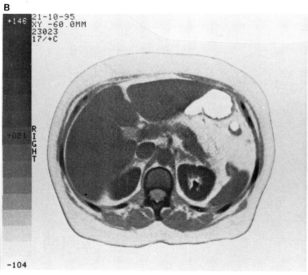

Figure 6.8. An abdominal scan displayed in negative (A) and positive (B) image polarity.

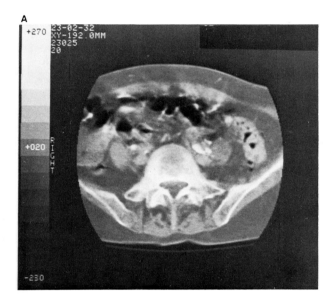

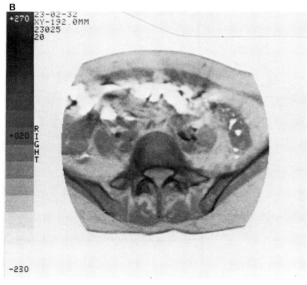

Figure 6.9. A scan through the lower spine displayed in negative (A) and positive (B) image polarity.

shades of gray on a black background. Denser structures are assigned lighter shades; less dense structures are portrayed in darker shades. Bone is displayed in white or lighter shades of gray; air and fat are in black and darker shades of gray. This provides a sense of continuity with more conventional radiological studies. It also engenders a feeling of familiarity in the individual who is a novice in CT or who does not routinely view CT images. The ease in changing the polarity, or mode, of the image in CT does not exist in conventional radiography. A polarity change can also be done easily in ultrasound. However, ultrasound images simply do not look like CT images (or HU), the lower limit in the normal scale is $-512 = -2^9$ (or $-1{,}024 = -2^{10}$) in order to accommodate all the available binary numbers. The upper end is similarly affected.

Extending the CT scale permits centering the CT display window at higher levels and increaasing the width of the window. Some examples of this are shown in Figure 6.7.

With an extended CT number scale a much wider range of tissue densities can be displayed.

Image Reversals

Image Polarity Conventionally, CT images have been displayed in a negative mode, the same polarity as radiographs, with the image displayed in conventional radiographs or scintigrams), and polarity reversals will not alter this dissimilarity. Scintigrams (the images from nuclear medicine obtained by counting radioactive emissions with a gamma camera) are also displayed in negative and positive modes. Generally, negative image scintigrams are printed on Polaroid film, and positive image scintigrams on transilluminated film.

A positive image mode display may be useful in CT examination devoted primarily to osseous structures. In the positive mode the bone appears dark; cortical bone often appears black and medullary bone in darker shades of gray. Many workers feel that the positive polarity increases the visual perceptivity of a bone lesion, and perhaps is also more aesthetically pleasing to view.

Examples of the reversal of image polarity are shown in Figure 6.8 for the abdomen and Figure 6.9 for the sacrum.

Although images will be routinely viewed and photographed in the negative mode, it is useful to have the capability of also viewing and photographing in the positive mode. Since the positive mode would routinely only be used in a limited number of studies, or in only a part of a single examination, it is important that the polarity change for viewing and photography be made with a minimal difficulty in adjustment. It is desirable to have a single polarity switch to reverse the image mode in the viewing monitor and another switch to reverse the polarity of the hard copy image. For convenience, there should be minimal or no changes in camera adjustments for hard copy photography after making a polarity reversal.

Image Position A CT image may be displayed as though the viewer were standing at the patient's head looking toward the patient's feet (Figure 6.10), or alternatively as though the viewer were standing at the patient's feet looking toward the patient's head (Figure 6.11). In the former case, organs or other structures on the patient's right side (e.g., liver) will be displayed to the viewer's right, and those organs and other structures at the patient's left side (e.g., the heart) will be shown on the viewer's left (Figure 6.12). This was the initial convention used in the early EMI head scanner (Mark I). In the alternative format, organs or other structures on the patient's right side will be displayed to the viewer's left, and

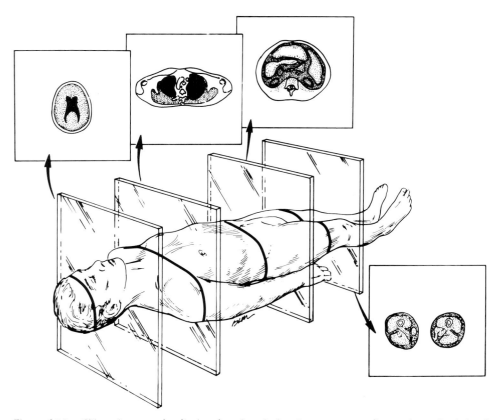

Figure 6.10. CT sections may be displayed as though the viewer were standing at the patient's head. The aortic arch and heart will be on the viewer's left, the liver on the viewer's right.

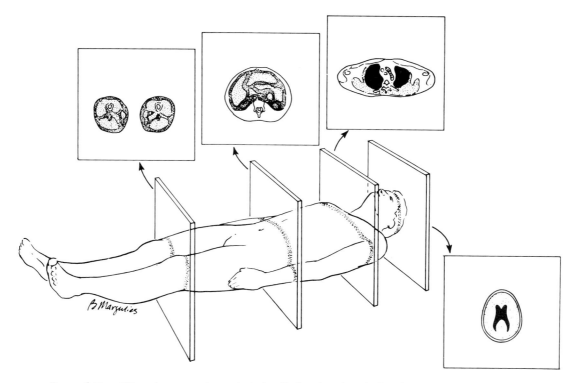

Figure 6.11. CT sections may alternatively be displayed as though the viewer were standing at the patient's feet. The aortic arch and heart will be on the viewer's right, the liver on the viewer's left. This is the standard convention.

those at the patient's left to the viewer's right (Figure 6.13). This format soon gained ascendancy in the torso and now has become the recognized convention for head and torso. This preference is due to the fact that the established convention in viewing and displaying radiographs is to consider the viewer, or reader, as facing the patient. Thus, in conventional radiology the radiographs are mounted on viewing boxes so that the patient's right is to the viewer's left. This convention has now been extended to CT and also to ultrasound.

A CT unit may incorporate a switch or set up

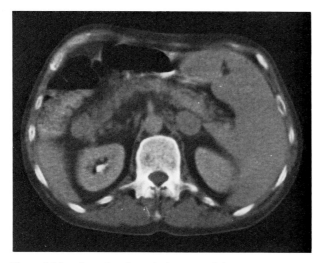

Figure 6.12. A section through the upper abdomen with the liver displayed on the viewer's right.

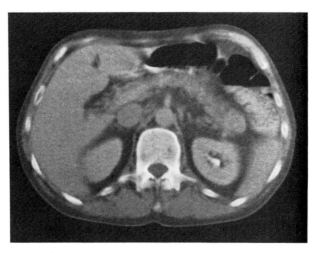

Figure 6.13. The same section through the upper abdomen shown in Figure 6.12, now displayed with the liver to the viewer's left.

instructions that may be typed in to reverse the side of left or right on the display monitor. In regions where there is anatomical symmetry, such as the head, it is not obvious which is the right and which is the left side. It is important to know the convention used and to label the patient's right and left sides appropriately.

Magnification

Magnification permits the viewer to enlarge part or all of the image on the monitor. This may be useful to enable the viewer to examine the image or a portion of the image more easily. For example, an image of a patient with a smaller torso who was scanned on a relatively larger (e.g., 42 cm) field of view may occupy significantly less than the total image space available. Magnification permits more of the image space on the monitor (and hard copy) to contain useful information. Magnification of the processed image, however, does not generally increase resolution; it merely makes the image larger by blowing up or magnifying the individual pixels comprising the image. An example is shown in Figure 6.14.

Scanning and reconstructing a smaller torso or body part on a smaller field of view (e.g., 35 or 25 cm) will allow the image to occupy more of the available image space on the monitor. Furthermore, this technique will also generally increase resolution, since it is not simply a process of magnifying a processed or finished scan image. However, it is fre-

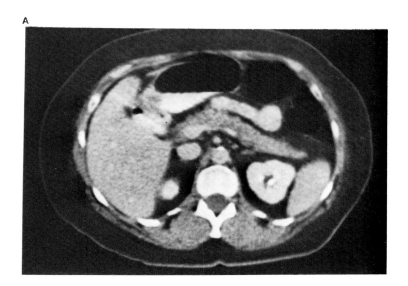
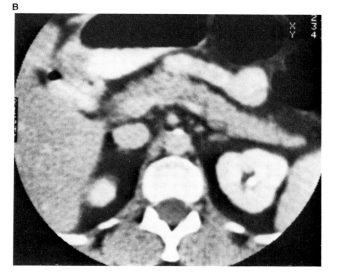
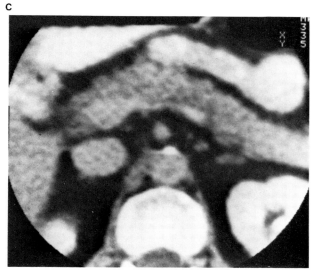

Figure 6.14. The scan through the upper abdomen in A is shown in B at 2× and in C at 3× magnification.

quently necessary to use a somewhat larger field of view for image reconstruction to be certain that all of the torso or area of interest is included in the reconstructed image.

Also, because in scanning a limb it may be difficult or impossible to center the limb in the gantry (especially a thigh or upper arm), a larger field of view may be necessary. This is not necessarily a disadvantage, since scanning both limbs permits a side-by-side comparison at the same levels. However, each limb may only occupy a relatively small part of the reconstructed area, and magnification of the post-processed image may make it easier to view the image. There is, of course, a large subjective factor in the value of magnification to a viewer.

Magnification is usually a keyboard control on the viewer's display console. One method for magnification involves calling up a cursor by typing in a command or depressing the appropriate key for the cursor. The cursor may then be centered in the region to be magnified with a trackball, joystick, or light pen. After typing in the magnification factor, the magnified image will be displayed on the monitor. An alternative method might involve typing in the coordinates of the center of the region to be magnified and the magnification factor. The coordinates might be located by superimposition of a coordinate grid or with a cursor whose coordinate position can be determined. Finally, a rectangle may be called up by a keyboard control. The magnification factor can be varied and may be sufficiently large to demonstrate the fundamental pixel structure (Figure 6.15).

Multi-Image Display

Multiple images or portions of multiple images can be displayed simultaneously on the console monitor. Variable formats are available. Figure 6.16 demonstrates simultaneous display of two, three, four, five, six, and nine different scans. Thus, a group of scans from a study may be simultaneously viewed on the monitor. This may be helpful in evaluating the anatomical relationships of normal and abnormal structures (Figure 6.17). This format also permits simultaneous viewing on the monitor of the same section scanned under two different circumstances, for example, before and after intravenous contrast enhancement (Figure 6.18). The same scan can also be viewed at different window settings with the two im-

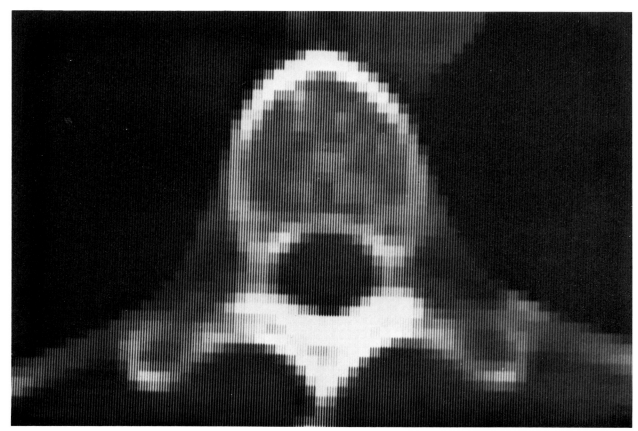

Figure 6.15. With sufficient magnification the pixel structure of the image may become more evident.

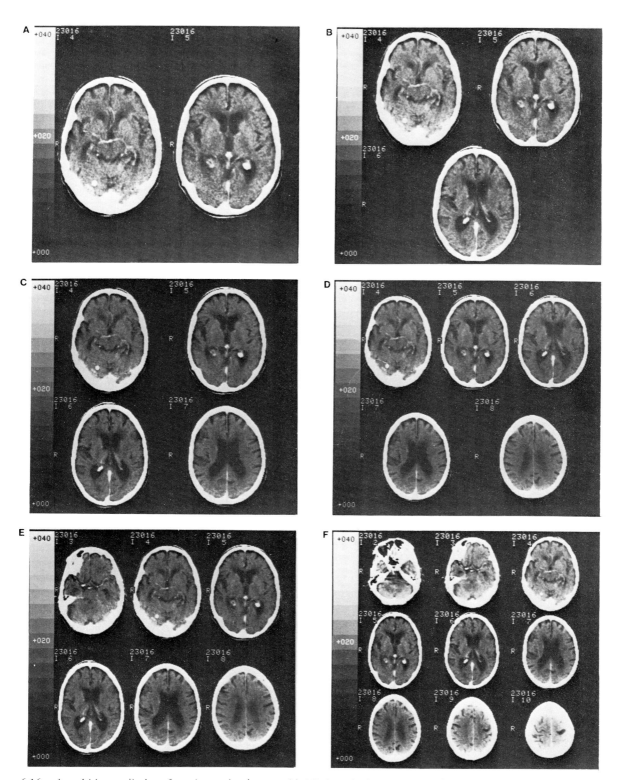

Figure 6.16. A multi-image display of contiguous head scans with (A) 2-on-1, (B) 3-on-1, (C) 4-on-1, (D) 5-on-1, (E) 6-on-1, and (F) 9-on-1 formats.

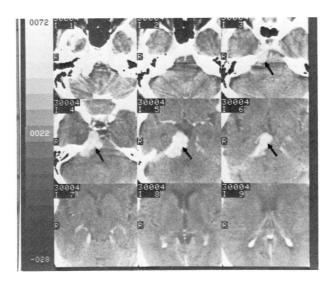

Figure 6.17. Contiguous head scans demonstrating a petrous ridge meningioma (arrows) on a 9-on-1 multi-image display format with magnification.

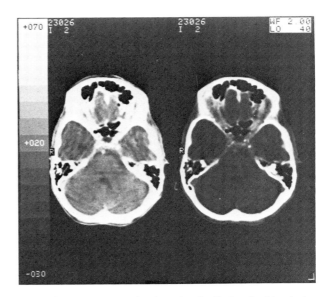

Figure 6.19. The same head section is displayed with window settings adjusted for brain detail and for bone detail on a 2-on-1 multi-image display formats.

ages side by side (Figure 6.19) on the monitor. This display format has shown some popularity for the display of consecutive sections scanned immediately one after the other using the technique of dynamic computed tomography (described in Chapter 9).

The multiple image format might have some economic value in reducing the number of pieces of film required for hard copy of a study, but at the expense of reduction of the image. This might be most useful when, for example, there are only spaces for 12 images on a film sheet and the study consists of 13 or 14 images (including perhaps a patient information picture). Then two of the images might be displayed together to save the expense of an additional sheet of film for a single image.

Color Display

An alternative to the conventional black-and-white television is the use of a color display. A color display was available with the first whole body scanner, the ACTA scanner. The actual color scale used is arbitrary. Advantages for a color display might include the capability of accentuating small changes in CT numbers in or about a particular tissue. Also, the CT values of widely separated structures might be compared more readily with a color display rather than with shades of gray. However, alternative methods of evaluating and comparing CT numbers are readily available, for example, the flashing technique described later in this chapter, in which a band of CT numbers is flashed on the monitor.

By and large, color displays have not been accepted in CT. The value of a color display is rather doubtful, and there does not appear to be any strong scientific or clinical evidence demonstrating its importance. Many viewers find the multiplicity of colors annoying and hard to read, particularly since they are used to looking at images in a gray scale. Small changes or differences in CT values may be overly accentuated. Also, the cost of color film is higher than that of black-and-white film.

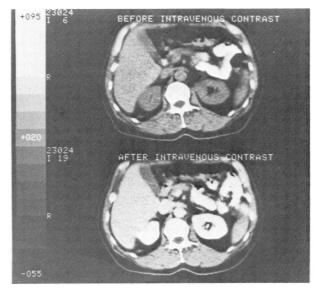

Figure 6.18. A 2-on-1 multi-image display format showing the same abdominal slice before and after intravenous contrast enhancement.

COMPUTER GRAPHICS AND MEASUREMENTS

Computer Graphics

Computer graphics is a technique for labeling or annotating images with alphanumeric symbols and for drawing lines, tracing outlines, and superimposing grids.

Cursor A cursor is an identifiable marker in the form of, for example, crosshairs, a dot, a dash, a rectangle, or a circle, which may be moved over the surface of a CRT by a joystick, trackball, or light pen. It can be used to alter, delete, or select instructions to the computer, to trace out areas, or to measure distances. A cursor thus permits communication of spatial information between an operator (or viewer) and the computer. A cursor may also be used to indicate the location on an alphanumeric of the position of the next character to be typed. A cursor may also serve simply to identify a particular structure. It may indicate the center of a region to be magnified, and if it is in the form of a box its dimensions may be enlarged to the area that is to be magnified.

Illustrations of cursors are shown in Figures 6.20 and 6.21.

Interactive Devices

Keyboard The keyboard on both operator and viewer display consoles is similar in layout to a typewriter keyboard except that only capital letters are customarily used. A return key permits transfer of data, instructions, or replies from the keyboard operator to the computer. The keyboard may also be used to annotate images.

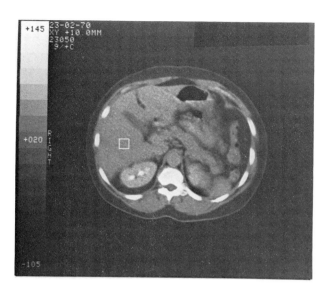

Figure 6.21. A rectangle or box cursor is positioned in the liver.

Joystick This is a stick on the operator or viewer display console which is freely moveable about a pivot, allowing the operator to move a cursor over a CRT. The cursor moves in the direction of displacement of the joystick away from its center or resting position. The rate of cursor movement may be either a constant velocity or a function of the amount of displacement of the joystick. The joystick may then be described as a directional (velocity) device. In a second mode of joystick operation, a slight displacement or bumping of the joystick permits the cursor to be moved just one element in the direction of joystick displacement. No further cursor movement will occur until the joystick is released and then either bumped again or displaced further. This second mode allows small incremental movements of the cursor for accurate positioning.

Trackball A trackball is a freely rotatable ball whose center is fixed in position on the operator or viewer display console. A trackball permits the operator to move a cursor. Trackballs are more expensive than joysticks.

Light Pen A light pen is applied directly to the face of the CRT by the operator. The pen may be used for moving the cursor on the image screen and for selecting or deleting instructions on another CRT.

Line A cursor may be used to identify two points on the image. The initial cursor position may be frozen or deposited in computer memory and the cursor moved to a new position and again deposited in the computer memory. A straight line can then be generated between these two points. An alternative

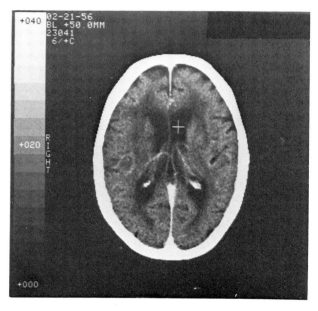

Figure 6.20. A crosshairs cursor is positioned in the anterior horn of the left lateral ventricle.

approach would be to have two different cursors that could be independently positioned. A line may be drawn from an organ or structure to a point on the screen outside the image where a label can be annotated. The distance or length of the line can also be measured.

Trace A cursor may be called up to trace a closed outline of arbitrary size and contour over the image. A trace is illustrated in Figure 6.22. The trace may be helpful in delineating a particular organ, structure, or other region which may be of interest, for example, the borders of a mass. It may also be used to enclose an area about which certain parameters of interest, such as the area or the average CT number, are to be determined.

Annotation Annotation refers to the labeling or annotation of information in the form of alphanumeric characters (letters, numbers, and symbols) on the CT image. Most units routinely include some standard annotation including information on the patient's name, the date, the sequence number, and the anatomical position of the scan. Some of this information is usually supplied by the operator or technologist prior to the scan sequence by typing it on the operator or control console keyboard. After initial positioning and identification of an anatomical landmark, the computer is able to update the information on the scan number and anatomical position. The positions for these standard annotations are fixed on the image. The CT numbers for the window settings are usually superimposed on the corresponding gray scale or gray bar. These numbers are updated as the viewer changes the window level and width at the console. The user may also have the option of deleting some of the routine annotation, or of adding information regarding the scan such as the kilovoltage or milliamperage.

Additional annotation may be added to the image at the discretion of the user. Normally this can be done at the viewer console by keying in the appropriate instructions for annotation, selecting the position on the image for annotation (usually with a cursor), and then typing the appropriate alphanumeric characters on the keyboard. This is illustrated in Figure 6.23. It may also be possible to store the annotated image on magnetic disk or tape for future reference.

Grid A grid may be superimposed on the image display by means of a single grid function key or by typing in an appropriate command on the keyboard. The distance between grid lines is generally fixed (8 cm on the General Electric CT/T 8800). This permits measurements of distances to be approximated. Additional 1-cm coordinate markers may be annotated along the main or central horizontal (X) and vertical (Y) axes as well. Figures 6.24 and 6.25 illustrate grids superimposed over head and body scans.

Measurements

CT Numbers There are several methods for measuring CT numbers. The measurements can be performed either throughout the entire image or in a localized area.

Blinker Function All the elements or pixels with CT values lying within a range or band of CT

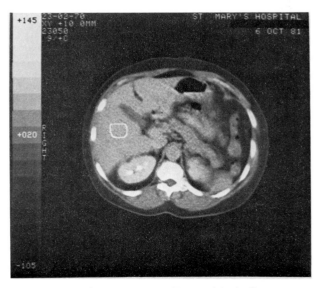

Figure 6.22. A trace is illustrated in the liver.

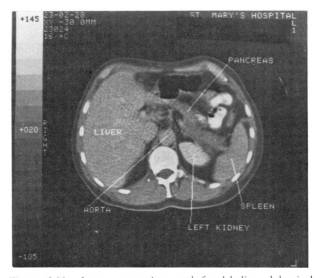

Figure 6.23. Image annotation used for labeling abdominal organs.

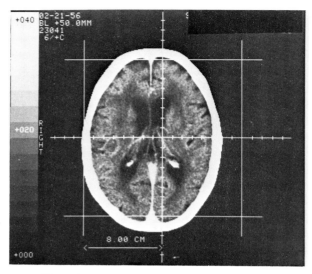

Figure 6.24. Grid superimposed on a head scan.

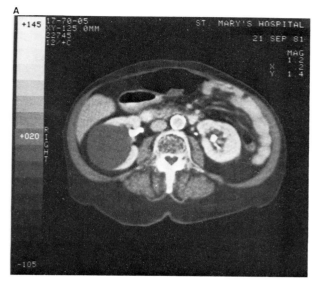

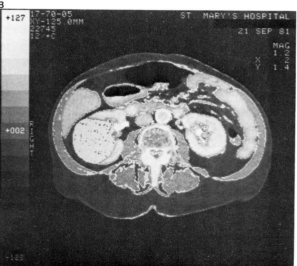

Figure 6.26. A, A right renal cyst is shown. B, The blinker function or identify control is used to flash the CT number of the cyst, seen to be equal to +002 EMI or old Hounsfield units.

numbers may be made to flash or blink at a set rate (Figure 6.26). This permits identification of the CT number of a particular normal organ or structure or an abnormal mass. Since the blinker identifies the range of CT numbers throughout the image, the CT values of widely separated areas can be compared. In the General Electric CT/T, the center of the range of blinking CT numbers is the current window level.

Measure Function This function can collapse the window width to a CT range as small as one. Thus, all pixels whose values are below the window level appear black, those at the window level are middle gray, and those above the window level are white. By changing the window level setting, the CT values of all organs and structures in the image can be measured. Similar to the blinker function, a measure function allows simultaneous examination of the entire image.

Cursor Box A cursor box or rectangle is positioned over the area whose CT value is to be measured, and the rectangle is expanded to an appropriate size. The average CT number within this area can then be established. Often the standard deviation of the average CT value for the pixels enclosed within the rectangle is also given. The CT value and standard deviation may be automatically annotated on the image (Figure 6.27). Unlike the blinker or measure

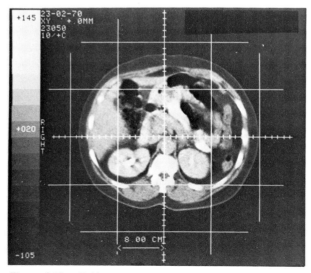

Figure 6.25. Grid superimposed on a scan of the abdomen.

The Image Display 145

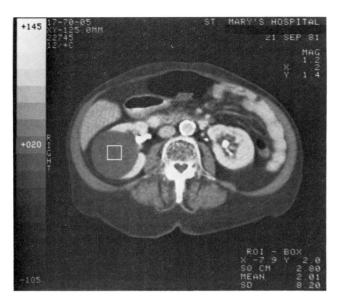

Figure 6.27. A cursor box is positioned in the right renal cyst. The notation in the lower righthand corner identifies the coordinates of the center of the box ($X = -7.9$, $Y = 2.0$), the area included in the box (2.80 cm^2), the mean CT number (2.01 EMI units), and the standard deviation associated with the CT number measurement (8.20 EMI units).

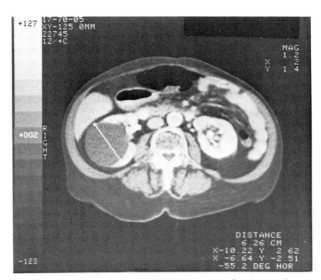

Figure 6.29. Measurement of the diameter of right renal cyst. Annotation in the lower right corner indicates the length of the line displayed (6.26 cm), the X and Y coordinates of the cursors positioned at the ends of the line, and the angulation of the line with respect to the horizontal axis.

functions, only the area within the rectangle is examined with the cursor box.

Tracer A cursor is used to trace or outline an area on the image. The average CT value for the pixels within this area can then be determined, as well as the standard deviation, and both may be automatically annotated on the image (Figure 6.28).

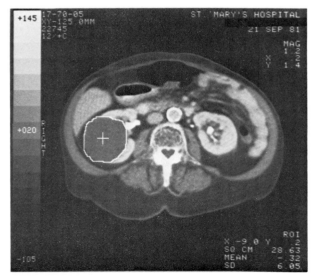

Figure 6.28. A trace approximates the borders of the right renal cyst. A crosshairs cursor is positioned in the area enclosed by the trace. The notation in the lower righthand corner identifies the coordinates of the cursor ($X = -9.0$, $Y = .2$), the area enclosed by the trace (28.63 cm^2), the mean CT number within the trace ($-.32$ EMI units), and the standard deviation associated with the CT number measurement (6.05 EMI units). The slightly negative CT value for the cyst is related to inclusion of some peripheral pixels containing fat.

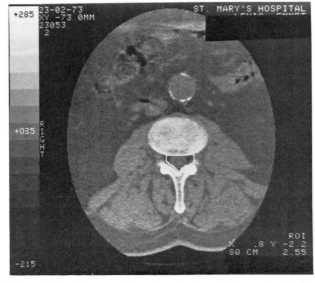

Figure 6.30. A trace outlines the spinal canal. Annotation in the lower right corner indicates the X and Y coordinates of the center of the trace and the area in square centimeters (2.55).

Spatial Measurements

Distance Measurement of distance entails drawing a line, as previously described, by identifying two points with a cursor or pair of cursors. A line can then be drawn between them and the length of the line, the distance between the two points, is measured. The distance is usually automatically annotated on the image (Figure 6.29).

Area An area is outlined by means of a trace function. The dimensions in square centimeters can be determined and are usually annotated on the image (Figure 6.30).

CONTRAST ENHANCEMENT

Although the use of contrast is a clinical decision, its significance for image display and information is considerable and appropriate to illustrate here. There are several types and methods of contrast enhancement.

Oral Contrast

Oral contrast is given primarily to opacify and identify bowel. Its importance can never be sufficiently stressed, since unopacified bowel can be one of the most confusing structures seen in the abdomen, as it can simulate abnormal masses, enlarged lymph nodes, or abscesses. Many bowel loops contain air, a natural negative contrast (less dense than the surrounding tissue) that is often sufficient to permit identification of bowel loops. However, many bowel loops contain only very small amounts of air or none at all. Not infrequently, a small amount of air in the bowel may be difficult to discriminate from air in an abscess. Particularly in patients with little intra-abdominal fat, the use of a positive contrast (denser than the surrounding tissue) enhances the diagnostic value of the image. This is shown in Figure 6.31.

Diluted water-soluble iodinated contrast agents have been frequently used, for example, Gastrografin (diatrizoate meglumine and diatrizoate sodium) diluted to several percent with water and a flavoring agent. More recently, less dense barium agents such as E-Z-CAT (E-Z-EM Company) have become available. Dense barium causes artifacts in the CT images and should not be used. Barium studies should be avoided prior to CT examinations of the abdomen or pelvis; otherwise a cleansing enema may be necessary.

Intravenous Contrast

Intravenous contrast may be administered as a bolus using an agent such as Renografin-60 (60% diatrizoate meglumine), as a longer infusion using an agent such as Reno-M-Drip (30% diatrizoate meglumine),

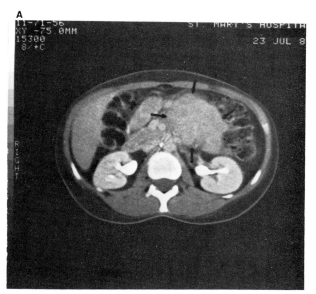

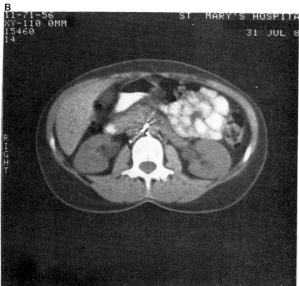

Figure 6.31. *A*, In the initial examination of this patient with lymphoma it was not certain whether the mass identified (arrows) represented poorly opacified bowel or lymphadenopathy. *B*, The examination was repeated a week later, at which time better bowel opacification permitted identification of the mass as bowel.

or as a combination of infusion and bolus. Intravenous contrast permits enhancement of the entire extracellular fluid compartment, both the intravascular and the extravascular or interstitial components. Enhancement of the intravascular component is more immediate.

Intravenous contrast enhancement permits identification of vascular structures, evaluation of the urinary tract, and frequently better contrast and spatial delineation of normal and abnormal structures.

A scan performed at the same level in the same patient prior to and following intravenous contrast is illustrated in Figure 6.18. The identification of cerebral blood vessels with intravenous contrast is demonstrated in Figure 6.32.

Intrathecal Contrast

Both positive (metrizamide) and negative (air) contrast may be introduced into the intrathecal space. Metrizamide CT examinations have been useful in evaluating the spine for disk disease or tumor and in studying the brain by better delineation of the cisterns and ventricles (Figure 6.33). Air contrast studies may be useful in studying the internal auditory canals or the sella turcica (Figure 6.34).

Biliary Contrast

A CT examination following intravenous or percutaneous cholangiography may permit more detail and information than the plain films. This may be especially true in intravenous cholangiography, where the positive contrast density is frequently very low. When there is only faint opacification of the biliary ducts, the capability of CT for detecting small differences in contrast may permit better identification of the ducts as well as surrounding soft tissues such as the pancreas. It is often possible to detect a stone in a duct (Figure 6.35).

Other Contrast Studies

CT following sialography, typically with ethiodol, may permit a detailed examination of the duct itself

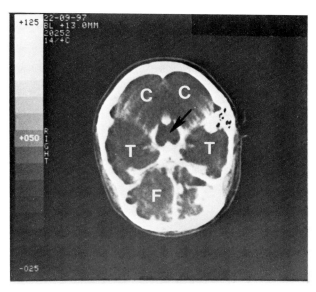

Figure 6.33. Metrizamide is seen in the cerebrospinal fluid, including the basal cisterns. The patient is prone. The cerebellar hemispheres (*C*), temporal lobes (*T*), and a frontal lobe (*F*) are identified.

and its relationship to surrounding structures (Figure 6.36). This may be useful to determine the extension of a tumor.

Positive contrast such as Cystografin (30% diatrizoate meglumine) diluted to a few percent and/or air may be introduced into the bladder in a retrograde fashion for examination of the bladder (Figure 6.37).

CT may also be used in conjunction with a sin-

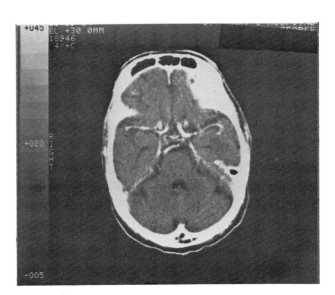

Figure 6.32. Following intravenous contrast the cerebral vessels at the level of the circle of Willis are well demonstrated.

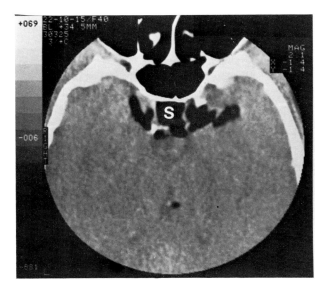

Figure 6.34. A large sella (*S*) is seen to fill with air (injected by means of a spinal tap), indicating an empty sella as opposed to a pituitary tumor. The scan plane is approximately coronal.

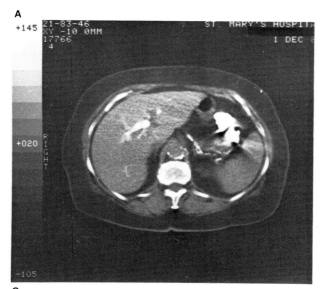
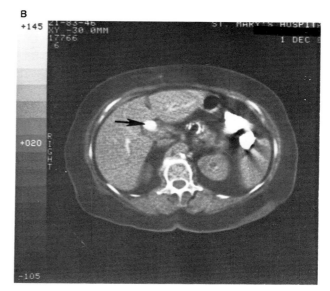
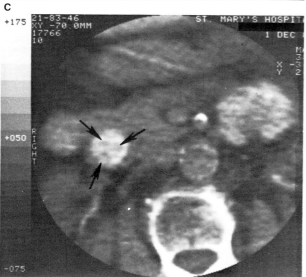

Figure 6.35. CT examination following intravenous cholangiography. *A*, The most cephalad scan shows dilatation of the opacified ducts. *B*, A scan caudal to *A* shows opacification of the dilated common duct (arrow). *C*, At the level of the pancreatic head this magnified scan demonstrates a stone (arrows) in the distal portion of the dilated common bile duct.

ogram (opacification of a fistulous tract draining to the skin).

FILTERING

The digital basis of CT permits computer manipulation of both the raw data accumulated during the scanning process and the final or postprocessed image. The manipulation can be performed immediately during the study or at an arbitrary later time by retrieving the appropriate data, either the raw data or the processed CT numbers, from storage on magnetic disk or tape. The algorithm used in virtually all CT units is filtered back projection, described in Chapter 5. A filter or convolution function is an essential component of this process. Different filter functions may be used to permit selective removal or enhancement of information of different spatial frequencies.

Smoothing

Smoothing is a technique for selectively removing the higher spatial frequencies in an image. Recall from Chapter 5 that any variation of a function or quantity (e.g., the linear attenuation coefficient or CT number) in space (e.g., over the spatial range or area of the image) may be expressed as a sum of sine and cosine waves, each of different frequencies, with appropriate amplitudes assigned to each frequency component. The higher spatial frequency components are necessary to demonstrate abrupt edges or sharp changes in the image. Removal of these higher spatial frequencies results in a loss of edge detail; the images appear smoother or blurred. The smoothed image therefore has decreased spatial resolution.

The smoothing reduces not only the fine spatial detail but also the graininess in the image. This image

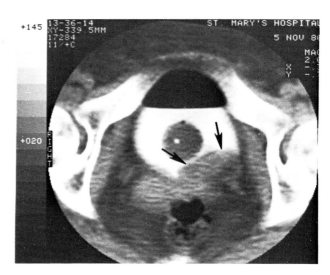

Figure 6.37. A bladder tumor (arrows) protrudes into the bladder lumen and invades the surrounding tissue. Both dilute positive contrast and air have been introduced into the bladder through a catheter. Intravenous contrast frequently causes the bladder lumen to be too dense. The water-filled balloon surrounding the opacified catheter lumen can be seen in the bladder.

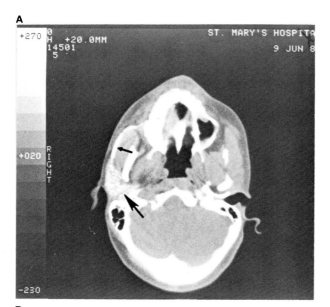

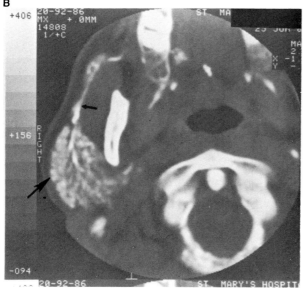

Figure 6.36. Unmagnified (A) and magnified (B) scans from two different patients on whom CT was performed following sialography. The parotid gland (large arrow) and duct (small arrow) are identified.

grain is present because of the finite number of x-ray photons (due, for example, to the limited dose) used to form the image, and it limits the accuracy with which the CT value of each pixel can be calculated. The picture grain therefore represents the random variation in the amplitude or CT value of the pixel elements.

Smoothing may be regarded as a method of filtering image noise (random or statistical variations in the CT values, as seen in picture grain) to improve the so-called signal-to-noise ratio (the ratio of the information amplitude to the noise amplitude). Smoothing may increase the ease in perceiving relatively large, low contrast structures that might otherwise be masked by image noise. The technique may be especially helpful in very noisy images.

Although smoothing has been utilized in scintigraphy, it appears to be more effective in reducing image noise in CT.

Smoothing of the CT image is accomplished by appropriate changes or modifications in the reconstruction algorithm. A smoothing function is incorporated as the filter function. The two possible technical approaches for smoothing of CT images involve either smoothing the final reconstructed image pixel by pixel, or smoothing the raw data (the digitized signal representing the intensity of x-rays entering the detectors) during the reconstruction by an appropriate mathematical filter.

Edge Enhancement

Edge enhancement is a technique for selectively enhancing the higher spatial frequencies of an image. This increases the sharpness of edges and boundaries; that is, abrupt changes in x-ray attenuation or CT numbers are portrayed more accurately. Inclusion of higher spatial frequency allows better spatial detail. This is done by using an appropriate edge enhancement function as the filter function in the reconstruction algorithm. Edge enhancement is the reverse of smoothing.

Edge enhancement accentuates the sharp differences between areas of high contrast such as between bone and soft tissue. Because of the restoration or enhancement of higher spatial frequencies, the high frequency noise is increased and the picture grain becomes more obvious; that is, the amplitude of the picture grain is increased. This increased high frequency noise and picture grain may obscure low contrast details. This may result in decreasing the perception of low contrast lesions (for example, a low contrast metastasis in the liver).

HARD COPY

The term "hard copy" refers to printed photographic images in contrast to the images viewed on a CRT monitor. The components of a hard copy system are a camera adapted for photographing images from a CRT monitor, and the film itself. In CT there are two common types of hard copy and photography systems: Polaroid positive print film and Polaroid camera mounted on the monitor of a CT display console, and transilluminated (radiographic) film and a multiformat camera system.

Positive Print Film (Polaroid)

Hard copy photography with Polaroid is a one-step process. Polaroid film is a direct positive print film. A print film is a nontransparent film viewed by reflected as opposed to transmitted light. A positive film is one in which the picture is a positive image of the original being photographed; that is, the image corresponds in light and dark tones (or light and dark gray shades) to the original. In a negative image the tones of the original are reversed, dark tones or gray shades becoming light and light tones or gray shades becoming dark. Polaroid film photography results in a direct positive print of the original (in CT, a monitor image) without having to go through the intermediate stage of obtaining a negative and then making positive prints from the negative.

The processing of Polaroid film begins immediately and automatically as the film is withdrawn from the camera. The only parameter that is controlled by the user is the time of development, and even this is not critical. The time of processing is typically 30 s or less. The most commonly used film size is 8.3 × 10.8 cm (3½ × 4¼ inches).

The Polaroid film pack is loaded into the back of the camera, which is mounted onto a CRT monitor on which the CT image is displayed. The film pack is kept at a fixed distance from the CRT monitor. The hard copy image is optimized by appropriate adjustments of the brightness and contrast of the CRT monitor as well as the lens aperture and shutter speed of the camera.

There are several advantages to direct positive print photography of the monitor. The photographic process is extremely rapid; an image can be viewed within 30 s after an exposure. The cost of the camera is a great deal less than the more complex multiformat type of cameras used with transilluminated radiographic films. Unlike transilluminated films obtained with multiformat cameras, or positive reflected prints obtained from an intermediate negative, darkroom facilities are not required. This also eliminates transportation of film cassettes to and from a darkroom, a time-consuming process in a busy CT suite. Errors in camera or monitor settings can be quickly identified. Polaroid film hard copy was commonly used in the early CT units such as the EMI Mark I and the ACTA scanner.

The advantages of Polaroid film are offset by some significant limitations. Polaroid film demonstrates a relatively short dynamic range, that is, a limited exposure latitude, compared to radiographic film. The cost of the Polaroid film itself is very high in terms of cost per image photographed compared to radiographic film. It is much more difficult to copy or duplicate Polaroid images than radiographic film; for practical purposes, copies of Polaroid images cannot be obtained routinely in a clinical setting. This necessitates making any additional copies at the time of initial photography. Alternatively, images archived on magnetic tape would have to be reloaded onto a magnetic disc and redisplayed on the monitor for photography. Most viewers regard the image quality of Polaroid prints as inferior to transilluminated hard copy. Radiologists in particular tend to have a strong subjective preference for transilluminated images. The Polaroid images usually have to be mounted on cardboard supports, and this presents a bulkier hard copy product for storage. Finally, the Polaroid prints are subject to tearing (an extremely rare occurrence in radiographic film) as well as to being scratched.

Transilluminated Film with a Multiformat Camera

Film Size and Format A multiformat camera is a photographic system which permts display of one or more images on a single sheet of radiographic film. The radiographic film is transilluminated; that is, it is examined with transmitted light from a view box on which the film is mounted.

The commonly used film sizes are 8 × 10, 11 × 14, and 14 × 17 inches. A specific camera is generally limited to one particular film size. However, companies frequently manufacture more than one camera model to provide the user with a choice in selecting a film size; some camera models may be adaptable to films of different sizes. Popular commercial models that have been interfaced to different CT units include the Dunn (Dunn Instruments Corporation) and the Matrix (Matrix Instruments Corporation). Different models from these two companies are available for use with 8 × 10 and 11 × 14 film.

Different formats are available with multiformat cameras, corresponding to the different numbers of images that may be displayed on a single sheet of film. Formats available include 1-on-1, 2-on-1, 4-on-1, 6-on-1, 9-on-1, 12-on-1, and 25-on-1. Some camera models are limited to a single format; others permit the user a choice between different formats on the same camera, usually by a single switch control.

As an example, the General Electric Company manufactures a multiformat camera for use with their CT/T systems. Their single standard camera will accommodate three different film sizes: 14 × 17, 11 × 14, and 8 × 10 inches. The camera is capable of recognizing the different cassettes associated with each film size. The most commonly used cassette is that for 14 × 17 inch film, followed in demand by one using 8 × 10 inch film. However, a cassette for 11 × 14 inch film is also available as a special order item. Each of these film sizes offers two different format options. A 12-on-1 and a 4-on-1 format are available on 14 × 17 inch film; both 4-on-1 and 1-on-1 formats are available for 8 × 10 inch film; the 11 × 14 inch film allows for 2-on-1 and 6-on-1 formats.

The actual size of the image on the hard copy is related to the size of the film and the format selected. For example, using 14 × 17 inch film the 12-on-1 format allows approximately 4¼ × 3⅞ inches for each image. A 4-on-1 format on this film increases this to about 5¾ × 6½ inches. By comparison, a 4-on-1 format on a camera model using 8 × 10 inch film allows approximately 4½ × 3½ inches per image. A 1-on-1 format on 8 × 10 inch film allows about 6½ × 8½ inches for the image.

Multiformat Camera Design Multiformat hard copy is obtained by photographing the video image on radiographic film from a CRT monitor. The CRT screen that is photographed is separate from any viewing monitor associated with either a display or operator console and is incorporated into a multiformat video camera system. This camera system includes the CRT monitor, a camera or lens/shutter assembly, a film holder, and a mechanical positioning mechanism. The CRT monitor in the multiformat camera system is electrically connected to the CT image display system via a coaxial cable.

A photograph made on radiographic film is a negative image of the original; that is, the film polarity is the reverse of the original on the CRT monitor. In a multiformat video camera system, the image on the CRT monitor within the camera system is the "reverse video," or inverted video, of the image that is seen on the CT display console. The CT image display system is designed with a video processing system that inverts the information to the multiformat camera. This results in a reversal of the gray scale or image polarity of the CRT image in the multiformat camera compared to the image on the CT display monitor. The photographic image on the radiographic film is a negative of this reverse video image. This double reversal will give a hard copy image on the radiographic film with the same polarity as that on the CT display console monitor.

The camera or lens/shutter assembly focuses the image on the CRT monitor onto the film. The exposure time is controlled electrically.

The multiformat camera system is designed to permit exposure of only one section of the film at a time. The number of such sections depends on the format used (4-on-1, 12-on-1, etc). A mechanical positioning mechanism is necessary to position the image from each exposure on the proper section on the film. This is commonly performed by shifting either the camera (lens/shutter) or the film between exposures. Dunn and Matrix camera systems shift the camera; the film is stationary. In the General Electric system the mechanical cassette containing the film is shifted between exposures and the camera is fixed in position.

Finally, to perform a "raster erase" (obliterate or minimize the appearance of individual raster lines on the photographic copy), identical interlaced fields may be very slightly offset from one frame to the next to fill out the spaces that otherwise would occur between scan lines. This field offset consists of a small displacement of each line in identical fields (all the odd numbered lines or all the even numbered lines for a frame). The displacement is a fraction of the distance between adjacent lines (e.g., an odd numbered line and an adjacent even numbered line).

Photography and Film Requirements The requirements for obtaining a good hard copy image from a video display include proper film selection, correct exposure, and appropriate adjustment of the video display monitor being photographed. There are five primary parameters, described by Schwenker (1979), to be considered in the selection of a film for a multiformat type of camera for CT (and ultrasound):

1. Contrast
2. Speed
3. Spectral sensitivity
4. Structure
5. Processing requirements.

A sixth parameter, base color, is not as significant.

The following discussion is based on Schwenker's work.

Contrast The selection of film contrast and speed characteristics should be based on the performance characteristics of CRT monitors. In a CRT a given variation in the electrical signal input will cause relatively greater change in the intensity of the optical output of the CRT for low signal voltages than for higher signal voltages. In other words, the optical contrast of a CRT is greater for weaker electrical signals than for larger voltages (i.e., there is contrast distortion). This has the following important effects: there will be more contrast in the anatomical detail at the dark end of a CRT monitor than at the bright end, and the gray scale will change more rapidly in going from black to mid-gray than from mid-gray to white.

These effects are seen on the viewing monitor, not on the film image. On the camera monitor the image is reversed in polarity (in gray tones), and it is this reverse image that is photographed. Any information near the black end of the viewing monitor will be near the white end of the camera monitor. However, on both the viewing and camera CRT monitors there is more contrast at the dark end than at the light end of the image, as described in the last paragraph. This means that although the image polarity is reversed between viewing and camera monitors, the contrast distortion is not reversed; instead, the contrast is greater at the dark end for both monitors.

If information is at the dark end of the viewing monitor, it will be seen with relatively high contrast. This same information will appear at the white end of the camera monitor, where it will be seen in relatively low contrast. The hard copy photograph of the camera monitor will reverse all the shades of gray and the contrast distortion on the camera monitor. The greater contrast seen at the darker end of the camera CRT will appear at the lighter end of the hard copy.

The image polarity or gray shades will have been reversed twice (from viewing monitor to camera monitor and from camera monitor to hard copy), but the contrast distortion will be reversed only once (from camera monitor to hard copy) in the photographic process. Thus, the image polarity (in terms of gray shades) will be identical for the viewing monitor and the hard copy. However, the contrast distortion will be reversed on the hard copy relative to the viewing monitor.

If a relatively low contrast film (for example, one with a film gradient of about 1.0) is used to photograph the camera monitor image, the hard copy image will demonstrate this reversed contrast distortion; and the film copy will appear quite different from the image on the viewing monitor. However, by photographing the camera monitor image with a relatively high contrast film (for example, one with a film gradient of about 2.0–3.0), the problems associated with contrast distortion can be minimized. This occurs because when a higher contrast film is used in photographing the camera monitor, a smaller portion of the CRT gray scale characteristic is used and the resulting film image gray scale transfer characteristic becomes more linear.

The use of a higher contrast film necessitates reducing CRT grid voltage by adjusting contrast and brightness controls on the camera monitor. A film with high contrast and high speed allows a more limited range of camera brightness to be used. This is achieved by decreasing the number of electrons in the beam striking the CRT phosphor. Decreasing the number of electrons in the beam decreases CRT spot intensity and size, with a concomitant increase in image sharpness.

Film Speed The film exposure is the product of the exposure intensity and the exposure time. The use of low intensities (low brightness) for the camera monitor, as discussed in the last subsection, necessitates the use of a relatively fast film and an appropriately long exposure time.

Short exposure times (less that .5 s) should generally be avoided in photographing a raster image with typically 30 frames or 60 fields per s. A multiformat camera may employ a raster erase technique as described earlier. The exposure time should be sufficiently long to integrate the effect of the different field offsets into a composite image. For example, in the General Electric CT/T system there are 16 different offsets to each pair of fields comprising a frame. Thus, in 16 frames the entire range of field offsets will be covered, and the exposure time should not be less than 16 frames.

A longer exposure time allows a lower camera monitor intensity, with improved image sharpness as well. Overly long exposure times may be an inconvenience to the user, however, and should be avoided. An appropriate exposure time is about 1–2 s.

The requirements relating to intensity and time necessitate the use of relatively high speed film.

Film Spectral Sensitivity Usually in CRT photography, film spectral sensitivity is important only in regard to the speed of the film with respect to the particular CRT phosphor being photographed. In multiformat cameras a P4 phosphor is generally used, and this particular phosphor also raises the problem of structure noise in the film image.

The P4 phosphor is a mixture of blue and yellow phosphors, providing a white appearance for black-and-white monitors. The two phosphors are heterogeneously distributed over the CRT face. The discrete areas of blue and yellow phosphor can be identified by direct visualization or with magnification.

If blue-sensitive film is used to photograph a P4 phosphor, only the areas containing blue phosphor will be exposed. Those areas on the film occupied by the yellow phosphor will be unexposed, resulting in a grainy appearance to the film. Orthochromatic film (green-sensitive film) has a spectral sensitivity that more nearly overlaps the light output of a P4 phosphor than does blue-sensitive film. The orthochromatic film displays some sensitivity to the yellow phosphor as well as the blue phosphors of P4. A panchromatic film would show even greater sensitivity to the yellow phosphor in addition to the blue phosphor, but this film would have to be handled and developed in total darkness, a great disadvantage. Both green-sensitive and blue-sensitive film can be handled in red light without being exposed. The use of orthochromatic film is thus a reasonable approach to reduce P4 structural noise.

Film Structure A single emulsion film should be used in CRT photography to maintain the resolution and sharpness of the monitor image. The use of a double emulsion film significantly reduces image sharpness. Although the diagnostic significance might not be great, the images would be less aesthetically pleasing.

Processing Requirements It would be very inconvenient not to be able to develop the CT films in the rapid automatic film processors used for other radiographic film. Strict quality control should be observed for the processor and processor solutions. Deterioration in film processing may be detected earlier in the single emulsion films used in CT imaging than in the double emulsion films used for conventional radiographic work. Particularly in busy CT facilities, it may be useful to have a processor devoted to CT use alone, or perhaps shared among CT, ultrasound, and nuclear medicine usages.

Base Color Traditionally, radiographs have been made on a blue base film. Supposedly this provides an intensity and color that minimizes fatigue during extended reading. Removal of the blue background has several effects, including an effective increase in viewbox brightness, a subjective increase in image contrast, and some apparent improvement of the visualization of detail in low density areas. The actual effects of the use of a clear base appear small, and there are apparently no quantitative data to support a significant clinical effect of base color. The choice between clear and blue bases seems to be aesthetic.

Summary The preceding discussion suggests that the following properties for film be used in medical video imaging:

High contrast (film gradient of 2.0–3.0)
High speed
Orthochromatic
Single emulsion
90-s processable
Clear or blue base optional.

REFERENCES AND SUGGESTED READINGS

Ackerman, L. V. Computed tomography scans on paper. Radiology 128:819–820, 1978.

Akutagawa, W. M., Huth, G. C., Levis, R. E., Drianis, G. C., and Davis, R. L. Increased tissue differentiation using color display of multiple-energy CT scans. Radiology 134:739–756, 1980.

Bentson, J. R., Mancuso, A. A., Winter, J., and Hanafee, W. N. Combined gas cisternography and edge-enhanced computed tomography of the internal auditory canal. Radiology 136:777–779, 1980.

Bergstrom, M., and Sundman, R. Picture processing in computed tomography. American Journal of Roentgenology 127:17–21, 1976.

Elliott, D. O. Data recording storage. *In* T. H. Newton and D. G. Potts (eds.), Radiology of the Skull and Brain: Technical Aspects of Computed Tomography, Vol. 5, Chap. 122, Part XVII, pp. 4200–4211. C. V. Mosby, St. Louis, 1981.

Glenn, W. V., Harlow, C. A., Dwyer, S. J., Rhodes, M. L., and Parker, D. L. Image manipulation and pattern recognition. *In* T. H. Newton and D. G. Potts (eds.) Radiology of the Skull and Brain: Technical Aspects of Computed Tomography, Vol. 5, Chap. 129, Part XVIII, pp. 4326–4354. C. V. Mosby, St. Louis, 1981.

Griver, J., and Perry, B. J. A graphic display system for

use with a computerized tomographic scanner. Computerized Tomography 1:167–178, 1977.

Hanafee, W. N., Mancuso, A., Winter, J., Jenkins, H., and Bergstrom, L. Edge enhancement computed tomography scanning in inflammatory lesions of the middle ear. Radiology 136:771–775, 1980.

Henrich, G., Mai, N., and Backmund, H. Preprocessing in computed tomography picture analysis: A "bone-deleting" algorithm. Journal of Computer Assisted Tomography 3:379–384, 1979.

Herman, G. T., and Coin, C. G. The use of three-dimensional computer display in the study of disk disease. Technical note. Journal of Computer Assisted Tomography 4:564–567, 1980.

Horton, J. A., and Kerber, C. W. The grain in the stone: A computer search for hidden CT patterns. Radiology 129:427–431, 1978.

Hounsfield, G. N. Picture quality of computed tomography. American Journal of Roentgenology 127:3–9, 1976.

Hounsfield, G. N. Potential uses of more accurate CT absorption values by filtering. American Journal of Roentgenology 131:103–106, 1976.

Huckman, M. S., and Ackerman, L. V. Use of automated measurements of mean density as an adjunct to computed tomography. Journal of Computer Assisted Tomography 1:37–42, 1977.

Joseph, P. M., Hilal, S. K., Schulz, R. A., and Kelcz, F. Clinical and experimental investigation of a smoothed CT reconstruction algorithm. Radiology 134:507–516, 1980.

Koehler, P. R., Anderson, R. E., and Baxter, B. The effect of computed tomography viewer controls on anatomical measurements. Radiology 134:189–194, 1979.

Kramer, R. A., and Janetos, G. P. Image manipulation in the detection of bone lesions with CT scanner. American Journal of Roentgenology 128:332–333, 1977.

Kramer, R. A., Yoshikawa, B. M., Scheibe, P. O., and Janetos, G. P. Statistical profiles in computed tomography. Radiology 125:145–147, 1977.

Larsen, L. E., and Evans, R. A. An off-line image processing system for digital display in computed tomography. Radiology 123:361–367, 1977.

Larsen, G. N., Glenn, W., Kishore, P. R. S., Davis, K., McFarland, W., and Dwyer, S. J. Computer processing of CT images: Advances and prospects. Neurosurgery 1:73–79, 1977.

Lee, K. R., Dwyer, S. J., Anderson, W. H., Betz, D., Faszold, S., Preston, D. F., Robinson, R. G., and Templeton, A. W. Continuous image recording using gray-tone, dry-process silver paper. Radiology 139:493–496, 1981.

McCullough, E. C. Factors affecting the use of quantitative information from a CT scanner. Radiology 124:99–107, 1977.

New, P. F. J., and Scott, W. R. General description of the EMI scanner: Operational notes. *In* Computed Tomography of the Brain and Orbit (EMI Scanning), Chapter 2, pp. 7–22. Williams & Wilkins, Baltimore, 1975.

Pullan, B. R., Fawcitt, R. A., and Isherwood, I. Tissue characterization by an analysis of the distribution of attenuation values in computed tomography scans: A preliminary report. Journal of Computer Assisted Tomography 2:49–54, 1978.

Reese, D. F., O'Brien, P. C., Beeler, G. W., Gerding, P. R., and McCullough, E. C. An investigation for extracting more information from computerized tomography scans. American Journal of Roentgenology 124:177–185, 1975.

Ritchings, R. T., Isherwood, I., Pullan, B. R., and Kingsley, D. Receiver operating characteristic curves in the evaluation of hard copies of computed tomography scans. Journal of Computer Assisted Tomography 3:423–425, 1979.

Schultz, G. W. Computed tomography displays. *In* T. H. Newton and D. G. Potts (eds.), Radiology of the Skull and Brain, Technical Aspects of Computed Tomography, Vol. 5, Chap. 121, Part XVII, pp. 4173–4199. C. V. Mosby, St. Louis, 1981.

Schwenker, R. P. Film selection for computed tomography and ultrasound video imaging. *In* A. G. Haus (ed.), Physics of Medical Imaging: Recording Systems Measurements and Techniques. Published for American Association of Physicists in Medicine by the American Institute of Physics, 1979.

Schwenker, R. P. Film selection considerations for computed tomography and ultrasound video photography. Appl. Opt. Instr. Med. VII, Proc. SPIE 173:75–80, 1979.

Shaffer, K. A., Volz, D. J., and Haughton, V. M. Manipulation of CT data for temporal bone imaging. Radiology 137:825–829, 1980.

Warren, R. C. Contrast and latitude of CT hard copy: An ROC study. Radiology 141:139–145, 1981.

Winter, J. Edge enhancement of computed tomography by digital unsharp masking. Radiology 135:234–235, 1980.

Zatz, L. M. General overview of computed tomography instrumentation. *In* T. H. Newton and D. G. Potts (eds.), Radiology of the Skull and Brain: Technical Aspects of Computed Tomography, Vol. 5, Chap. 116, Part XVII, pp. 4025–4057. C. V. Mosby, St. Louis, 1981.

Chapter 7
A PRACTICAL COMPUTED TOMOGRAPHY SYSTEM

THE CT SYSTEM: COMPONENT PARTS

    Patient Table and Gantry Components
        The Patient Table
        The Gantry
    X-Ray Generator
    Data Processing and Storage System
        Disk Unit
        Central Processing Unit
        Magnetic Tape Unit
        Array Processor
        Ramtek
        Software
    Line Printer
    Display Terminals
    Operator Terminals
    Multiformat Camera

SCANNING PARAMETERS

    Tube Kilovoltage
    Tube Current and Exposure Time
        Tube Current
        Exposure Time
        Total Exposure
    Field of View for Reconstruction

ENVIRONMENTAL REQUIREMENTS

    Physical Space and CT Suite Design
    Ambient Conditions
    Patient Environment

REFERENCES AND SUGGESTED READINGS

In this chapter the component parts, scanning parameters, and environmental requirements of a CT system are discussed, based on the example of one of the most commonly used commercial CT units, a General Electric CT/T system. Thus, the specifics of design, operation parameters, and nomenclature are described in this chapter for a particular third generation unit (rotating tube and detector array). However, many of the basics of design, operation, function, and environment are widely applicable to CT systems in general. It is hoped this illustrative approach will clarify and reinforce much of the previous discussion in this book.

THE CT SYSTEM: COMPONENT PARTS

The component parts of a CT system are illustrated in schematic form in Figure 7.1 and in the drawing in Figure 7.2. The diagrams are based specifically on General Electric CT/T systems but are applicable to other CT systems as well.

The initial General Electric CT/T system was the 7800 model. This was replaced by the CT/T 8800 model. The most recent addition to this family of CT units was the CT/T 9800. The author's experience has been with the two prior models, and the discussion will be based on the features and specifications of these, unless otherwise stated.

Patient Table and Gantry Components

The patient table and gantry are shown in Figure 7.3.

The Patient Table The patient table functions both as a means for supporting and positioning the patient and as a transport system for moving the patient into and through the gantry. A concave cradle containing cushions or pads on which the patient rests is placed on top of the table. The cradle is concave in order to help position the patient in the center of the reconstruction circle. A control panel for directing the position and the motion of the table is located on the side of the table (Figure 7.3).

A number of table accessories that are part of the system are illustrated in Figure 7.4. These include a foot rest (for patient comfort and to help maintain patient position on the table), a patient shaper (sometimes useful in helping to mold the contours of obese patients so that loose amounts of superficial soft tissues can be included within the circle of reconstruction), an arm injection board to assist in starting intravenous injections, an arm restraint strap for agitated patients, a knee cushion (for supporting the patient's knees and reducing the lordotic curvature of the lower back in patients undergoing lumbar spine studies), a head holder and restraint straps (for centering and stabilizing the position of the head during a head study), body restraint straps (to help maintain the body position during the examination), cradle pads (to provide a cushion for the patient on the metal cradle top), and calibration phantoms and a phantom holder for periodic calibration of the CT unit.

There are a number of controls and panel lights at the side of the table. Functions governed by these controls include raising and lowering of the tabletop, tilting of the gantry in either direction (15° in the 7800 and 8800, 20° in the 9800), cradle traversal into or out of the gantry aperture at different speeds, internal external alignment lights, and an emergency power switch for the x-ray tube, gantry, and table.

The internal alignment light is a red colored beam which indicates the slice plane location in the center of the gantry. Two external alignment lights, one on the ceiling and one on the wall, project red colored laser beams onto the patient as a cross pattern on the same section or slice of the patient. The section indicated by the external alignment lights lies 47 cm from the center of the gantry aperture. These external alignment crosshairs help to center the patient within the circle of reconstruction and to define reference positions (e.g., the xiphoid) on the patient. After external positioning of a patient reference position, a fixed movement of 47 cm of the cradle into the gantry aperture will move the patient so that the reference level is in the center of the gantry aperture.

In addition, various panel lights at the side of the table indicate when the tabletop may be lowered

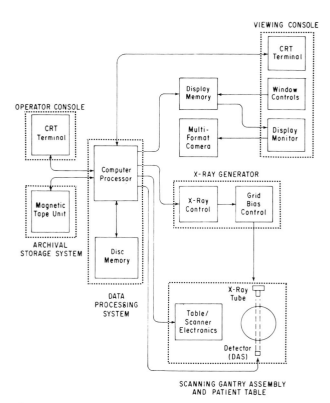

Figure 7.1. Schematic diagram of a CT system. This is based on a General Electric CT/T system but is applicable to other CT systems as well.

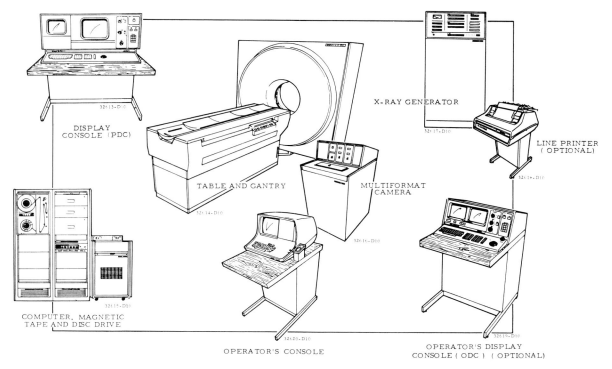

Figure 7.2. Drawings of the components of a CT system. (Courtesy of General Electric Medical Systems.)

for positioning, when the gantry may be tilted, when the patient is outside the circle of reconstruction, when the cradle is unlatched from the tabletop, and various other conditions. The cradle may be unlatched from the top of the table so that it is free to move in or out of the gantry aperture by physical maneuvering. This feature facilitates the emergency removal of the patient out of the gantry aperture when the table drive is not functional.

The Gantry

Gantry Mechanics The gantry contains the x-ray tube (including filtration and collimation), the data acquisition system (DAS), and associated electronics. This is illustrated in Figure 7.5. The gantry also contains oversize lights, which indicate when a patient is too large, and motors for rotating the x-ray tube and DAS either clockwise or counterclockwise and also for tilting the gantry.

In the scanning process there is an initial sector of angular acceleration until the tube and DAS achieve a constant angular velocity. After 360° of data acquisition at this constant angular velocity, there is a final sector of angular deceleration. Alternate scans are performed with the gantry rotating in the clockwise and then in the counterclockwise direction.

For the 7700 and 8800 models the gantry aperture through which the cradle holding the patient passes is 60 cm (24 inches) in diameter. The distance from the x-ray tube focal spot to the center of the gantry aperture is 78 cm. The distance between the center of the gantry aperture to the detector array is 32 cm. The 9800 model has been modified and has a 70-cm aperture.

X-Ray Tube General Electric CT/T 7800 and 8800 systems have used Maxiray 125B and Maxiray 100-CT rotating anode x-ray tubes, both manufactured by General Electric. The Maxiray 125B was the original tube used, particularly in the 7800 systems. The Maxiray 100-CT, a later tube, was designed especially for application in CT and used in the 8800 system. A larger heat storage capacity and a greater heat dissipation rate are the primary advantages of the Maxiray 100-CT compared to the earlier Maxiray 125B tube. This increased heat storage capacity and heat dissipation rate facilitate large exposure factors (mAs) and shortened intervals between scans without overloading the tube. The Maxiray 125B is now out of production.

Both the Maxiray 100-CT and the earlier Maxiray 125B are housed in shockproof cast aluminum lined with lead to minimize radiation leakage. Tube cooling has been provided by means of an internal oil circulator coupled to an external forced air heat exchanger.

In the computer-controlled pulsed operation the maximum ratings at 60 Hz are 120 kVp at 600 mA for a maximum pulse duration of 3.3 ms, with a pulse repetition rate of 60 per s and a pulse train duration of 9.6 s. At 50 Hz the maximum ratings are 120 kVp at 500 mA for a maximum pulse duration of 4.0 ms, with a pulse repetition rate of 50 per s and a pulse train duration of 11.5 s. The maximum duty cycle (on or pulse time compared to total time) is 20%.

The Maxiray 100-CT tube has a target (anode) diameter of 4 inches and a 7° target angle. The focal spot size is 1.2 mm × 1.2 mm.

In a rotating anode x-ray tube the power that causes the anode to rotate is supplied by a magnetic field produced by stator coils which surround the neck of the x-ray tube outside the glass envelope of the tube. The stator coils produce a rapidly varying magnetic field which also intercepts the copper rotor of the induction motor, inducing an electrical current in the rotor. The induced current supplies the power to rotate the anode assembly. This was illustrated in Figure 3.3. In the Maxiray 100-CT tube (and the earlier Maxiray 125B) the stator and rotor are designed so that the rotor attains a rotational speed of not less than 10,000 rpm in 3.0 s with power supplied from a rapid acceleration rotor controller. At the end of the anode acceleration time, the voltage is reduced

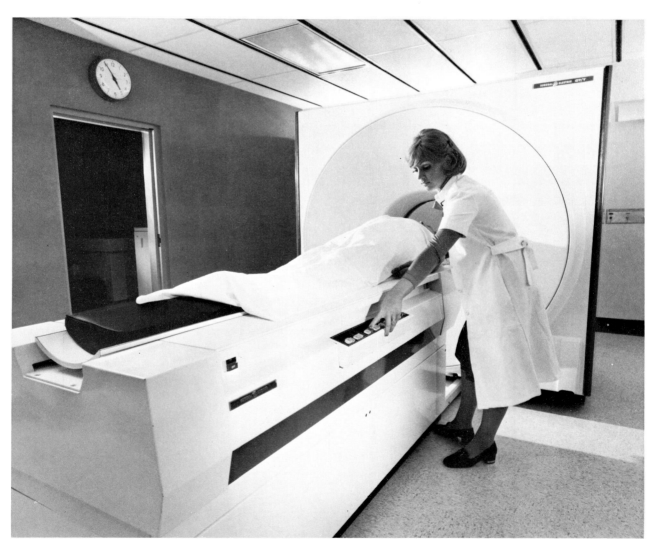

Figure 7.3. Table and gantry of a General Electric CT/T 8800 system. (Courtesy of General Electric Medical Systems.)

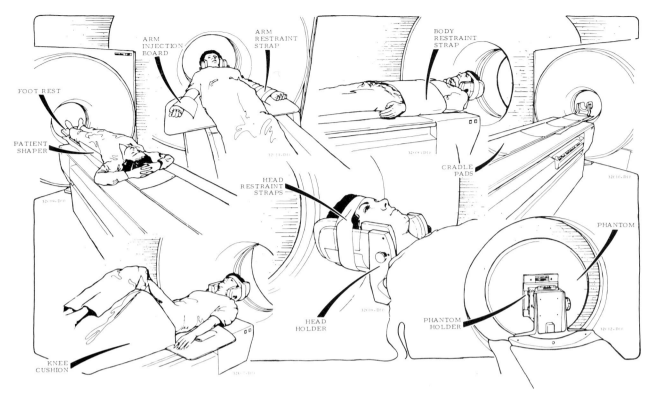

Figure 7.4. Associated table accessories for a CT system. (Courtesy of General Electric Medical Systems.)

to a value sufficient to maintain 10,000 rpm with minimal heat buildup within the tube. At the end of the exposure a braking voltage is applied for 4.5 s to decelerate the rotor to near 0 rpm.

The heat storage capacity of a tube represents the total amount of heat that can be stored in the x-ray tube. This heat energy is an accumulation of heat dissipated from the electron beam striking the anode, from rotation of the anode, and from cathode heating. The heat storage capacity is expressed in terms of heat units. A heat unit is defined for three-phase or constant potential circuits as:

$$\text{heat units} = 1.35 \text{ kVp} \times \text{mA} \times \text{exposure time}. \quad (7.1)$$

For a pulsed x-ray tube, the exposure time for a single scan is the actual time during which the x-ray tube is pulsed and emitting x-rays. It is equal to the product of the scan time, the pulse repetition rate, and the pulse duration; that is,

$$\text{total exposure time per scan} = \text{scan time}$$
$$\times \text{ pulse repetition rate} \times \text{pulse duration}. \quad (7.2)$$

Both the tube anode and the entire tube unit (including tube and housing) have specified heat storage capacities, which should not be exceeded; otherwise the tube would be ruined. The heat accumulated, according to Equation 7.1, depends on the operating parameters of the tube, a larger mA or exposure time resulting in the accumulation of more heat units per x-ray exposure or scan. The heat within the tube is dissipated by the cooling system. When the scanning parameters (mA and exposure time) are increased, the minimum time between scans must be decreased to prevent overloading of the tube.

The computer contains a program which assimilates the data relating to tube heating during the scans. This includes the mA and exposure time per scan (as defined in Equation 7.2), the number of scans, the time between scans, and the time since the last scan. This permits an accurate calculation of the total heat load in the tube and in the tube housing at any time. The computer will delay further scanning if the heat buildup within the tube is excessive. In addition, there is a temperature-sensitive probe within the tube casing near the anode to monitor the temperature and indicate when this temperature has become excessive.

The heat storage capacity of the Maxiray 100-

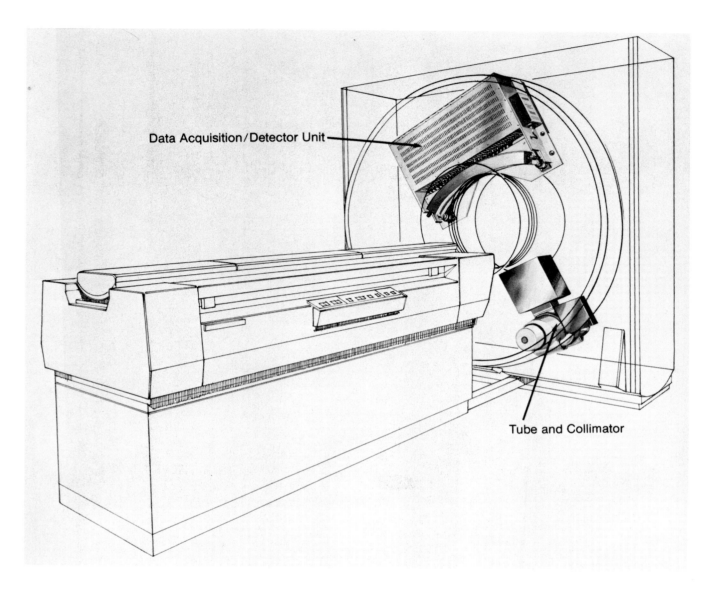

Figure 7.5. Drawing of the patient table and gantry, including the x-ray tube, collimator, detectors and data acquisition electronics. (Courtesy of General Electric Medical Systems.)

CT tube is 700,000 heat units for the anode and 2,000,000 heat units for the entire tube unit. The maximum heat dissipation rate is 150,000 heat units per min for the anode and for the tube unit (with the internal pump and the external blower operating).

The x-ray tube has three electronic assemblies or systems controlling the production of x-rays. The rotor controller rotates the tube anode up to the required 10,000 rpm, as previously described, before x-ray production. After attaining this rotational speed, the tube grid becomes biased (turned on), so that x-ray production begins. The pulse bias tank supplies the appropriate signals for biasing the grid. Each bias of the grid is equivalent to a single pulse of the tube in the CT/T 7800 and 8800 systems. Each tube pulse results in a single data view, that is, simultaneous measurements in each detector of the array.

The high voltage transformer produces the high voltage required between the anode and the cathode.

The rotor controller, pulse bias tank, and high voltage transformer are contained in large boxes that are located near the scanner in the CT suite. They can be conveniently enclosed within a storage area and in close proximity to the main x-ray tube power supply.

At the beginning of the workday, or whenever more than 2 h have elapsed since the last scan, a series of test exposures must be performed to warm up the tube anode.

In contrast to the pulsed emission of x-rays in the CT/T 7800 and 8800 systems, the CT/T 9800 employs a rotating anode x-ray tube, which continuously emits x-rays during the scan. A discrete measurement time is designated during which a set of x-ray transmission readings is collected by all the xenon cells in the array.

Filtration and Collimation The filters and collimators are both housed in a box in front of the x-ray tube along with the collimator (Figure 7.5). The minimum inherent filtration for the Maxiray CT-100 used in the CT/T 8800 is 2.7 mm aluminum equivalent at 150 kVp. This results from .8 mm aluminum equivalent at 150 kVp from the tube insert (the glass part of the x-ray tube), .4 mm aluminum equivalent at 150 kVp from the insulating oil and x-ray port (made of Lexan) of the tube housing, and a 1.5-mm aluminum fixed external filter in the collimator adapter. In addition, individual concave (bowtie) shaped filters are preselected to accommodate head or body examinations.

The collimator adjusts the aperture for the desired slice thickness as well as collimating the x-ray beam to the correct geometry and safety standards for CT. Both the filter and slice (collimator) thickness are selected automatically under computer control when the operator calls up the appropriate scan program (head or body) and are driven into place by a servomechanism.

The operator has a choice of three slice thicknesses: 10 mm, 5 mm, and 1.5 mm. An additional 3-mm slice thickness is available in the CT/T 9800 system. Most often 10 mm will be adequate. The thinner slices are often helpful in obtaining better spatial detail, particularly in smaller structures where high contrast resolution is present (e.g., posterior fossa detail, coronal scans of the sella turcica). Also, a thin section may give a more accurate estimate of the CT value in smaller structures by minimizing partial volume errors.

Data Acquisition System The DAS consists of the array of xenon gas detectors and associated electronics. Its position in the gantry is shown in Figure 7.5. As described in Chapter 3, during each pulse of the x-ray tube each xenon cell or detector element in a CT/T 7800 or 8800 system, examines a single ray originating from the tube and traversing the patient along a specific path (see Figure 3.16). The angle that the detector array subtends from the x-ray tube focus is 30°. The set of measurements made by all the cells or elements in the array during a single pulse time constitutes a view in this third generation geometry.

There are 289 individual data cells and 12 reference cells in the CT/T 7800 system, hence 289 data measurements or rays in a view. The CT/T 8800 has 511 data cells and 12 reference cells, hence 511 data measurements or rays in a view.

Since the overall length of the xenon detector array is the same for the CT/T 7800 and 8800 systems, the spacing between the individual xenon cells is reduced in the 8800 to accommodate the larger number of cells. This results in a reduction of the aperture width of each cell or individual detector element. In the 7800 the aperture width is 1.83 mm; in the 8800 it is .90 mm. The smaller aperture width of the 8800 accounts for its improved spatial resolution.

Successive x-ray pulses during the simultaneous rotation of the tube and DAS permit the collection of additional independent views (see Figure 3.15). This data acquisition process continues through a 360° rotation (Figure 7.6). A fast scan can be performed in 4.8 s and results in the collection of 288

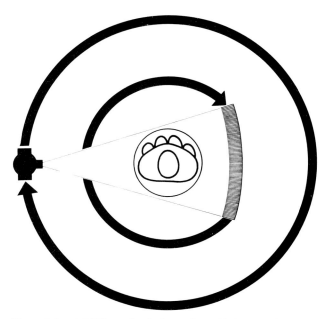

Figure 7.6. A 360° rotation is shown for a third generation scanner. The tube and detector rotate about the isocenter of the system. (Courtesy of General Electric Medical Systems.)

views. A slow scan requires 9.6 s but permits the acquisition of 576 views. As described in Chapter 3, the total number of measurement data obtained during a scan is the product of the number of views in a scan and the number of measurements made in each view (the latter being equal to the number of detectors).

Both fast and slow scans involve the same 360° rotation. In a slow scan the angular rotation and the spacing between consecutive views are one-half that for the fast scan.

The ions formed in each xenon cell or detector element are collected as an analog electrical data signal and then converted into digital data by appropriate electronic boards (analog-to-digital converters) in the DAS.

The CT/T 9800 system has a total of 742 xenon cells (detector and reference cells). The number of views obtained may range from 1240 to 7880. A view represents the set of x-ray transmission readings made during a designated measurement time by all the xenon cells in the array.

X-Ray Generator

The x-ray generator used in the General Electric CT/T 7800 and 8800 systems is an MSI 850 x-ray generator. It controls the kVp (120 kV), the mA (typically 100–600 mA), and the pulse width duration (1.1, 2.2, and 3.3 ms). The kVp and mA are selected directly on the x-ray generator; the pulse time is selected by the operator through the control console and central processing unit (CPU). The generator allows a range of mA selections from 20–600. It is a three-phase, 12-pulse generator manufactured by General Electric.

The generator also has a TEST mode of operation, which is utilized when the system is turned on in order to check the x-ray tube.

Data Processing and Storage System

The computer is an integrated system of hardware components which performs various control functions and data processing under the direction of appropriate software or programs. Although theoretically tomographic image reconstruction is possible without a computer, practically the vast amount of data that must be collected and processed to obtain satisfactory diagnostic images necessitates a computer system. Each of the separate hardware components in the system plays an important, and in most cases an indispensable role in the performance of the computer system. The computer system in the General Electric CT/T 7800 and 8800 systems is based on Data General Company components.

Disk Unit The disk unit consists of a Data General disk drive and a disk pack that stores the programs the computer uses in patient scanning and in image reconstruction and display. The disk pack is basically a stack of individual magnetic disks, all of which can be addressed simultaneously. This permits a significant expansion of the storage capacity compared to a single disk. Both the raw data and the reconstructed scans are stored on the disk pack on a short-term basis. A disk pack system used in the General Electric CT/T systems, for example, contains 10 platters or disks and has a storage capacity of 89.5 Mbytes, permitting storage of around 300 reconstructed slices. The only interfacing that the operator has with the disk drive is to turn it off and on.

Central Processing Unit The CPU, sometimes referred to (but not entirely correctly) as the "computer" or the "mainframe," is responsible for handling all the calculations involved in image reconstruction as well as the management of command/data flow.

The mainframe or CPU capability of both the General Electric CT/T 7800 and 8800 systems is based on a Data General S/140 Eclipse system. This has been updated from the earlier Eclipse S/200. The S/200 initially had a 48K (48-kilobyte) memory, later increased to 96K. The S/140 has a 128K memory.

The CPU is manipulated by the operator under the following circumstances:

system morning startup or warmup
system down, as indicated on operator terminal by the word DOWN
failure of the system to respond normally to the operator terminal
system in a halt condition, i.e., the lights on the front panel are brightly lit and not flashing
after the specific computer communication HELP ROSEBUD has occurred and the file causing the problem has been renamed.

Under these circumstances, rebooting the CPU allows the computer to escape from a trapped location and start again at the first location in its operating program.

Magnetic Tape Unit In the General Electric CT/T systems, a Data General magnetic tape drive for archival storage uses 2,400-foot magnetic tapes, each capable of storing 140 images (processed images based on a 320 × 320 matrix). The processed data (CT numbers comprising a scan), and raw data when

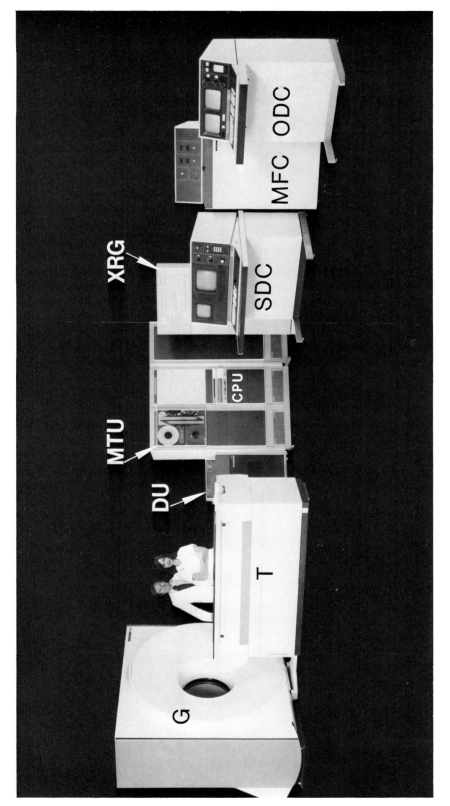

Figure 7.9. Photograph of the components of a General Electric CT/T system. From left to right: gantry (*G*), patient table (*T*), disk unit (*DU*), computer system including the magnetic tape unit (*MTU*) and the central processing unit (*CPU*), x-ray generator (*XRG*), system display console (*SDC*) multiformat camera (*MFC*) and operator display console (*ODC*). (Courtesy of General Electric Medical Systems.)

Tube Current and Exposure Time

Tube Current The anode pulse current can be varied in the range from 20–600 mA. Lower values of mA (less than 120 mA) do not provide a sufficient number of x-ray photons at the detector array. An insufficient photon flux at the detectors results in poor contrast resolution. Larger values (500–600 mA), especially with larger pulse times, result in a greater heat load to the tube, necessitating a longer cooling time between scans.

Exposure Time For a single scan the exposure time is described by Equation 7.2. In a CT/T 7800 or 8800 system operating with 60 Hz power, the pulse repetition rate is 60 per s. The scan time is either 4.8 or 9.6 s. The total number of pulses or the number of views obtained during a scan is the product of the scan time and the pulse repetition rate; that is,

$$\begin{aligned}\text{total number of pulses per scan} &= \text{Total number of views per scan} \\ &= \text{scan time} \times \text{pulse repetition rate} \\ &= \text{scan time} \times 60/\text{s} \quad (7.3)\\ &= 288 \text{ views (for a 4.8-s scan)} \\ &\text{or } 576 \text{ views (for a 9.6-s scan).}\end{aligned}$$

By combining Equations 7.2 and 7.3, the total exposure time per scan can be expressed as the product of the number of views per scan and the pulse duration:

$$\begin{aligned}&\text{total exposure time per scan} \\ &= \text{total number of views per scan} \times \text{pulse time.} \quad (7.4)\end{aligned}$$

The pulse time (pulse duration or pulse width) is usually referred to in terms of the pulse width code (PWC). There are usually three values of the PWC that the operator can select. These are assigned the numbers 1, 2, and 3, corresponding to pulse times of 1.1, 2.2, and 3.3 ms, respectively.

The duty cycle (fraction of the time that the tube is on or pulsing) is expressed as

$$\text{duty cycle} = \text{pulse time/pulse cycle time,} \quad (7.5)$$

where the pulse cycle time is the time from the beginning of one pulse to the beginning of the next pulse. This is the inverse of the pulse repetition rate and is equal to $\frac{1}{60}$ s, or $16\frac{2}{3}$ ms.

For pulse times of 1.1, 2.2, and 3.3 ms, the respective duty cycles are .066, .132, and .198 (approximately 20%).

For those countries using 50 Hz power, longer scan times are required to obtain the same number of views. A scan composed of 288 views requires 5.76 s; a scan with 576 views requires 11.52 s. The pulse durations are increased to 1.3, 2.7, and 4.0 ms.

The pulse repetition rate is fixed; however, the operator can vary the scan time and the pulse time. Both of these factors are selected at the operator terminal. An increase in either of these factors with the other one held constant would cause a corresponding increase in the exposure time. An increase in the exposure time results in an increased total number of x-ray photons and patient dose for a fixed mA.

The exposure time may be doubled by doubling either the pulse time or the scan time. There is a significant difference between these two approaches, however. Doubling the pulse time doubles the number of photons in each ray; that is, each detector will measure twice as many photons. If the mA is constant, the photon flux (number of x-ray photons crossing a unit area in a unit time) is constant. Therefore, by doubling the pulse time, the constant x-ray flux is measured twice as long, resulting in twice as many photons entering the detector cell during a measurement. However, the total number of individual measurements (the product of the number of views and the number of detectors) is unchanged.

On the other hand, doubling the scan time doubles the number of views. This means that the total number of individual measurements is doubled. However, the number of photons in each measurement, as determined by the photon flux and the pulse time, is unchanged.

Increasing the pulse time improves the statistical reliability of each individual measurement but not the number of measurements. Increasing the scan time increases the number of measurements without improving the statistical reliability of the individual measurements. An increase in the pulse time and/or the mA is especially helpful in larger patients or body sections, where significant x-ray attenuation results in a marked reduction in the number of photons available for measurement at the detector.

Total Exposure A certain amount of compromise is necessary in adjusting exposure factors (mA, pulse time, scan time). Raising the mA increases the photon flux but also increases tube cooling time and patient radiation dose. Increasing the scan time increases the number of views or data measurements but requires the patient to be immobile for a longer period. A longer pulse time increases the number of photons in a single measurement and thus the statistical reliability of the measurement, but also increases the patient radiation dose and the measurement time (during which the detector array is moving).

As a general rule it is prudent to increase the exposure factors at the risk of a somewhat higher radiation dose in order to obtain the maximum information from the diagnostic study. However, unusually high factors may be more likely to improve the aesthetic rather than the diagnostic quality of the images. There must obviously be a tradeoff between radiation dosage and image noise. Larger patients or body sections will require higher exposure factors. Exposure factors may be reduced in smaller patients, for example, small children, without compromising diagnostic image quality. Individual judgment and experience will obviously play an important role in these decisions.

In scanning adult heads, typical exposure factors with a General Electric CT/T 8800 might be 250 mA with a PWC of 3 (3.3 ms), or 320 mA with a PWC of 2. In the posterior fossa, with its greater amount of bone, 320 mA with a PWC of 3 may be needed to overcome the increased bone attenuation. An infant head might be adequately imaged with 125–160 mA and a PWC of 2. Adult body scans generally require greater exposure factors, typically 250–320 mA with a PWC of 3. Extremities require less exposure, perhaps about 125 mA with a PWC of 2 or occasionally 1. More often than not, a 9.6-s scan time is preferable over the 4.8-s scan time.

In estimating the mAs for a scan in a pulsed tube unit (third generation) the duty cycle of the tube must be taken into account:

$$mAs = mA \times scan\ time \times duty\ cycle. \quad (7.6)$$

Thus, if a scan is performed at 250 mA in 9.6 s with a PWC of 3, the total mAs during the scan is

$$250\ mA \times 9.6\ s \times .20$$
$$= 480\ mAs,$$

since a PWC of 3 in the CT/T system has a duty cycle of .20.

Field of View for Reconstruction

The operator has a choice of several different fields of view for image reconstruction (or circle of reconstruction). Appropriate files are present for the head, for the body, and for infants. The head file performs an image reconstruction for a 25-cm field of view, which is somewhat ovoid (to match the general shape of the head) in appearance. There are two body files available, one with a 42-cm and one with a 35-cm field of view. The infant file is a 25-cm field of view and is more circular in appearance than the head file.

The two body files are each calibrated with respective body phantoms of the appropriate size. The head and infant files are calibrated with a common smaller phantom.

ENVIRONMENTAL REQUIREMENTS

Physical Space and CT Suite Design

One of the most common mistakes in the design of many earlier CT suites involved the allocation of an inadequate amount of floor space to the new CT suite. Floor space is nearly always at a premium in a hospital, and it is especially hard to come by in a radiology or imaging department. A new service frequently acquires its required space at the expense of preexisting services. Too often the question has been posed: what is the minimum amount of space required for a CT suite? A more appropriate question to ask is rather: what is the optimum amount of space in a CT suite for efficient operation and for a comfortable patient and work environment?

Another serious problem that often arises involves the internal allocation or distribution of space among the different component work areas within the CT suite. These different work areas include the scanning room, operator control room, computer room, image viewing room, storage area for electrical transformers, and storage closets or areas for medical supplies, magnetic tapes, and other materials.

It is easy to underestimate the optimal space required for the entire CT suite and its individual component work areas. In the scan room itself the patient table and gantry occupy a large area. There must be sufficient area around the sides and ends of the table/gantry system to accommodate efficient movement of personnel and equipment. Not uncommonly, very sick patients or individuals with fractures need to be transported in hospital beds. The corridors leading to the scan room and the door of the scan room must be large enough to accommodate hospital beds efficiently. Life support systems such as respirators, when required, must be positioned near the patient. Cabinets and drawer space are needed for a wide variety of medical supplies, including contrast materials, intravenous sets and fluids, drugs, and syringes. The CT scan room should not serve as a general storage area for supplies not directly and immediately pertinent to the scanning process and the patient's safety and comfort. However, a minimal storage space for necessary medical supplies is usually required.

The operator control room or area should be large enough to permit the technologist(s) a relatively comfortable working area and facilitate ready access to the scan room and the computer room. The operator terminal, x-ray generator, and not infrequently a work desk for handling paper work and scheduling must be included. The number of personnel in the control room may vary considerably in the same CT suite, especially if a visiting or student technologist must be periodically accommodated. The actual working area in the control room may be further reduced if initial planning inappropriately provided access to the scan room from the viewing room or other areas through the control room.

The image viewing room usually has the most frequent and largest variations in the number of individuals that must be accommodated. Commonly, large groups of physicians, students, and others have to be accommodated simultaneously in the viewing area. The viewing room or area must provide space for the display terminal, multiformat camera, viewing boxes, film cassette holders, and a work desk or top.

The computer room must be readily accessible to the technologist(s) operating the system. This facilitates changing magnetic tapes, booting the computer, and turning off and on the disk drive. There should also be adequate room for personnel to check, repair, or alter the equipment.

A storage area, preferably enclosed, is needed as part of or immediately adjacent to the scan room for electrical transformers and equipment (e.g., the pulse bias tank and the high voltage transformer in the General Electric CT/T system).

There should be sufficient floor space for efficient movement between the different work areas without interrupting or disturbing personnel in the operator control and image viewing areas.

Of considerable importance is the maintenance of patient visualization by the operator during the entire scan procedure. A large glass window (with appropriate lead shielding) is placed between the control and scan rooms. This permits direct visualization of the patient table and gantry. To facilitate direct visualization of the patient's face as the patient is advanced into the gantry, the patient table and gantry are often obliquely oriented in the scan room with respect to the long axis of the room. Television cameras may be used for better visualization when the patient's face is partly obscured by the gantry. A two-way audio system is also necessary to permit verbal communication between operator and patient.

As in any radiographic room, lead shielding is required to minimize possible radiation exposure to working personnel and others in the area of the CT suite. The tube must also satisfy appropriate requirements dealing with permissible radiation leakage.

Ambient Conditions

The most stringent ambient conditions apply to the computer room. The importance of maintaining proper conditions of temperature and humidity for the computer environment is discussed in Chapter 4.

In the General Electric CT/T system, the temperature in the computer room must lie within the range of 65–80° F (18–27° C). The optimal temperature range is 72–74° (22–23° C), with a maximum variance of ±5° F (2.8° C) per hr.

For the CT/T systems the humidity must lie within the range of 20–70%. The optimal humidity range is 40–60% with a maximum variance of ±5% per hr.

The computer room should also be clear of dust. As described in Chapter 4, accumulated dust within the solid-state devices can interfere with heat transfer and therefore affect the local ambient temperature. More importantly, small dust particles can damage the playback heads in the disk drive. Cigarettes are a frequent and hazardous form of dust contamination, and so smoking in the computer room should be forbidden.

Outside of the computer room the temperature and humidity conditions are not as critical in the rest of CT suite. Optimal cooling of the x-ray tube unit could be inhibited by an excessively high local temperature (greater than 91° F or 33° C). Ambient conditions in the scan room and the control room should be adjusted for patient and technologist comfort, respectively.

Spillage of fluids into the computer parts, including peripheral devices, may result in an equipment malfunction. The keyboards in operator and display terminals are at a particularly high risk for fluid contamination from accidental beverage spills. Technologists and physicians should be particularly alert to the potential dangers associated with beverage cups on console tables adjacent to keyboards.

Patient Environment

Another facet of the environment that is receiving increased attention is the appearance of the scanning room that is presented to the patient. Professional industrial designers are being employed in the medical industry in increasing numbers to help develop more patient-oriented environments.

Many hospitals and medical offices have become more aware of the importance of establishing an attractive, or at least a nonthreatening appearance to their facilities in an increasingly consumer-oriented society. However, too frequently the main efforts are limited primarily to lobbies, waiting rooms, administrative offices, patient rooms, the building facade, and external grounds. Although these are commendable efforts in themselves, decorative lobbies and waiting rooms may provide more pleasure to visitors than to patients undergoing extensive diagnostic examinations and treatment. It is even more important to provide a more patient-oriented environment during actual examination or therapy, thus allaying or at least decreasing patient apprehension and anxiety.

Several factors contribute to the establishment and maintenance of an appropriate environment for the patient undergoing diagnostic testing or therapy. The personal appearance, dress, and communication and understanding of the medical team—physicians, nurses, and technologists and support personnel—are obviously of paramount importance. The decorum of the examination or therapy room can alter a patient's fear of being in an uncomfortable or foreign environment. The appearance of diagnostic or therapeutic equipment with which the patient is being interfaced may be threatening, neutral, or even pleasing.

Although features of the physical clinical environment that are psychologically discomforting to the patient may be identified and modified, it is usually better, simpler, and in the end less costly to try to anticipate and avoid these problems. The establishment of this patient-oriented environment therefore requires the efforts of many different groups including the medical team, hospital architects, interior designers, industrial engineers, and equipment manufacturers. The initial and ongoing efforts in engineering and manufacturing a piece of medical equipment such as a CT scanner should incorporate design features that permit the patient to interface with the equipment without undue fear or discomfort. As an example, many early CT units had gantries that often resembled gigantic meat slicers to the patient. This initial perception was not improved when the patient heard the physician or technologists discussing what "cuts" or "slices" they should take.

Human engineering features, such as mechanical systems that facilitate loading and unloading of immobile patients onto the CT table, can improve efficiency, patient throughput, and employee job satisfaction.

The decorum of the scanning room may appear alienating to the patient. The room may appear small and cramped; cabinets and medical paraphernalia, such as needles and drug boxes, may be scattered about the room; the color scheme may be either too bright or too drab (the latter often lending a sterile, "institutional" appearance to the room).

Appropriate architectural design and interior decoration commencing with the planning stages, not merely after the fact or as an afterthought, will result in a better room decorum.

To coordinate efforts in achieving this common goal of a more patient-oriented environment, there must be an initial commitment on the part of all involved and cooperation from the planning stages through to the installation. The key is to be able to strike an appropriate balance between a proper and necessary clinical appearance and an environment of human warmth and comfort.

REFERENCES AND SUGGESTED READINGS

General Electric CT/T Operator Manual.

General Electric CT/T Technology Continuum. Technical Performance of the CT/T system. General Electric Publication No. 4870.

General Electric Company. Computed Tomography. A Comprehensive Guide for Evaluating CT Systems. General Electric Publication No. 4873.

Haaga, J. R., Miraldi, F., MacIntyre, W., LiPuma, J., Bryan, P. J., and Wiesen, E. The effect of mAs variation upon computed tomography image quality as evaluated by in vivo and in vitro studies. Radiology 138:449–454, 1981.

Matsuda, H. Design of the medical environment. Radiology/Nuclear Medicine Magazine. CT Forum Update 81. October, 1981, pp. 6–9. W. G. Holdsworth and Associates, Mt. Prospect, Ill.

McCullough, E. C. X-ray transmission CT scanner survey, January 1982. Journal of Computed Assisted Tomography 6:423–428, 1982.

CHAPTER 8
IMAGE QUALITY, RESOLUTION, AND DOSAGE

IMAGE CLARITY (VISIBILITY) IN RADIOGRAPHY

Sharpness and Spatial Resolution
 Sharpness and Blur
 Spatial Resolution
Contrast
 Subject Contrast
 Film Contrast
 Radiation Scatter
Noise
 Film Grain
 Intensifying Screen Mottle

SPATIAL RESOLUTION IN COMPUTED TOMOGRAPHY

Geometric Limitations (Beam Size)
 Focal Spot Size
 Collimation
 Geometric Scale Factor
 Detector Aperture Size
Sampling
Image Reconstruction
Display Parameters
Mechanical Factors
 Mechanical Accuracy of Scanner
 Scan Speed
Measurements of Spatial Resolution
 Point Spread Function
 Line Spread Function
 Edge Response Function
 Modulation Transfer Function

CONTRAST RESOLUTION AND NOISE IN COMPUTED TOMOGRAPHY

Contrast Resolution
 General Description of Contrast
 Factors Determining Contrast
Noise
 Types of Noise
 Noise Power Spectrum (Wiener Spectrum)
 A Formula for Statistical Noise
Relationship between Noise, Matrix Size, Dose, and Section Thickness

Picture Grain (Noise)
Spatial Resolution (Matrix) and Grain
Patient Dose
Section Thickness

PATIENT DOSAGE IN COMPUTED TOMOGRAPHY

Basics of Radiation Exposure and Dosage
Parameters Affecting the Patient Dosage
Scanning Time
Scanner Geometry (Generations)
Scan Rotation Angle
X-Ray Beam Geometry
Detectors
Radiographic Factors
Image Quality Factors
Dosage Measurements (Dosimetry)
Dosimeters
Conditions and Techniques

ACCURACY AND RELIABILITY OF CT NUMBERS

CT Numbers and Linear Attenuation Coefficients
Basic Relationship
Contrast Scale
Basic Definitions
Accuracy of CT Numbers
Precision of CT Numbers
Linearity of CT Numbers
Spatial Uniformity
Factors Affecting the Reliability of CT Numbers

CT PHANTOMS

REFERENCES AND SUGGESTED READINGS

IMAGE CLARITY (VISIBILITY) IN RADIOGRAPHY

The quality of an image in computed tomography depends upon several parameters: spatial resolution, contrast, noise, and artifacts. Each of these in turn is determined or affected by a number of different factors. Some of these limiting factors are identical to those determining image quality in conventional radiography, for example, x-ray tube focal spot size. Other factors limiting the CT image quality may have analogues in conventional radiography, for example, detector or receptor limitations to spatial resolution. Other factors, such as image reconstruction artifacts and limitations, are peculiar to CT.

A knowledge of the basic concepts and problems associated with image clarity in conventional radiography provides a useful starting point for understanding the basic factors determining image quality in CT. Furthermore, many of the concepts, terms, and measurement parameters associated with radiographic image clarity are very pertinent to CT image quality.

The author has drawn on several excellent sources listed in the references, including the texts by Christensen, Curry, and Dowdey (1978) and by Sprawls (1977), and the classic papers of Rossman (1969a, 1969b).

Sharpness and Spatial Resolution

Sharpness and Blur Sharpness can be defined as the ability of an imaging system (x-ray recording film or a film-screen combination) to define an edge. The image of an edge on an x-ray film is not distinct but rather has a gradual change from the dark to the light area on each side. Sharpness and contrast (as discussed later) are interrelated, since even a sharp edge may not be well identified if the contrast is low, whereas both sharp and unsharp edges may be readily apparent if contrast is high.

Blur or blurring refers to the spreading of the image of a point. Blur generally causes two deleterious effects: the image of a point is "smeared out" or spread over a surrounding area of the film, and contrast is reduced. In the presence of significant blur the image has an unsharp appearance.

Another term used in describing an image is detail. This is basically a subjective characteristic of an image that describes its ability to show small objects or structural features. Image detail depends on three quantitative factors: blurring, contrast, and noise. Blur and noise reduce detail, as does poor contrast.

Focal Spot Blur (Geometric Blur) This arises because of the finite size of the x-ray tube focus. Since the focal spot is not a point but has a finite nonzero area, the x-rays originate from all points within the area of the focal spot. This leads to an "edge gradient" or "penumbra," which is a zone of blur or unsharpness that occurs at the edge of a shadow image.

If the object is in direct contact with the film, the blur associated with the focal spot disappears. When the object is moved away from the film toward the tube, the blur increases directly with the distance from the film.

Motion Blur Motion blur is almost invariably due to motion of the patient rather than of the imaging system (e.g., the x-ray tube). It is usually seen on examinations requiring longer exposure times, for example, on abdominal films rather than on chest films. This motion blur or unsharpness may be reduced by decreasing the exposure time and concomitantly increasing the x-ray tube current or mA for a given mAs.

Receptor Blur (Screen Blur) Radiographic film is much more sensitive to optical or light radiation than to x-rays. Intensifying screens are used to obtain an adequate film exposure or density with a reduced patient x-ray exposure or dose. The screens capture part of the incident x-ray beam and then convert a fraction of the captured beam into optical radiation, or light, which then exposes the film directly.

Luminescence describes the process of light emission by a substance, typically after absorption of a higher energy radiation such as x-rays or ultraviolet. A chemical reaction may also provide the stimulus. Fluorescence refers to the type of luminescence in which light emission occurs within 10^{-8} s after the stimulation, as in absorption of x-rays. Phosphorescence is used to describe the type of luminescence in which light emission is delayed beyond 10^{-8} s.

The term fluorescence as used in radiology refers to the capability of crystals of certain inorganic salts called phosphors to emit light after absorbing x-rays. The fluorescent material consists of small crystals suspended in a base material with a typical thickness of .1–.2 mm. Until the 1970s, the screens most commonly employed used calcium tungstate as the fluorescent material. Since the 1970s other materials, including rare earth salts, have replaced calcium tungstate because of their greater efficiency in converting x-rays to light.

The film and intensifying screen are contained in a cassette, which presses the film and screen together, maintaining good uniform contact between them. The finite or nonzero thickness of x-ray screens is a cause of blur because of light diffusion in the fluorescent layer of the screen. This is exacerbated by poor film-screen contact.

Usually the blur profile associated with the receptor is Gaussian in nature.

The amount of blur is a function of the thickness of the fluorescent layer of the screen. If the object is magnified by placing it closer to the tube and farther from the film, the absolute value of the receptor blur does not change, but its value relative to the magnified image decreases.

Absorption Blur Absorption blur occurs because most tissue borders within a patient are not sharp edges, particularly in curved surfaces. Absorption blur is not related to any limitation in the imaging process or system; rather, it is an inherent physical property of the object being imaged.

Parallax Blur This is a phenomenon seen only with double emulsion films. An image is present on each emulsion. The two images are separated by the thickness or width of the film base (typically .007 or .008 inches). These two images will overlap if they are viewed straight on; however, if the film is viewed from an angle the two images will not overlap exactly. Parallax blue is a negligible effect, making no significant contribution to image unsharpness.

Composite Blur Total blur in an image is a composite of the different types of blurring.

A generally accepted relationship for the composite or total blur is

$$B_C = \sqrt{B_G{}^2 + B_M{}^2 + B_R{}^2 + B_A{}^2 + B_P{}^2} \quad (8.1)$$

where B_C is composite blur, B_G is geometric blur, B_M is motion blur, B_R is receptor blur, B_A is absorption blur, and B_P is parallax blur. One source of blur may predominate, for example, the focal spot size. In this instance the composite blur is essentially equal to the predominant blur component.

Spatial Resolution

Relationship to Sharpness Sharpness refers to the capability of an imaging system to record sharply defined borders or abrupt edges. Spatial resolution refers to the capability of an imaging system to record a distinct image of two or more closely spaced, high contrast objects. As the distance separating two objects is decreased, the unsharp or blurred edges of the two objects begin to merge into one. The spatial resolution or resolving capability of the system is usually defined in terms of the minimum distance between the two high contrast objects at which they may be detected or identified as separate objects in the image.

The image resolution within any region in a radiograph is a measue of the sharpness of structures displayed in that region. The margins of small pointlike objects and edges are blurred in the imaging process. The spatial resolution is inversely related to this blurring. An increase in the blurring results in a decrease in the resolving capability. For small, pointlike objects, the minimum distance for which spatial resolution can be achieved is approximately equal to the width of the blur.

The spatial resolution is specified in terms of the number of line pairs per millimeter that can be resolved by the imaging system (in conventional radiography, a film-screen combination). A line pair consists of a line and a space. One lead strip and one adjacent space constitute an appropriate test object for the purpose of measuring the spatial resolution of an x-ray system. The test object consists of alternate opaque (lead) and radiolucent strips or bars of varying separations, the different spatial separations corresponding to different spatial frequencies.

Point Spread Function In a perfect imaging system, that is, one in which the image is an exact or perfect replication of the object, the radiant energy (x-rays in radiography) emanating from a point source in the object plane would be concentrated entirely in a corresponding point in the image plane (the ideal image point). In practical imaging systems the radiant energy associated with an object point produces a "smearing out" of the energy around the ideal image point. This results in a blurred or unsharp image of the object point source.

The point spread function is an indication of the blurring or degree of film exposure about the ideal image point. The maximum film exposure of a pointlike object is concentrated at the ideal image point. The relative film exposure as a function of the radial distance from the ideal image point (or from the center of the finite, nonzero area of a very small circle having the same size as the very small object circle) is an indication of the blurring. The more gradual the dropoff in film exposure, the wider the blur, and the more imperfect is the corresponding imaging system. The point spread function is an exposure profile that shows how the radiation passing through a single point (or, more practically, a small, pointlike object) in the object is spread over the surface of the film.

The point spread function or exposure profile of point may often be described in terms of a Gaussian function.

If the point spread function possesses rotational symmetry (in other words, it looks the same in any angular direction), it is termed isotropic. An anisotropic function lacks rotational symmetry (it is different in different angular directions).

The first suggested definition for resolution is the Rayleigh criterion, proposed by Lord John William Strutt Rayleigh (1842–1919). Point sources of light which underwent diffraction by lenses were being studied. There is a point spread function associated with the diffraction of such a point source, and this is characterized by a central peak surrounded by alternating concentric dark and light bands. Rayleigh's criterion states that two adjacent point sources (objects) can be resolved if the peak of the point spread function of one point source occurs at the first minimum of the point spread function for the other point source.

Line Spread Function A line spread function may also be defined to describe quantitatively the blurring or unsharpness associated with the image of an abrupt or sharp edge. The line spread function represents the radiation intensity distribution in the image of an infinitely narrow and infinitely long slit (line source). In a perfect imaging system, the radiant energy emanating from a line source in the object plane would be concentrated in a line in the image plane; that is, a line would be imaged as a line. In practical imaging systems there is a smearing out or blurring of the radiant energy (and film exposure) around the ideal line image, causing an unsharp or blurred image of the line source. The line spread function is a method of describing this unsharpness quantitatively.

In actual practice, the line spread function is determined by approximating an ideal line source by a long narrow slit formed between the two jaws of a metal that is highly opaque to x-rays. The width of the slit is typically 10 microns (.01 mm), and the metal jaws are about 2 mm thick. The slit is placed in contact with the film-screen combination and an exposure performed. The spread or blurring of the image line can be measured by determining the optical density or photographic effect on the film as a function of the linear distance from a line in the center of the slit image.

It can be demonstrated mathematically that the direct measurement of the line spread function is equivalent to scanning the point spread function with a narrow slit that is long compared to the point spread function. This is greatly simplified when the point spread function is isotropic. In this case the line spread function is independent of the orientation of the line source or narrow slit in the object plane (it is symmetric or independent of orientation). If the point spread function is anisotropic, the shape of the line spread function depends on the direction in which the point spread function is scanned.

Point spread functions describe the spreading or blurring of points, whereas line spread functions describe the spreading or blurring of lines. Although they may differ in shape, generally they have similar widths.

Modulation Transfer Function The modulation transfer function (MTF) is a means of providing a quantitative or graphical description of the blur and spatial resolution characteristics of an imaging system or of the individual components of the system. The term "modulation" refers to a change in the size (amplitude, intensity, or amount) of a signal. The MTF describes the response of an imaging system (or a component of an imaging system) to different spatial frequencies. As described in Chapter 5, any signal in either a time or a frequency domain may be expressed as a summation of a finite or infinite number of different frequency components. These frequency components are sinusoidal waves. They may be discretely separated (e.g., f_0, $2f_0$, $3f_0$, etc., where f_0 is a primary or fundamental frequency), or the frequencies may form a continuous spectrum. (Figure 5.9 illustrates this concept for a square wave.)

The spatial frequency components that define an object are determined by the shape of the object. Spatial frequencies are associated with the rate or abruptness of the change of an object's thickness. Consider a large, flat object of uniform thickness but with sharp edges or borders. Low spatial frequency components describe the large uniform portion of the object, but high spatial frequency components are required to define its sharp edges created by the abrupt changes in thickness. Small objects of a particular cross-sectional shape generally have higher frequency components than do large objects. An object in which the cross-sectional thickness varies abruptly will require more high frequency components for an adequate description than an object in which the cross-sectional thickness changes more gradually.

Any object being imaged may be described in terms of a group of spatial frequencies, and these are related to the changes in thickness that are responsible for producing image contrast. To form an accurate image of an object, the imaging system must be able to provide sufficient contrast for all the spatial frequencies describing the object. If certain spatial frequency components are lost or inadequately represented, the image will be distorted. For example, if the imaging system does not record the high frequency components, or if these high frequency components are reduced in amplitude relative to the low frequency components, the image will be blurred.

The MTF is a graph demonstrating the fractional contrast of a number of test objects or patterns. Each of these test patterns is a sinusoidally varying thickness of a radioopaque object of a given spatial frequency (the spatial repetition rate of the sinusoidally varying thickness of the object). The spatial frequency is expressed in cycles (of the sine wave) per millimeter. The fractional contrast, or contrast modilation, is the difference in x-ray transmission, or film exposure, between the thickest and thinnest parts of the phantom (the trough and crest of the sine waves). The fractional contrast of a test object is plotted against the spatial frequency of the test object.

Practically, the MTF is obtained by first measuring the line spread function for the imaging system and then performing a Fourier transformation. The line spread function actually represents the description of the response of the imaging system in the spatial domain, whereas MTF is the description in the frequency (spatial frequency) domain. The line spread function describes an intensity distribution in the spatial coordinate domain; the MTF characterizes this intensity distribution in terms of the amplitudes of its spatial frequency components. The Fourier transformation is the means for translating between these two languages (spatial coordinates and spatial frequencies).

Each component of an imaging system can be characterized by its own individual line spread or point spread function or MTF. Calculation of an output (the image) from an input (the object being imaged) in the spatial domain requires the application of a complex mathematical process called convolution. The image is obtained by convolving the object with the line spread function or the point spread function. Convolution essentially involves multiplying each point in the object intensity distribution by the system line spread (or point spread) function and summing over the entire object distribution.

In Fourier transformation theory, a convolution in the spatial domain becomes a simple multiplication in the spatial frequency domain, and the amplitude of each frequency component is simply multiplied by the value of the MTF for that frequency. Furthermore, the MTF for a complex imaging system is merely the product of the MTF of each component of the system. For each spatial frequency the individual MTFs at that frequency are multiplied to obtain the system MTF at that frequency. The MTF thus provides a convenient method for analyzing each component of a complex imaging system and estimating the effect of the system. Figure 8.1 illustrates component and composite MTFs.

The MTF of a complex system is determined by the component or components with the smallest individual MTFs. In a film-screen combination the resolution capabilities of x-ray film are far superior to those of intensifying screens. Therefore, the MTF of a film-screen combination is essentially equal to the MTF of the intensifying screens.

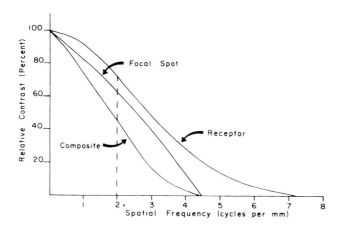

Figure 8.1. A composite MTF obtained by multiplying the MTFs associated with the focal spot and receptor. For example, at 2 cycles per mm, the MTF for the focal spot is 62% and that for the receptor is 72%. At this frequency the total system will have a composite MTF of 44%. (Reproduced by permission from P. Sprawls, Jr., The Physical Principles of Diagnostic Radiology. University Park Press, Baltimore, 1977.)

In addition to the contribution from the film-screen combination, the other significant MTFs contributing to the total system MTF are those associated with the focal spot size, magnification, and motion. The MTF is essentially independent of the x-ray beam quality (kVp).

Contrast

Contrast is one of the most important characteristics defining an image. Radiographic contrast is the difference in the film density or darkening in different regions of the radiograph. It is, of course, this difference in density or film darkening that constitutes the image.

The image contrast is the result of two components: subject contrast and film contrast. Subject contrast is the amount of contrast in the x-ray beam when it reaches the receptor. It is the difference in the x-ray intensity transmitted through one part of the subject (the patient) compared to the transmitted intensity through another part. Subject contrast may also be referred to as radiation contrast.

Film contrast is a photographic property of the x-ray film or of the film-screen combination. The x-ray film essentially converts subject contrast to radiographic contrast. The appropriate x-ray film and exposure conditions will amplify or increase subject contrast. Some film and exposure conditions, however, may decrease subject contrast.

Contrast is reduced by blurring because the image is spread over the surrounding background area.

Subject Contrast The factors determining subject contrast include differences in thickness, differences in mass density, differences in atomic number, and the x-ray photon energy or kVp.

Differences in Thickness As described in Chapter 2 and illustrated in Figures 2.4 and 2.5, the amount of attenuation of an x-ray beam is related to the thickness of the object through which the x-ray beam passes. If two objects composed of the same material but of different thicknesses are irradiated by the same x-ray beam, the thicker object will cause a greater attenuation of the x-ray beam.

Differences in Mass Density A very significant factor for increasing subject contrast is difference in mass density. The mass density is the amount of mass (usually expressed in grams) per unit volume (usually expressed in cubic centimeters). An illustrative example that has been used by Christensen et al. (1978) is that of water and ice. Ice floats in water and so is less dense; water in fact is about 9% denser than the ice. An equal thickness of both water and ice will result in 9% more x-ray attenuation by the water than by the ice; hence there will be subject contrast between them. The strong dependence of x-ray attenuation on tissue density was illustrated earlier in Figure 2.6.

Differences in Atomic Number The photoelectric effect described in Chapter 2 is the most important factor contributing to subject contrast. The effect depends upon the third power of the effective atomic number Z of a material, as described earlier in Equation 2.5, so that it is extremely sensitive to even small differences in the effective atomic number. Contrast material containing elements with high atomic numbers such as iodine ($Z = 53$) and barium ($Z = 56$) are used to provide high subject contrast for structures or organs in which they become localized.

X-Ray Photon Energy or Radiation Quality The radiation quality, or kVp, is a very significant factor in the penetrating capability of the x-ray beam. For a higher kVp more of the x-ray photons possess a higher energy. If the kVp is high enough, relatively little x-ray attenuation occurs; there is little subject contrast. If the kVp is decreased, more of the x-ray beam is attenuated, particularly by bone. Subject contrast is improved by low kVp, providing the kVp is sufficiently high to provide enough penetration for adequate film exposure.

The maximum effect of radiation quality occurs when the average value of the photons in the x-ray beam is just above the threshold for a photoelectric effect. This is described by Equation 2.4.

Film Contrast Radiographic film produces an image which is to be viewed as a transparency (light passing from a viewbox through the film to the viewer's eyes) rather than as a print (light reflected off the film to the viewer's eyes). There are a number of significant parameters characteristic of the film itself which affect the contrast as well as the overall clarity of the radiographic image.

Density (film density) is a quantity used to describe the degree of opacity of a film (i.e. the film darkening). Light penetration P through the film may be defined by the expression

$$P = \frac{I}{I_0}, \quad (8.2)$$

where I_0 is the incident light intensity entering the film and I is the light transmitted by the film. The definition of density is given by

$$D = -\log P = -\log \frac{I}{I_0} = \log \frac{I_0}{I}. \quad (8.3)$$

The penetration may also be expressed in terms of the density, by solving Equation 8.2 for P

$$P = 10^{-D}. \quad (8.4)$$

From Equations 8.2 and 8.3, if a region of the film only transmits 10% of the light incident on it ($I = .1\,I_0$), then the penetration is .1 and the density of the film in that region is 1 ($\log I_0/I = \log 10/1 = 1$). If a region of the film only transmits 1% of the light, the penetration is reduced to .01, and the film density in this region is 2.

Thus, a change in the film density by 1 unit corresponds to a change in the light penetration (and brightness) by a factor of 10. Higher values of film density correspond to blacker regions on the film. Typically, the density in radiographic film ranges from about .2 to more than 3. For higher values, normal viewbox light will not adequately penetrate the film, and brightlighting the film is required.

There are several reasons for expressing film density on a logarithmic scale. First, logarithms are a convenient way of expressing large differences in numbers or values. Second, the subjective response to changes in brightness, or, more accurately, the physiological response of the eye to different light intensities, is logarithmic. Finally, the use of logarithms permits single addition of superimposed densities. If films are superimposed, the total density is the sum of the density of each film.

During an exposure, the individual silver halide crystals (90–99% silver bromide, 1–10% silver iodide) suspended in a layer of gelatin as an emulsion absorb some of the incident photons. Since intensifying screens are normally employed, most of the absorbed photons are light photons; a small fraction (about a couple of percent) of the absorbed photons are actually x-ray photons that have penetrated the screen and are absorbed directly by the film.

The silver halide molecules are contained in small crystals called grains, which are of the order of .001 mm in size. Larger grains increase the sensitivity of the film to light but also increase the film graininess (noise) in the final radiography, especially with magnification.

The photographic or radiosensitive emulsions of silver halide crystals is coated on a transparent plastic sheet or base. Single emulsion films coat only one side of the base; double emulsion films coat both sides.

During exposure, silver ions may be converted into clumps of metallic silver in one or more centers in a crystal grain. These clumps constitute latent image centers. This latent image is not a visible image; film processing is required.

The exposed film is immersed in a developer solution that converts other silver ions into silver atoms in those grains that have received sufficient exposure and contain latent image centers. The silver atoms in each such grain combine to form an opaque speck. The developing process increases the number of free silver atoms in the latent image in a speck by a factor approximating 10^8. On the final processed film, the radiographic contrast is the density difference between image areas in the radiograph.

The film density is a function of the x-ray intensity to which the film-screen combination is subjected. Variations in the incident x-ray intensity are responsible for the differences in the film density or contrast.

Since the number of photons in the x-ray beam is determined by the exposure, the film density can be related to the exposure. The change in the film density with exposure can be plotted as the characteristic curve, or Hurter and Driffield (H and D) curve, of the film. This curve is named after F. Hurter and V. C. Driffield, who published the first such curve in England in 1890.

A characteristic curve, as illustrated in Figure 8.2, has three different sections. The end at lower exposure values is horizontal, having zero slope. The density in this portion of the curve is a combination of the inherent density of the film base material and a slight amount of fog caused by development of unexposed grains of silver halide in the emulsion. This is referred to as the base plus fog. The steep midline portion is the portion corresponding to the maximum transfer of contrast. The steeper the curve (the greater the slope) in this region, the greater the contrast of the film. The uppermost portion, where the curve again becomes horizontal, corresponds to the maximum density the film can produce. Maximum image contrast (subject or radiation contrast converted to film contrast) is achieved by using an exposure such that the object being imaged as well as the background lie on the steep mid-portion of the curve.

A density range of .25 to 2.0 above base plus fog is generally felt to be the useful for normal viewing on a viewbox. This range can be extended by brightlighting (Figure 8.2).

Useful parameters to describe the contrast characteristic of a film are the gamma value and the average gradient. The gamma value is the maximum slope of the characteristic curve. The average gradient is the average slope between two designated densities, usually .25 and 2.0. Another useful film parameter is the latitude, which is the range of exposure values corresponding to the useful density range (Figure 8.2). Generally, the latitude of a film varies inversely with the film contrast.

The sensitivity and contrast characteristics of a film also depend on the processing. The degree of film processing is generally determined by the chemical activity of the developer solution, the developer temperature, and the time of film immersion in the developer. Close adherence to the recommended values of these factors is necessary if the ultimate potential image quality and contrast are to be realized.

Radiation Scatter Radiation scatter is produced primarily by Compton scatter. This scattered radiation intercepting the film or film-screen combination causes film blackening without providing any signal or image information. There is an unwanted increase in film density without any concomitant increase in the contrast. Scatter actually reduces the contrast which comprises the image.

Radiation scatter is increased with increasing subject thickness, the size of the field of exposure, and a higher kVp of the x-ray beam, because the number of photoelectric interactions will decrease relative to the number of Compton interactions at

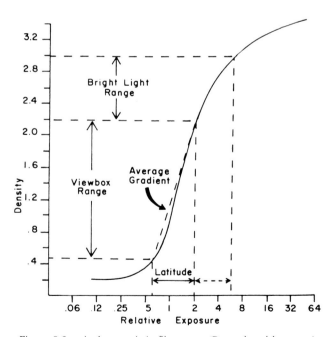

Figure 8.2. A characteristic film curve (Reproduced by permission from P. Sprawls, Jr., The Physical Principles of Diagnostic Radiology. University Park Press, Baltimore, 1977.)

higher kVp. The scatter may be decreased by collimating the x-ray beam so that a smaller field is exposed. The use of grids or air gaps also decreases scatter, but at the cost of a higher exposure or dose.

Noise

The random variation in the film density or darkening is referred to as noise or mottle. Noise is an undesirable effect. It would be preferable to have the film density uniform except for changes or variations related solely to the formation of an image. Other factors, however, will contribute an irregular mottled appearance to the film that is easily visualized. Radiographic noise or mottle may arise from one of three causes: graininess is a property of the x-ray film; structure mottle and quantum mottle arise from the radiographic intensifying screens.

Film Grain In the processes of exposure and development, the silver halide crystals of the film exposed to radiation are converted to silver crystals. Usually the film graininess is not detectable with the naked eye, except perhaps in situations such as cineradiography where the image is enlarged, but the individual silver crystals or grains may be detected with magnification. Even in these circumstances, film graininess is not the major factor contributing to the total noise, and in conventional radiographs the grain of the film is not seen.

Intensifying Screen Mottle

Screen Structure Mottle Variations in the size or distribution of the individual small crystals in the intensifying screens, or defects such as varying thickness or physical imperfections in the phosphor screens, can contribute to the radiographic mottle or noise. Because of the strict quality control in the manufacture of intensifying screens, this effect is usually negligible.

Quantum Mottle (Photon Fluctuation) The third and only really important cause of image noise or radiographic mottle is quantum mottle (quantum noise). This type of noise is due to the random variation in the number of photons absorbed by the intensifying screens. In other words, quantum mottle is the statistical photon fluctuation in the number of x-ray quanta absorbed per unit area by the intensifying screen.

The x-ray beam is not a homogeneous or uniform flow of x-ray energy. Rather, it is composed of individual discrete x-ray photons or quanta. The intensifying screen is then being showered by a stream of particles. There is a random variation in the number of photons striking each small area of the screen, similar to the random variation in the number of raindrops striking different adjacent areas during a rainstorm. Superimposed on this background pattern of noise are the larger fluctuations in the number of incident photons over larger areas due to variations in the absorption or attenuation of x-rays by intervening objects.

The number of photons impinging on equal areas will fluctuate about an average or smear value. The standard deviation or magnitude of the random fluctuation about this mean value is governed by statistical law (a Gaussian probability). The standard deviation is equal to the square root of the average number of photons, or

$$\sigma = \sqrt{N}, \quad (8.5)$$

where σ is the standard deviation and N represents the average number of photons striking equal areas. Most of the areas (68% by Gaussian statistics) will then be struck by a number of photons in the range $N - \sqrt{N}$ to $N + \sqrt{N}$. Thirty-two percent of the areas will be outside this range. Ninety-five percent will be within 2 standard deviations of the average. For example, if 100 photons on the average strike each area of the screen, 68% of the areas will intercept from 90 ($100 - \sqrt{100} = 100 - 10$) to 110 ($100 + \sqrt{100} = 100 + 10$) photons. Ninety-five percent of the areas will intercept from 80 ($100 - 2\sqrt{100} = 100 - 20$) to 120 ($100 + 2\sqrt{100} = 100 + 20$) photons.

Now consider the percent fluctuation in the number of photons striking each small area. This is equal to

$$\frac{\sqrt{N}}{N} \times 100 = \frac{1}{\sqrt{N}} \times 100. \quad (8.6)$$

This means that as the average number of photons striking each area of the screen increases, the percent or relative fluctuation will decrease. This is illustrated in Table 8.1, which shows that the relative fluctuation

Table 8.1. Change of fluctuations with increasing number of photons

N	$\sqrt{N}$	$\dfrac{1}{\sqrt{N}} \times 100$
10	3.2	32
100	10	10
1000	32	3.2
10,000	100	1

or noise is decreased with an increasing flux of photons.

SPATIAL RESOLUTION IN COMPUTED TOMOGRAPHY

The main factors determining spatial resolution in CT are listed in Table 8.2.

Geometric Limitations (Beam Size)

Focal Spot Size The x-ray photons used to create a CT image do not arise from a point source but from a finite area. Analysis of the effect of the size of the focal spot on the resolution of the final image is further complicated by the fact that the emitted x-ray intensity along the focal spot is not homogeneous. To simplify the description of the effect of focal spot size on spatial resolution, it is often helpful to assume a uniform distribution of x-ray intensity arising from the focal spot.

The effect of the focal spot size on image distortion is modified by a number of factors, including the x-ray intensity distribution along the focal spot, the collimator width, the size of the object being imaged, the relative position of the object between the focal spot and the detector aperture (the ratio of focus-detector distance to focus-object distance), the size of the detector aperture, and the detector response profile (the response of the detector along its area). Thus, there is an interdependence of the different geometric factors in the determination of spatial resolution (and of the geometric factors with the other nongeometric contributions of spatial resolution). The effective dimensions of the focal spot size are further determined or limited by entrance collimation between the x-ray tube and patient.

Table 8.2. Factors limiting spatial resolution in CT

Geometric limitations (beam size)
    Focal spot size
    Collimator width (section thickness)
    Geometric scale factor
    Detector aperture size
Sampling
Image reconstruction
    filter function
    reconstruction matrix
Display parameters
Mechanical factors
    Mechanical accuracy of scanner
    Scan speed

A simple example that helps to explain the effect of focal spot size (and other geometric factors) in determining spatial resolution is to consider a single point object which is to be imaged. The point object is located between the tube focus and the detector. The point object will intercept a ray or straight line corresponding to the path of x-ray photons originating from each point of the x-ray focus. There will be a theoretically infinite number of such straight lines. Each line arises from a different point on the x-ray tube focus and passes through the object point before striking the detector. Since the rays or lines arising from different points on the x-ray focus strike different points along the detector, the point object becomes spread out or "smeared" over the detector. A point is no longer imaged as a point. The larger the focal spot area, the larger the area over which rays passing though the point object will originate, and the greater the resulting spread of the image of the point object.

Several other properties related to the focal spot will influence the image. The size, shape, and intensity distribution of the image of the point object will be modified not only by the size of the focal spot, but by its shape or configuration and the x-ray intensity profile distribution of the focus. Actually, the radiation arising from every point on the focus follows the inverse square law (the intensity or energy flux per square centimeter), so that there is a variation of intensity with the length of the different paths through the point object.

Collimation Narrow collimation for thin sections further limits the effective size of the x-ray focal spot that is used in the dimension corresponding to the scan section thickness. Decreasing the section thickness also permits improved imaging of fine spatial detail. Structures occupying only a small part of the total thickness of a section may show deterioration in image detail related to partial volume effect. The voxels of a thicker section may include not only the small structures of interest but also the overlying separate tissues. Even if the structure of interest occupies the entire section thickness, the detail of rapid or abrupt variations in the structure over the section thickness may be lost. An example is the middle ear, where the fine spatial detail of the small structures in question requires the use of thinner sections.

Geometric Scale Factor Both the x-ray intensity distribution of the x-ray focal spot and the response profile of the detector must be appropriately scaled by an amount depending on their geometric projections at the position of each point to be imaged.

Consider again the imaging of a single point object. If the point to be imaged lies against the detector, all rays drawn from the different points of the tube focus through the point object will fall on the same point on the detector. As the point object is brought closer to the tube focus, the different rays from the points of the x-ray tube focus through the point object will diverge more and the point object will become more smeared.

The magnification M of a finite object (not a point) is equal to the focal spot-detector distance divided by the focal spot-object distance. The focal spot-detector distance is equal to the sum of the focal spot-object and the object-detector distances. The focal spot size is divided by a scaling factor which is equal to the focal spot detector distance divided by the object-detector distance. This is equal to a value of $M/(M - 1)$. The detector aperture is divided by a scaling factor equal to M.

Detector Aperture Size The detector aperture size is typically the most significant of the geometric factors determining spatial resolution in CT. Its closest analog in conventional radiography is receptor blurring.

The measurement of the spatial variation of a physical parameter (e.g., x-ray intensity) is limited by the size of the detector used in measurement. Rapid or abrupt spatial variations that occur over only a fraction of the dimension of the detector will be averaged out, with a resulting loss of spatial detail. A smaller detector will measure and record the parameter in question over smaller distances and is better able to identify more rapid spatial changes.

As an example, consider a row of metal pins irradiated by a flux of x-rays (Figure 8.3). The pins are of equal size, and the spacing between their centers is constant. The row of pins is constructed so that the distance between their centers equals twice the width of the pins; that is, the space between two pins is equal to the width of a pin. The incident x-rays will be assumed to be parallel. The row of pins produces a variation in the spatial distribution, or a

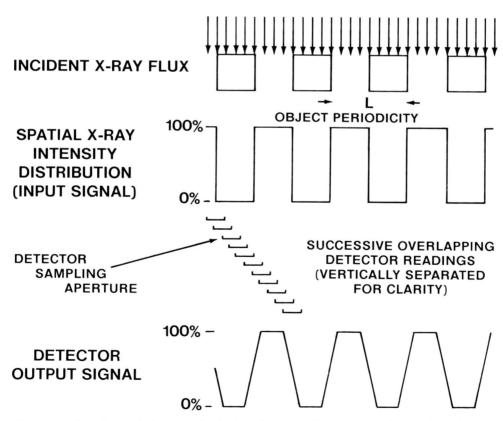

Figure 8.3. Sampling of the intensity distribution of x-rays incident on a row of pins, using a detector with an aperture much smaller than the pin spacing. (Reproduced from General Electric Publication No. 4870, with the permission of General Electric Medical Systems.)

modulation, of the x-ray beam. It is assumed that the x-rays are completely absorbed by the pins and pass without any attenuation through the spaces between the pins. The minimum value of the spatial x-ray intensity distribution is 0%, and the maximum value is 100%.

In Figure 8.3 this spatially varying or modulated x-ray intensity is being sampled with a detector whose aperture is small compared to the spacing L between the pins. A normally important consideration is the spacing or incrementation between samples. To eliminate this important (and practical) factor, the sampling will be performed at extremely small increments. A small increment is one that is significantly less than the aperture size. All other factors, including focal spot size and scaling factor, will be considered negligible. Under these circumstances, the output signal approximates the input signal (an even closer approximation would be achieved by sampling more frequently, at smaller increments, but this would of course necessitate more separate measurements and a greater exposure). There is a minimal broadening of the signal. The amplitude of the output signal is equal to the amplitude of the input signal. The output signal or image closely resembles the input or spatial x-ray intensity distribution; it has a square wave appearance.

Now suppose that the detector aperture is increased so that it is now about equal to about half the spacing between the pins; in other words, the aperture size is increased to approximately $L/2$. This is illustrated in Figure 8.4. The larger aperture distorts the image associated with each pin, so that the output more nearly approximates a sawtooth appearance rather than a square wave. The effect of widening the aperture is to remove the higher spatial frequencies that are required to reproduce the sharp or abrupt edges associated with a square wave. The larger aperture has resulted in a broadening of the individual pins. There is also a reduction in the amplitude of

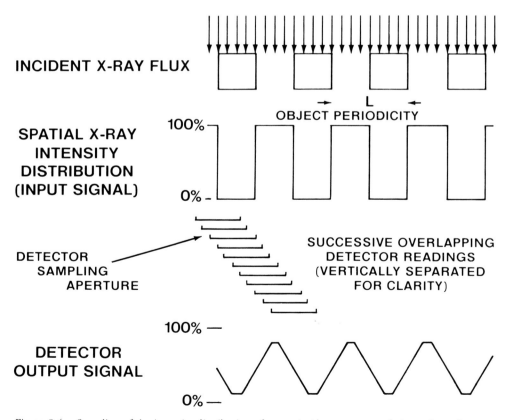

Figure 8.4. Sampling of the intensity distribution of x-rays incident on a row of pins, using a detector with an aperture approximately half the size of the pin spacing. (Reproduced from General Electric Publication No. 4870, with the permission of General Electric Medical Systems.)

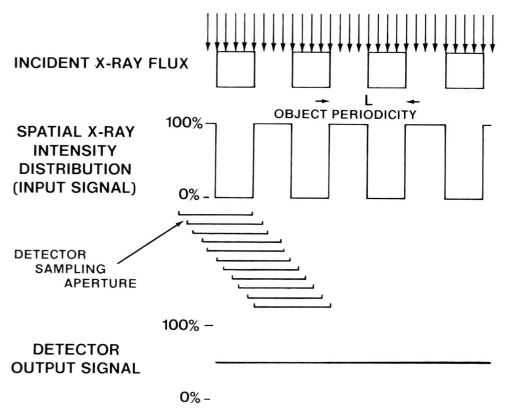

Figure 8.5. Sampling of the intensity distribution of x-rays incident on a row of pins, using a detector with an aperture equal to the pin spacing. (Reproduced from General Electric Publication No. 4870, with the permission of General Electric Medical Systems.)

the output signal, so that the modulation is less than 1. The increasing detector aperture width has introduced a significant distortion in the image.

When the detector aperture is increased so that it is equal to the pin spacing, or the primary object spatial frequency, the output signal becomes flat, as shown in Figure 8.5. There is no modulation to the output, regardless of how or where the measurements are performed, because wherever the detector is positioned, 50% of the detector aperture intercepts x-rays and 50% does not. The image distortion has been further increased.

A further increase in the detector aperture size will again result in modulation, but it will be reversed in polarity compared to the incident x-ray intensity distribution. This introduces another significant distortion.

Thus, the image distortion is increased as the detector aperture size is decreased, until a critical aperture size is reached, at which point no modulation is detected. In the example shown in Figures 8.3–8.5, this occurred when the detector aperture became equal to L, the periodic spacing of the pins. From the viewpoint of the spatial frequency domain, increasing the detector aperture size corresponds to distorting or eliminating entirely higher spatial frequency components greater than $1/A$, where A is the aperture size. When the aperture is increased to L, the primary frequency $1/L$ of the square wave represented by the pins is distorted and no longer present in the image.

Consider now a detector aperture of fixed size, a more realistic situation for a practical CT scanner. Typical aperture sizes are of the order of 1–4 mm. The aperture size places an upper limit on the spatial frequencies that can be displayed. The upper limit or critical frequency f_c is $1/A$, where A is the aperture size.

The discussion on detector aperture size has assumed that other factors determining spatial resolution, in particular, the sampling frequency, were negligible. The incrementation between samples has

Image Quality, Resolution, and Dosage

been taken as significantly less than the detector aperture size. From the previous discussion it is obvious that a high sample rate will not increase f_c. Theoretically, however, a deconvolution of the measured data in an attempt to undo the convolution effect of a wide aperture may eliminate some of the effects of the wide aperture widths. This involves the application of a mathematical filter that emphasizes the high spatial frequencies to compensate for high resolution loss in the measurement system due to the wide aperture. Noise considerations, however, may limit this technique.

Sampling

The data sampling rate or frequency refers to the spacing between the rays (individual data measurements) in each view (profile or projection). It is a spatial rate or frequency referring to the distance or spacing incrementation between data samples, that is, the number of data samples performed per unit of distance. The Nyquist sampling theorem states that an adequate reproduction or imaging of an object can be achieved if the spacing between data samples is less than half that associated with the highest spatial frequency contained in the object; that is, the spatial sampling frequency must be more than twice the highest spatial frequency in the data being measured. The maximum frequency that can be demonstrated is the Nyquist frequency.

The Nyquist sampling theorem can be grasped intuitively, without the need of a sophisticated mathematical derivation. If a sine wave spatial frequency is to be portrayed, the sinusoidal wave should be sampled at least once in both the positive and negative parts of the cycle (the crest and the trough of the wave). That is, a minimum of two samples per spatial cycle must be performed, so that the minimum sampling rate must be twice the frequency of the highest spatial frequency that is to be identified. The limit to spatial resolution from sampling, as determined by the Nyquist theorem, is equal to twice the spacing or distance between data measurements or rays. The corresponding Nyquist spatial frequency is one-half the sampling frequency.

The data sampling rate is often the ultimate limiting factor in spatial resolution for third generation scanners, in which both the tube and the detectors rotate. In these units the ray spacing or distance between data samples that represents the Nyquist sampling limit is fixed; it is the distance between the centers of the detector element. Twice this distance is equal to twice the sum of the detector aperture width and the intervening cell wall (the electrode). Thus, the detector aperture is less than half the distance which represents the Nyquist sampling limit to spatial resolution.

In translational-rotational units (first and second generation scanning geometries) and in rotating tube-fixed detector systems (fourth generation scanning geometry), the sampling frequency can be changed by acquiring more data. In translational-rotational units this is achieved by taking more measurements (more closely spaced rays) during each translation. In rotating tube-fixed detector systems, more measurements or rays are obtained during the rotation. In both cases the spacing between rays or data samples is decreased. This is done because units employing first, second, and fourth generation scanning geometries usually have larger detector apertures than do third generation units.

When the detector aperture and x-ray focus size are extremely small so that they do not contribute significantly to broadening effects in the image, then the limit to spatial resolution is usually determined by the sampling rate (i.e., the Nyquist frequency).

If there are spatial frequencies in the object greater than the Nyquist frequency, these frequencies are responsible for an artifact termed "aliasing." The sampled values for two waves whose respective frequencies are just below and just above the Nyquist frequency are identical. The two waves are thus completely indistinguishable. The higher frequency wave seems to have the appearance of the lower frequency as an "alias." This is the basic effect of the aliasing artifact: the high spatial frequency (greater than the Nyquist frequency) information in the object appears as low frequency information in the image. This is false information resulting from undersampling. Aliasing artifacts are decreased in theory and in practice by decreasing the sample spacing (increasing the spatial frequency). Aliasing is discussed further in Appendix I, which deals with artifacts.

Image Reconstruction

Image reconstruction algorithms using the technique of filtered back projection involve two operations. The first employs the use of an appropriate mathematical function called a convolution kernel or filter to perform a convolution or filtering of the projection data. The second process is the back-projection and summation of the convolved data.

As described in Chapter 5, two frequently employed convolution kernels are those described by Ramachandran and Lakshminarayanan in 1971 and by Shepp and Logan in 1974. These convolution kernels are proportional to the spatial frequency for lower spatial frequencies. They eliminate or reduce the contributions from frequencies above a cutoff value, usually selected as the Nyquist spatial sampling frequency.

Details of convolution kernels employed in commercial CT scanners are proprietary. Variations in these kernels and in the cutoff frequency can change the resolution and noise characteristics.

Following convolution, back-projection is performed onto a two-dimensional matrix of pixels. As a general rule, the pixel size approximates half the width of the point response function determined by the scanner geometry and convolution kernel.

The field of view or reconstruction circle is the area in which reconstruction is to be performed. It is usually circular, sometimes ovoid, and contains the object to be reconstructed. The field of view and the pixel size are the fundamental quantities in the reconstruction matrix.

Interpolation techniques are used to estimate the contribution of a particular ray to a specific pixel when the ray does not line up with a pixel in the reconstruction matrix. These have been described as zero-order and first-order.

Further improvement in spatial resolution can be achieved by a process called "target reconstruction." A portion of the image, not the entire body, is reconstructed in a smaller field of view. This is not simply magnification or image enlargement. The spatial frequency response of the convolution kernel is extended to match a new smaller display pixel size. The back projection is carried out on pixels as small as .25 mm. This is illustrated in Figure 8.6.

Display Parameters

Limitations in the video display or in the hard copy format may degrade the spatial resolution. Generally, video systems are well designed and are not a limiting factor in spatial resolution.

The video display and its associated memories should be capable of adequately displaying the pixel matrix. Sometimes a coarser display matrix may be used in a monitor not requiring as accurate a display. For example, the operator display console of a General Electric CT/T 8800 system reproduces the image

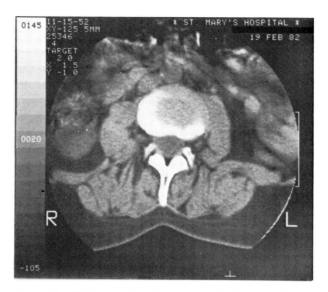

Figure 8.6. High resolution CT scan of the lumbar spine for soft tissue detail.

on a 160 × 160 matrix rather than the 320 × 320 matrix used in the viewer system display console.

Mechanical Factors

Mechanical Accuracy of Scanner The mechanical accuracy of the scanner relative to the position of rays and views may also contribute to spatial resolution. Whether the spatial resolution determined by geometric, sampling, reconstruction, and display factors is realized depends upon the accuracy with which the data are collected.

Scan Speed A result of increasing scan speed is to eliminate or reduce some of the effects associated with patient motion. With a reduction in scanning time, the effects of patient breathing during scanning can usually be eliminated entirely. Involuntary or uncontrolled motions of the head or torso, as well as peristalsis, may still cause image deterioration. However, with faster scanning times it is easier to confine these motions to the time between scans, or even to repeat selected scans that are unsatisfactory.

Although the image deterioration and problems associated with motion are more properly described as artifact, there is a loss in spatial resolution associated with many of these motion artifacts. For that reason this type of image deterioration is analogous to motion blur in conventional radiography.

Motion artifacts are discussed in Appendix I.

Image Quality, Resolution, and Dosage

Measurements of Spatial Resolution

In CT as in conventional radiography or any other imaging technique, spatial resolution specifies what the minimum distance between two small, high contrast objects must be in order to detect them as separate objects. A high contrast difference of the objects from their background is necessary so that noise does not affect the recognition and delineation of the corresponding images of the objects.

The point spread function, line spread function, and MTF used in conventional radiography provide useful means for describing the spatial resolution characteristics in CT as well. An edge spread function may also be useful in characterizing a CT system.

Point Spread Function The most commonly used criterion for the spatial resolution of an imaging system in terms of its point spread function is the width of the point spread function at half its maximum value. This is referred to as the full width at half-maximum (FWHM).

As discussed earlier, the point spread function may be anisotropic, that is, lacking in spatial symmetry so that it changes appearance when viewed from different directions. It may also vary from the center to the edge of the image. In well designed CT systems, the point spread function should be isotropic (spatially symmetrical) and independent of position.

The point spread function for a CT system may be measured by scanning a dense narrow wire aligned perpendicular to the scanning section. The use of a wire rather than a small, dense, pointlike object will assure that the object being measured occupies the full thickness of the scanning section. This will minimize partial volume effects by distributing the density of the object throughout the entire thickness of the portion of the scanning section that the object occupies. The wire diameter must be smaller than a pixel. If it is sufficiently dense and narrow, the wire will approximate a point object. The image of this pointlike object will then approximate the point response or point spread function of the CT scanner. A number of wires should be placed at different locations in the scan section so that the relative position of the wire in the pixel (or overlapping adjacent pixels) can be randomized and then averaged.

Line Spread Function The line spread function is a description of the distribution of radiation intensity that results from imaging a straight line object of infinitesimal width by an imaging system that creates two-dimensional images. This function may be obtained from the point spread function by performing a mathematical integration over the point spread function. The line spread function may also be measured directly by scanning a phantom in the form of a thin object in a water bath. A valid estimate of the line function using this method requires that the object be thin compared to the resolution of a CT scanner.

The line spread function may also be obtained indirectly from the measured edge response or step response function, as described below.

Edge Response Function The edge response function, or step response function, describes the image of a straight boundary between adjacent regions of high and low x-ray transmission. A dense plate with a perfectly planar edge should be used, oriented so that the plane of the edge is exactly parallel to the x-rays and perpendicular to the scan section. If the edge is not exactly perpendicular to the scan section, partial volume effects will influence the measurement. If metal is used, sampling artifacts may occur which can affect the measurement.

The line spread function is a spatial derivative (a mathematical function indicating the x-ray intensity) of the edge response function along the direction perpendicular to the edge. If the edge is lined up exactly perpendicular to the direction of the rows or columns of pixels, the entire change from maximum to minimum might occur in a few pixels. This may not provide enough information to calculate an accurate line spread function. By aligning the edge at a slight angle to the direction of either the pixel rows or columns, so that the boundary is shifted by one pixel in 10 or 20 rows or columns, there is some magnification of the edge response through a partial volume effect. This permits a more accurate measurement of the edge response and therefore the line spread function.

Modulation Transfer Function The MTF is a useful concept for describing spatial resolution in CT as well as in conventional radiography. The amplitude of the output signal is measured for a sinusoidal wave input signal as a function of the sinusoidal spatial frequency of the input. The output modulation, or ratio of the output amplitude to the input amplitude, is plotted against the input frequency. The ratio is normalized or adjusted so that its value at zero frequency is equal to 1. Figure 8.7 illustrates MTF curves for General Electric CT/T 7800 and 8800 systems.

The point spread function and line spread function are spatial coordinate descriptions of the re-

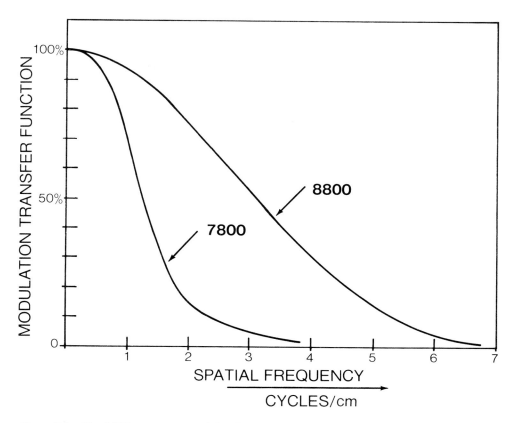

Figure 8.7. The MTF curves measured for the General Electric CT/T 7800 system and CT/T 8800 systems, by M. Trefler, University of Miami, and E. Goodenough and K. Weaver, George Washington University, respectively. The CT/T 7800 MTF was measured using 1.3-mm pixels, and the CT/T 8800 MTF was measured using 0.8-mm pixels. (Reproduced from General Electric Publication No. 4870, with the permission of General Electric Medical Systems.)

sponse of an imaging system. The MTF is a spatial frequency description. As discussed earlier, Fourier transform techniques provide the means for translating back and forth between these two languages.

The MTF is usually calculated from the point spread function or line spread function rather than measured directly. It is also possible to attempt an approximate direct measurement of the MTF by using phantoms containing periodic structures at different spatial separations (corresponding to different spatial frequencies). One example is the Siemens type of star or sunburst phantom. This consists of tapered wedges, typically of Lucite or nylon, which converge toward a common center. Air, water, or another fluid may fill the spaces between consecutive wedges. The spaces are equal to the wedges. The farther the distance from the center of the circle or segment of wedges, the greater the spacing between the wedges. Thus, the phantom is a periodic structure of decreasing spatial frequency as a function of distance from the center. The resolution is determined by measuring the diameter of the circle within which the structure blurs and cannot be distinguished. The total number of wedge/space pairs divided by the circumference (or portion of the circumference if only a segment is used) at the radius at which the structure blurs represents the frequency of disappearance.

The MTF is defined for sinusoidally varying input signals. Such signals are difficult to obtain for imaging systems, unlike in electric or audio systems. More typically, square wave or bar patterns (periodic structures characterized by abrupt edges or boundaries) are used. The transfer function obtained with this type of phantom or spatial pattern is called a contrast transfer function (CTF). It is related to but not identical to the MTF. Thus the true MTF is not usually measured.

This type of bar or square wave pattern is often used in practice to measure spatial resolution in CT scanners. Phantoms of this type have been built to the specifications of the American Association of Physicists in Medicine and the Bureau of Radiological Health. Typically, the phantom contains water-filled bars or holes in Plexiglas at different periodic spacings (spatial frequencies).

An important feature of the MTF is the method by which the individual MTFs of different components of an imaging system are cascaded together by simple multiplication to give the composite MTF for the imaging system, as described earlier in this chapter. In contrast, a composite point spread function for an imaging system entails the relatively complicated mathematical technique of convolution of the individual point spread functions associated with each component of the system. This situation occurs because of a mathematical theorem which states that a convolution in the coordinate description becomes a multiplication in the spatial frequency description.

An imaging system with high spatial resolution will be characterized by a narrow point spread function (small FWHM) and a broad MTF (good or nonzero response) at higher spatial frequencies.

CONTRAST RESOLUTION AND NOISE IN COMPUTED TOMOGRAPHY

Contrast Resolution

General Description of Contrast Contrast resolution refers to the capability of the CT scanner to detect an object with a small difference in the linear attenuation coefficient in relation to a homogeneous background. Contrast resolution is a function of both the size and the shape of the object. Phantoms designed to measure contrast resolution usually employ objects with circular images, either spheres or cylinders, that extend through part or all of the tomographic section.

Contrast resolution is typically expressed in one of two ways: as the smallest difference in x-ray attenuation that can be discriminated for an object of a particular diameter, or as the smallest diameter of an object with a particular contrast that can be detected. Usually the primary limitation in detecting a small difference in contrast between an object and its background is determined by noise. The threshold for contrast resolution or detection of circular objects in a homogeneous background occurs when the contrast of the signal is about 10 times the amplitude of the pixel noise (Zatz, 1978). Signal contrast and size vary inversely at the detection threshold. A low contrast object (relative to a homogeneous background) can be identified only if it is large, whereas small objects can be identified if they have high contrast.

In comparison to conventional radiography, CT is much more sensitive to small differences in x-ray attenuation. Thus, a smaller contrast difference may be measured by CT than by conventional radiography; in other words, CT has greater contrast resolution than conventional radiography. It is this capability for high contrast resolution, as in delineating soft tissue structures, that is perhaps the most important single characteristic of CT. A higher degree of spatial resolution, on the other hand, can be achieved with conventional radiography than with CT because of the high spatial resolution characteristics of film-screen combinations.

Factors Determining Contrast Factors determining contrast in CT are listed in Table 8.3.

Subject (Inherent) Contrast CT, like conventional radiography, is an imaging technique in which the images are based on the detection and recording of contrast differences. The fundamental parameter measured in both conventional radiography and CT is the intensity of an x-ray beam incident on the imaging receptor (detector). The differences in the x-ray intensity recorded by the receptor over the time of the measurement constitute the contrast differences or signals, which form the basis for the image. Differences in measured x-ray intensity are the result of differences in the attenuation of the x-ray beam through different paths within the subject being imaged. The same fundamental factors responsible for the difference in x-ray attenuation through the subject in conventional radiography are therefore the basic or inherent factors determining contrast in CT. They include the parameters discussed earlier in contrast in conventional radiography: differences in thickness, differences in mass density, differences in atomic number, and the x-ray photon energy or radiation quality (kVp). As in conventional radiography, the natural or inherent contrast contributed by these factors can be enhanced by the appropriate use of contrast media of high atomic number, which localizes in specific organs or body compartments.

Table 8.3. Factors affecting contrast in CT
Subject (inherent) contrast
Collimation and scatter reduction
Detector sensitivity
Signal processing and reconstruction
Image display
Photography

Collimation and Scatter Reduction Scatter radiation constitutes a large part of the transmitted x-ray intensity in conventional radiography. The scattered radiation is responsible for a significant amount of the film blackening or density but makes no contribution to the contrast or signal information. In fact, scatter significantly reduces contrast.

In conventional radiography, scatter can be decreased by collimation of the x-ray beam, and by the use of grids or air gaps. However, the amount of collimation is limited by the minimum size of the field of view that must be imaged.

In CT, tight collimation is a basic and necessary feature of the imaging technique. The x-ray beam is finely collimated in both its height (corresponding to the section thickness) and its width (which usually approximates the pixel dimension). Furthermore, the narrow aperture detectors only intercept those x-ray photons that remain within the finely collimated cross-sectional area of the primary beam. Photons scattered out of the primary beam do not intercept the detector. In contrast, the wide aperture receptor of conventional radiography (all or part of a sheet of x-ray film) may intercept x-ray photons scattered out of the primary beam, although this may be decreased by the use of grids.

Detector Sensitivity A prerequisite for a practical CT system is a detection system of sufficient sensitivity to detect small differences in the intensity of the transmitted x-ray beam. These small differences comprise the signal or information from which an image is to be reconstructed. Film contrast resolution is of the order of a few percent; many of the natural contrast differences in soft tissues are of the order of 1% or less. Thus, the detectors used in CT must be significantly more sensitive to fine differences in x-ray intensity than film. The detectors used in CT must also be capable of performing multiple repetitive independent measurements of the x-ray intensity without any decrease in their sensitivity.

Signal Processing and Reconstruction Noise introduced into the electronic circuits and in the reconstruction process must be kept sufficiently small so that the signal-to-noise ratio does not deteriorate significantly. Appropriate filtering techniques during reconstruction, for example, smoothing, may enhance the perceptibility of low contrast lesions such as liver metastases.

Image Display The digital basis of the CT image permits adjustment of the contrast of the image display. This important feature is not available in conventional radiography, where only a hard copy film image derived directly from the incident x-ray beam is available.

The viewer's perception of a lesion can be greatly enhanced by optimizing both window level and width settings. For low contrast lesions this frequently necessitates narrowing the CT window width about an optimal window level. The brightness and contrast settings of the monitor should also be adjusted for optimal viewing.

Although hard copy is a practical necessity, it does not substitute for direct examination of the image on the display monitor at different window settings. The clinical value of this direct physician-display monitor interaction cannot be overemphasized. Frequently, significant lesions such as low contrast liver metastases can be detected only by careful examination at an appropriate low window width. In contrast, detection of a bone lesion may be more apparent at a higher window level and with a greater window width.

Photography The hard copy or film image should replicate as closely as possible the optimized image presentation on the display monitor. In particular, there should be no significant loss in contrast resolution in this final stage. This necessitates selection and adjustment of a video photography system, for example, a multiformat camera. An appropriate film, optimized for photography of video image displays, should be used as well. These points have been discussed in Chapter 6.

Noise

Contrast resolution is degraded by noise, which often represents the ultimate limiting factor to image quality. Noise represents that portion of the signal that contains no information. Its presence tends to mask or obscure the information-containing portion of the signal. There are several sources of noise. These may originate at any point in the chain of processes that comprise the total CT system. However, the ultimate limiting type of noise is the random statistical noise that has its basis in the finite number of x-ray quanta utilized in the imaging process.

Types of Noise Several sources or types of noise are of relevance to CT, as shown in Table 8.4.

Table 8.4. Sources of noise in CT
Statistical
Electronic
Roundoff errors
Artifactual
Filter (reconstruction algorithm)

Statistical Noise (Quantum Noise) The response of any image receptor or detector depends upon the number of quanta of energy that it intercepts. In CT this is the number of x-ray quanta or photons. Even under exactly the same conditions, individual detectors of the same type will measure different numbers of x-ray quanta. The same individual detector will vary in the number of x-ray quanta detected from one measurement to the next. Even if it were possible to construct a "perfect" detector (one that accurately counted all the x-ray quanta it intercepted and that introduced no noise of its own in the system), this random variation in the number of quanta measured would occur.

Statistical noise in CT occurs because of the inherent statistical fluctuations that arise from the detection of a finite number of x-ray quanta. It is caused, therefore, by an insufficient number of photons arriving at the detector after penetrating the body. Statistical noise may also be called quantum noise. It has the same source as the quantum mottle of conventional radiography.

For a particular radiation dose, CT systems are very efficient (especially compared to conventional radiographic systems) in detecting photons; the capture rate varies from 30% to as high as 90% (Hounsfield, 1979). Therefore, there is little hope for any significant reduction in noise by improving the efficiency of detectors; rather, a reduction in noise will necessitate an increase in the radiation exposure or dose.

Electronic Noise Each of the electronic circuits associated with the CT imaging system is capable of introducing some noise into the system. Generally, circuits in the initial or early stages of any complex electronic system may be particularly bothersome, since the noise introduced in the initial stages of signal processing may be more difficult to separate from the basic data and is often amplified with the signal information in later stages.

Analog electronic circuits, which handle continuously varying signals, are especially susceptible to noise. This is exaggerated in CT since the analog processing of data occurs in the early part of the image processing chain, at a point where the electronic signal is small. However, from the work of Cohen (1979) it appears that the analog electronics are sufficiently well designed that the electronic noise contribution is only a fraction of that of the statistical noise.

Roundoff Errors An analog-to-digital converter turns an analog signal into a digital signal. The signal is then channeled through digital circuits, such as a digital computer, which are characterized by the processing of discrete (as opposed to continuous) signals. Digital computers generally do not introduce electronic noise into the system; however, they may introduce noise in the process of reconstruction through roundoff errors. The basis of roundoff errors is the limited number of bits that are used to represent numbers in a digital computer. As an example, whenever two numbers are multiplied, their product must be rounded off to the least significant bit that the computer uses in the representation of that number. Roundoff errors may be reduced by using a larger number of bits per word or through programming.

Artifactual Noise An artifact may be considered as a type of noise, since it represents a part of the signal or image that contains no information and obscures the information present in the image. Artifacts affect overall image quality and detail, including contrast and spatial resolution. There are numerous sources and types of artifacts, and these are discussed in Appendix I.

Filter Noise (Reconstruction Algorithm) The initial purpose of filtration was to eliminate the blur artifact associated with simple back projection. The filter function is also used to modify the final image and can have an important effect on image quality.

The application of the appropriate convolution kernel can introduce either smoothing or edge enhancement. In the case of a smoothing filter, both high frequency signal components and high frequency noise can be reduced. This modifies not only the appearance of the image but the appearance or quality of the noise as well. Thus, the filter can affect the noise. In the case of smoothing, the higher frequency components of the noise become selectively attenuated compared to lower frequency components. In contrast, a filter for edge enhancement will retain and even emphasize the high frequency components of both the signal and the noise.

Noise Power Spectrum (Wiener Spectrum) The noise power spectrum, or Wiener spectrum, in CT as in conventional radiography is a measure of the frequency distribution of noise. The Wiener spectrum is to contrast resolution and noise what the MTF is to spatial resolution.

The noise power spectrum is obtained by examining an image consisting only of noise. The noise image is broken down into its different frequency components. The amplitude of each frequency component is squared. This is done because the power associated with each frequency component is proportional to the square of the amplitude. The peak amplitude (in a negative or positive direction) is used in this process, since the average amplitude of a sine wave frequency is zero. The results may be averaged from those from other similar noise images for greater reliability or accuracy. The plot of the square of the amplitude of each frequency component against the frequency represents the noise power spectrum. The noise power spectrum is a complicated but accurate description of noise.

In conventional radiography the noise power spectrum is fairly constant over a wide frequency range. This is referred to as "white noise," as an analogy to white light, which contains light of all frequencies in the visible spectrum.

A power spectrum of white noise means that the noise occurring at one image point is independent of the noise at another image point; that is, the noise is uncorrelated. This occurs in conventional radiography because separate x-rays are intercepted at different points. This lack of correlation or independence of the noise at different image points assumes that the points are sufficiently well separated; in other words, there is no "cross-talk" between the image points. When the points are close enough, the noise begins to correlate. A consequence of this is that the noise power spectrum decreases and eventually becomes zero at higher spatial frequencies (corresponding to small distances between adjacent points).

Thus, both the MTF and the noise power spectrum fall to zero for higher frequencies. The necessity for this to occur can be understood intuitively. Imaging systems have finite resolution capabilities, determined by the component with the least resolution, for example, screen unsharpness in conventional radiography and aperture size or sampling rate in CT. Spatial frequencies corresponding to smaller spatial distances will be lost. In the case of the noise power spectrum, if the power were to be nonzero for all frequencies extending to infinity, the total noise power would be enormous, perhaps approaching or equal to infinity. Thus there must be a cutoff of power beyond a certain frequency.

The power noise spectrum of CT is not that of white noise. There is a decrease in noise at lower frequencies in CT. This is a bit complicated but is based on a long range negative correlation of noise in CT. This is a result of the image reconstruction algorithm used in CT. The noise at each point in the image, even at wide separations, is correlated or influenced to some extent by noise at all the other points. The negative correlation implies that if there is a strong positive noise fluctuation at one point, the noise fluctuations at nearby points (but beyond the spatial resolution dictated by the algorithm) will tend to be negative. The negative correlation decreases as the distance between the points increases.

A Formula for Statistical Noise Statistical (quantum) noise is variation in the number of photons intercepting different small areas of the detector. This variation represents a deviation about some average value. Some small areas on the detector see more photons than the average, whereas others see fewer. The amount of this deviation will vary over the detector. It is useful to define a quantity that represents an "average" variation or deviation. This quantity is an indication of the amount of statistical noise in the system.

The quantity used is called the standard deviation (root-mean-square deviation, or RMS). The amount of statistical noise present is proportional to the standard deviation.

The standard deviation is equal to the square root of the average number of photons in an area; that is,

$$\text{standard deviation} \propto \sqrt{N}, \quad (8.7)$$

where N is the number of photons (the symbol $\propto$ means "is proportional to"). Equation 8.7 is the same as Equation 8.5 for quantum mottle.

A more useful expression is the standard deviation as a fraction of the average:

$$\sigma = \frac{\sqrt{N}}{N} = \frac{1}{\sqrt{N}}, \quad (8.8)$$

where σ is the fractional standard deviation. Generally, the term standard deviation is taken to refer to σ.

The standard deviation is a much simpler description of noise than the noise power spectrum. However, it is also a less complete description, since it does not show the frequency distribution of the noise.

In CT it is useful and more practical to relate the standard deviation to appropriate and measurable CT parameters. Such a formula for the standard deviation has been derived by Brooks and Di Chiro (1976):

$$\sigma^2 \propto \frac{1}{w^3 h D}, \quad (8.9)$$

or alternatively as

$$\sigma \propto \frac{1}{w^{3/2} h^{1/2} D^{1/2}}, \quad (8.10)$$

where w is the effective beam width, or the spatial resolution element (the pixel size), h is the beam height (equal to the slice thickness), and D is the radiation dose. The complete equation would include constant factors and appropriate parameters, including the photon energy, a beam spreading factor, a linear attenuation coefficient, and an average depth-dose factor. These have been omitted in Equation 8.9 for simplicity.

In deriving Equation 8.9, several assumptions were made. These have been listed by Zatz (1981):

1. The width of the spatial resolution element, w, was determined by the ray sampling interval. The spacing in the reconstruction matrix and the size of the display pixel were considered to be less than or equal to the ray sampling interval.
2. Filtering or smoothing of the profiles (views) was not considered in the reconstruction process.
3. Postprocessing smoothing was ignored.

Consider the effect of the different parameters shown in Equations 8.9 and 8.10 on the standard deviation σ. If the dose D is doubled, the standard deviation will be reduced by $\sqrt{2}$, or 1.4. The dose might be doubled in practice, for example, by doubling the mAs from the x-ray tube.

If the height h of the beam is doubled, the standard deviation would be reduced by $\sqrt{2}$. This would be done in practice by doubling the slice thickness, that is, decreasing the collimation in the direction of the beam height.

If the pixel size (the length of one side of the pixel) were doubled, the standard deviation would be reduced by a factor of $\sqrt{8}$, or 2.8. Thus, changing the pixel size has the most dramatic effect on the standard deviation. Although the noise (as measured by σ) can be reduced by increasing the dose, it would require a large increase in the dose to yield a significant decrease in the noise. However, by increasing the pixel size by 2, it is possible to reduce noise by 2.8. Alternatively, for the same level of noise, an increase in pixel size by 2 permits a reduction in the dose by a factor of 8.

Relationship between Noise, Matrix Size, Dose, and Section Thickness

It would be useful at this point to correlate some of the concepts discussed earlier and describe how they interrelate to influence picture quality. The following discussion is based on the published work of Hounsfield.

Picture Grain (Noise) Picture grain refers to the effect of statistical noise on the picture. The random variation of the amplitude of the matrix points is the picture grain. This grain can be described in terms of its amplitude and coarseness (Figure 8.8). An example of picture grain is shown in Figure 8.9.

It is an interesting feature of CT that the presence of fat generally improves image quality by providing contrast to delineate borders of organs, for example, the liver and pancreas in the abdomen. Without a certain amount of fat, contrast suffers. However, excessive fat actually causes some deterioration in picture quality. The strong attenuation of the x-ray beam by the large amount of adipose tissue reduces the signal size. This results in the increased prominence of the picture grain seen in Figure 8.9 as the size of the noise is increased relative to the decreased signal.

There is an analogy to this effect in conventional radiography as well. Some intra-abdominal fat is helpful in delineating organs; for example, the perinephric fat outlines the kidneys. An excessive amount of fat, however, increases scatter, which decreases

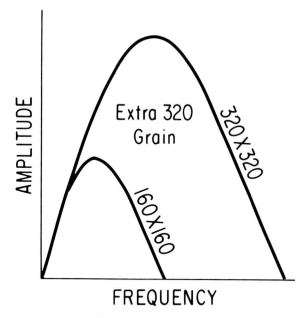

Figure 8.8. Plot of frequency spectrum of x-ray photon noise after modification by algorithm for application to picture matrix. The peak amplitude of the noise occurs at a frequency well below the maximum frequency applied to the matrix. The 320 × 320 matrix curve peaks at twice the frequency of the 160 × 160 matrix, so that a finer grain by a factor of 2 is expected, as well as a greater amplitude. (Reproduced by permission from G. N. Hounsfield, Picture quality of computed tomography. American Journal of Roentgenology 127:3–9, 1979.)

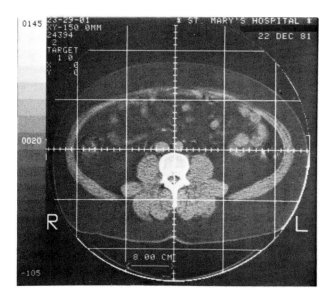

Figure 8.9. Some picture grain is evident in this scan of the abdomen of an obese patient.

contrast, and may even result in inadequate penetration of the x-ray beams.

Spatial Resolution (Matrix) and Grain An improvement in the spatial resolution may be important if variations in the shapes of certain organs have to be better delineated. This obviously entails increasing the number of picture points, that is, the number of pixels, in the same area. Thus, a larger matrix size is required. This in turn requires scanning with a narrower beam and obtaining more samples (readings or measurements) across the body. However, as the matrix size is increased, the amplitude of the picture grain is increased, since the same amount of information must now be shared among a larger number of pixels (it is assumed that the dose is kept constant).

Hounsfield (1979) has expressed the relationship in the following way:

$$(\text{inaccuracy})^2 \propto (\text{resolution})^3, \quad (8.11)$$

or in other terms:

$$(\text{grain})^2 \propto (\text{matrix size})^3. \quad (8.12)$$

Hounsfield has used the term "inaccuracy" to refer to the inaccuracy of the value of each pixel point (grain). This limits the accuracy with which the attenuation value of each pixel can be calculated.

Equation 8.12 of Hounsfield may be related to Equation 8.9 of Brooks and DiChiro when it is re-alized that the standard deviation is related to the grain or inaccuracy, and the beam width approximates the pixel size, which is inversely related to the matrix size. In other words,

$$\text{grain} \propto \sigma \quad (8.13)$$
$$\text{matrix size} \propto \frac{1}{\text{pixel size}} \propto \frac{1}{\text{beam width}}.$$

Thus, if the matrix size is doubled from 160 × 160 to 320 × 320, the grain will increase in amplitude by 2.8, but the additional grain will be of a finer nature (Figure 8.8).

Patient Dose Picture grain will vary in the following way with dose:

$$\text{grain} \propto \frac{1}{\sqrt{\text{dose}}}. \quad (8.14)$$

This is seen to be consistent with Equation 8.10, considering that σ is proportional to grain. By increasing the dose, the picture grain improves.

When accurate readings of CT numbers on large structures (e.g., brain or liver metastases) are required, a coarse matrix to reduce picture grain is appropriate. However, when shape or spatial detail is of prime importance, for example, in the spine or middle ear, a fine matrix should be used. Figure 8.10 demonstrates the relationship between picture resolution (matrix size) and grain for optimal viewing of different body parts.

Patient dose is discussed in greater detail later in this chapter.

Section Thickness The use of thinner sections may permit less spatial detail, especially in small structures which would occupy only a fraction of a thicker section. There may even be some improvement in contrast resolution for a structure significantly smaller than a thicker section. However, this is offset in part by an increase in image noise, which makes picture grain more obvious. This is shown in Figure 8.11. To offset this effect it would be necessary to have the same total number of x-ray quanta in the thinner slice as in the original thicker slice. This would markedly increase the dose, as the same amount of radiation would now irradiate a thin body slice. The x-ray tube output would have to be increased so that the more finely collimated beam would contain the same number of photons as the thicker original beam. The mAs of the tube may be increased somewhat for thinner sections, but there is a practical limit to this increase.

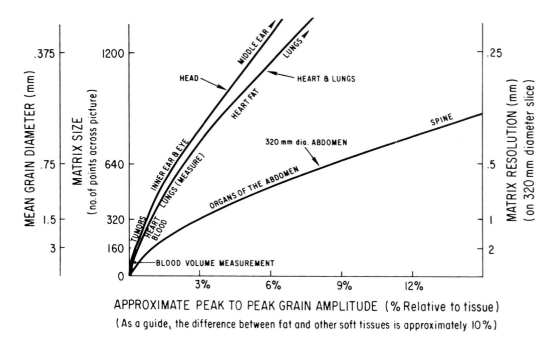

Figure 8.10. Relationship between picture resolution (matrix size) and picture grain amplitude. (Reproduced by permission from G. N. Hounsfield, Picture quality of computed tomography. American Journal of Roentgenology 127:3–9, 1979.)

PATIENT DOSAGE IN COMPUTED TOMOGRAPHY

CT, like conventional radiography, involves the use of ionizing radiation. The patient dosage, the amount of radiation absorbed by the patient, is related to the basic image quality factors of the CT unit, namely, noise, spatial resolution, and section thickness, according to Equation 8.9. It is also related to the fundamental radiographic factors kVp, mAs, filtration, and collimation as well as to the spatial relationships between the x-ray tube, collimators, and detectors. The scanner geometry (generation) and the scanning further modify the patient dosage. The scanning angle influences the distribution of the dosage. Finally, the patient dosage can be significantly modified by the method or techniques employed by the physician in performing a CT examination. McCullough and Payne (1978) have investigated many of these factors in their evaluation of different CT units in their published work. An excellent discussion of dosimetry in CT has also been written by Pentlow (1981).

Basics of Radiation Exposure and Dosage

The basic unit to describe radiation exposure is the roentgen (R), which is defined as the amount of radiation that will produce a quantity of ions of one sign (positive or negative) with a total electrical charge of 2.58×10^{-4} coulombs per kg of air. A single roentgen approximates the surface exposure required for an anteroposterior view of the abdomen.

Radiation exposure is not equivalent to the energy in the x-ray beam, although the two are related. The relationship depends on the average energy of the individual photons. The energy flux, or fluence, of an x-ray beam is the product of the number of photons crossing a unit surface (e.g., 1 cm^2) in a unit time (e.g., 1 s) and the average energy of the individual photons. For lower average photon energies, the absorption rate is relatively high and fewer photons are needed to produce a specific amount of ionization in a volume of air. For higher energies the photon absorption rate in the volume of air is lower, but each absorbed photon loses more energy and thus produces more ionization and exposure.

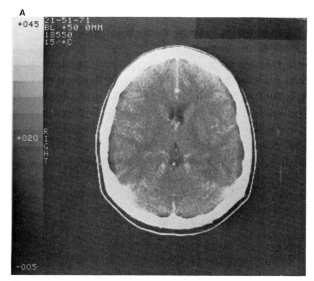

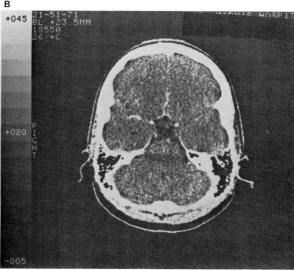

Figure 8.11. Head scans of the same patient using (A) 10-mm and (B) 1.5-mm section thicknesses. More noise is evident in the thinner section.

The advantage of exposure as a radiation parameter lies in the fact that it is relatively easy to measure. The exposure, as determined by radiation-produced ionization in air, can be measured with an ionization chamber.

The basic unit of absorbed dose is the rad (radiation absorbed dose), defined as the absorption of 100 ergs of energy per g of material. Generally, a gram of soft tissue occupies about 1 cc of volume.

Exposure describes the amount of radiation passing through an area; absorbed dose describes the amount of energy removed from the x-ray beam by the absorbing material. The roentgen and the rad are different units measuring different quantities. These quantities, exposure and absorbed dose, are related. The absorbed dose in rads per R of exposure depends on the energy of the x-ray beam and the composition of the absorbing substance. This relationship may be expressed as

$$\text{dose (rads)} = f \times \text{exposure (R)}, \qquad (8.15)$$

where the f factor is in units of rads per R.

In soft tissues in the diagnostic energy range, the f factor is relatively constant within a few percent, with a value of about .95 rads per R. This is related to the fact that the radiation absorption is primarily due to the Compton effect, which is fairly constant with energy in the diagnostic range. In bone, on the other hand, the f factor changes dramatically, decreasing from a value of 4 to 5 rads per R at lower energies, where the photoelectric effect predominates, to values closer to 1 rad per R at the upper end of the diagnostic range, where the Compton effect is the dominant absorption mechanism.

The rad is the unit of absorbed dose in the traditional cgs (centimeter-gram-second) system. Its value of 100 cgs per g is equivalent to .01 joules per kg. In the newer SI (Système Internationale) system of units for science and medicine, the unit of absorbed dose is the gray (Gy), which is defined as the absorption of 1 joule of energy per kg of material. Therefore, 1 Gy = 100 rads, and 1 rad = 1 centigray (cGy). There is no separate unit for exposure in SI.

A quantity used to describe the biological impact or effectiveness of radiation is the dose equivalent. The basic unit for the dose equivalent is the rem. The dose equivalent is obtained by multiplying the absorbed dose in rads by the quality factor (QF) of the radiation:

$$\begin{aligned}\text{dose equivalent (rem)} \\ = \text{absorbed dose (rads)} \times \text{QF}. \qquad (8.16)\end{aligned}$$

The dose equivalent is a means of describing not only the dose but the different biological effectiveness of various types of radiation, whether x-rays, gamma rays, beta particles, protons, slow and fast neutrons, or alpha particles. The dose equivalent also depends upon the energy of the specific radiation. The QF for diagnostic x-rays is essentially equal to 1. The QF for alpha particles, on the other hand, is about 20. Thus, in soft tissues an exposure of 1 R produces an absorbed dose of about 1 rad, which would correspond to about 1 rem.

The relative biological effectiveness (RBE) is a quantity used to express the impact of a radiation in producing a specific biological effect, rather than general biological damage. Its unit is the rem, the same as for the dose equivalent. The RBE dose is obtained by multiplying the absorbed dose in rads by a factor that describes the relative effectiveness of the particular radiation in producing the specific effect. The factor is called the RBE of the radiation and may vary for the same radiation if different biological effects are examined. The RBE for diagnostic x-rays and most biological effects has a value of about 1. RBE is usually reserved for laboratory investigation.

The linear energy transfer (LET) is the amount of energy deposited per unit length of travel and is expressed in keV per micron (10^{-6} m). A larger particle such as a proton encounters more "friction" in its path than a smaller particle such as an electron or a photon, and so transfers more energy to the absorber per unit of path length. It therefore has a higher LET radiation.

Another radiation measurement quantity is the integral dose (ID). This is the total amount of energy absorbed by the body. The basic unit of ID is the gram-rad, which is equivalent to 100 ergs of energy. The ID is the sum total of the absorbed dose of each gram of tissue in the body. It may be the most important radiation quantity when dealing with biological effects that are not limited to small critical organs (e.g., eyes, gonads).

The surface integral exposure (SIE) is the product of the exposure in roentgens by the exposure area in square centimeters ($R \cdot cm^2$). SIE is a measure of the total amount of radiation delivered to a surface area. It is a means of expressing the higher total radiation delivered to the surface of a patient by increasing the area when the exposure in R is constant.

Parameters Affecting the Patient Dosage

The patient dosage in CT is related to several different parameters, which have been discussed in detail by Pentlow (1981).

Scanning Time Significant increases in scanning time with first generation units are usually not practical because of the already long scanning time of a few minutes. However, in later generation scanners, particularly in third and fourth generation units, where typical fast scan times of 1–5 s are routine, it is quite practical to use a slower scan mode. This may increase the scan time and patient dosage by a factor of 2 or more. This is usually done in the interest of improving image quality by decreasing noise and obtaining higher contrast resolution. All other factors being equal, the patient dosage will vary directly with the scan time.

Scanner Geometry (Generations) In addition to the effect on scanning time described above, later generation scanners may introduce the possibility of image degradation by the acceptance of larger amounts of scatter radiation in the larger arrays of detectors. The seriousness of the problem varies with the scanner design, and sometimes an increased dose is required to maintain image quality.

First and second generation scanners generally use smaller scanner rotation angles than third and fourth generation units, and this also influences the dosage and its distribution as described below.

Scan Rotation Angle This has a significant effect on the distribution of radiation dose to the patient.

When data acquisition is done over 180° (as in first and second generation scanners), the isodose curves (corresponding to areas of equal radiation absorption) will be U-shaped, with considerable gradients (changes) over the skin. The ratio of the maximum to the minimum skin dose is of the order of 10 to 1. This wide variation occurs because only half of the body surface in a section is receiving an entrance dose, whereas the other half receives only an exit dose. The dose to the center of the patient in the scan section will be intermediate between the entrance and exit skin doses. When acquisition is done over 360° (a typical scan in third and fourth generation units), the isodose curves will generally follow the body contours. The dose is more or less uniform over the skin surface. The dose to the center of the patient in the scan section is less than the skin dose. Scan angles between 180° and 360° (overscanning beyond 180° in a first or second generation unit, or scanning less than 360° in a third or fourth generation unit), result in dose distributions that are intermediate between those described.

The point receiving maximum dose is situated at the midpoint of the scanning for a 180° scan angle. It is at the center of the overscan region (if any) for a 360° scan.

X-Ray Beam Geometry Geometric considerations are an extremely important factor in determining x-ray dose. They are also a significant factor in establishing the efficiency of the dose, that is, how much of the radiation that passed through the patient, and is responsible for the patient dose, is captured by the detector. Geometric factors include the size collimation (including the aperture or collimation size and its relative distances from the x-ray tube focus and the patient), and details of the postpatient collimation and the detectors. To minimize the patient dose, or increase the efficiency of the dose, the primary x-ray beam should approximate the detector aperture as closely as possible.

There is considerable variation in the size of x-ray tube focus. First and second generation scanners employ larger tube focuses or focal lines, typically of the order of 2 × 15 mm, whereas third and fourth generation scanners usually employ smaller tube focuses, typically of the order of 1 × 1 mm. A long focal line results in a large penumbra (shadow) perpendicular to the scan section (the Z direction). This penumbra is wasted dosage; the patient is irradiated by radiation that is not intercepted by a detector.

Penumbra is primarily a problem in the direction perpendicular to the scan section (Z dimension). Penumbra is less of a problem in the X and Y dimensions (in the scan plane), since the focal spot size is no more than 2 mm. There are a number of approaches for minimizing penumbra in the Z direction. These have been described and illustrated by Pentlow. Basically, the problem is one of attempting to match the width of the dose profile (the distribution of the x-ray beam including its penumbra) at the patient to the width of the sensitivity profile (the detector's sensitivity across the slice thickness). The dose profile width will ideally match that of the sensitivity profile, and both should have the appearance of square waves. A dose profile curve for the General Electric CT/T system is shown in Figure 8.12.

Another important geometric factor is the overlap of successive slices. The dose profile curves should be immediately contiguous, but there should not be significant overlap, since this would result in unnecessary increased dosage to the patient. The effect of a multiple contiguous or a cumulative dose profile is shown in Figure 8.13 for a General Electric CT/T system.

Detectors The efficiency of detectors in both capturing and absorbing incident radiation, as described in Chapter 3, is determined as follows:

total detection efficiency

$$= \text{capture efficiency} \times \text{absorption efficiency}. \quad (8.17)$$

Generally, solid-state scintillation detectors (e.g., sodium iodide, calcium fluoride, cesium iodide, and bismuth germanate) coupled to photomultiplier tubes or photodiodes have very high efficiencies (e.g., 90–99%) for absorbing the radiation which they capture. Xenon ionization chambers are less efficient in

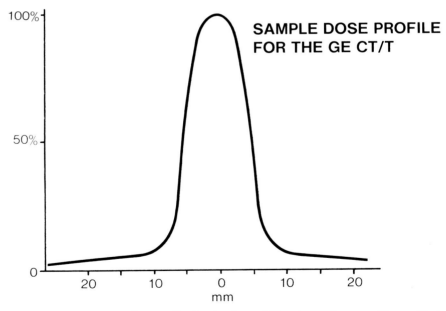

Figure 8.12. Sampling dose profile for the General Electric CT/T system. The profile is similar for phantoms of different diameter; however, the peak dose differs in these different cases. The profile has been normalized to 100%. (Reproduced from General Electric Publication No. 4870, with the permission of General Electric Medical Systems.)

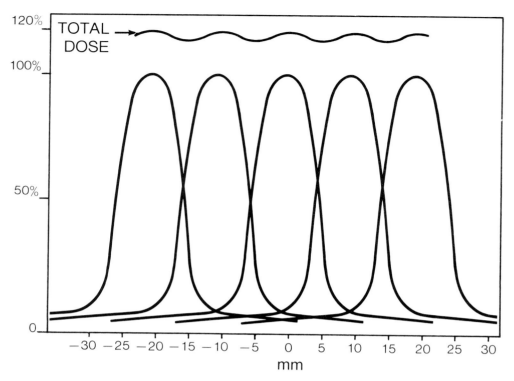

Figure 8.13. The effect of multiple slices in the General Electric CT/T system. The individual dose profiles can be summed in order to give the total dose produced by multiple slices. The exact value for the total dose depends on the distance between slices. In the figure above, the distance between slices is taken to be 10 mm, equal to the slice thickness. This increases the dose by approximately 20%. (Reproduced from General Electric Publication No. 4870, with the permission of General Electric Medical Systems.)

absorption (e.g., 50–60%), because some of the captured x-rays are not absorbed or because some of the fluorescent radiation produced after absorption is not recaptured.

However, in fourth generation scanners, the capture efficiency may approximate only about 50%, whereas that of the xenon detector commonly used in third generation scanners is greater than 90%. This is the result of the large amount of detector or post-patient collimation used in fourth generation scanners; the xenon detectors of third generation units have no detector collimation other than the plates separating the individual xenon cells.

As an example (McCullough and Payne, 1978), if 600 detectors in a fourth generation unit are located in a circumference of 3–3.5 m, then the center-to-center distance is about 5 mm. When reflected back to the patient, this becomes a separation of 3–4 mm; that is, the detector aperture is 3–4 mm at the patient. If a spatial resolution approximating mm is desired, there must be some reduction in the effective width of the detector. This is most easily accomplished by blocking out some portion of the detector (usually about 50%).

Methods of increasing the total detection efficiency include the use of solid-state detectors in third generation scanners (e.g., Siemens Somatom), removal of the collimating pins in fourth generation scanners (which would result in reduced spatial resolution), or precollimation of the beam to block out some of the radiation that would otherwise fall on the lead pins between detectors.

Radiographic Factors The patient dosage is directly proportional to the x-ray tube current, or mA, since the number of x-ray photons irradiating the patient is increased the same way as the mA.

The dosage is also proportional to the scan time. There may be some variation from an absolute direct proportionality, however. In translational-rotational scanners, an increase in scan time involves an increase in the time for translational motions, during which the patient is being irradiated. The rotational time, during which the patient is not being irradiated, is not increased proportionally and becomes a smaller fraction of the scan time. Thus, the dose goes up by slightly more than the factor by which scan time is increased. In some purely rotational systems the image noise levels can vary with scan time for a given mAs, since the electronics may be optimized for a specific scan time (Pentlow, 1981).

In pulsed systems (most third generation scanners), the dose is proportional to the product of the pulse duration and the number of pulses. This product is also equal to the duty cycle (fraction of the time the tube is emitting x-rays) times the scan time, so the dose is proportional to the total scan time in pulsed tube systems. Allowing for the variations described above, the patient dosage is proportional to the mAs.

An increase in the kVp or beam quality results in higher energy photons, with increased penetration and more photons arriving at the detectors, improving statistical accuracy. With a lower kVp the relatively lower energy photons can give better contrast or differentiation between soft tissues, assuming there is adequate penetration. In large bodies higher kVp are generally needed for the penetration. Therefore, in some scanners higher kVp and/or additional filtration may be used in body scans compared to head scans. In practice, the kVp (for a fixed mAs) increases the dose and improves statistics. This may be understood better by realizing that an increase in the kVp (with mAs and filtration fixed) not only increases the average and peak photon energies, but results in more total energy emission as well (there are in fact more photons at all energies).

An increase in the kVp also increases the ratio of the dose in the center of the patient to the entrance surface dose, since the beam has better penetration. An increase in filtration will also increase this dose ratio (patient center to entrance surface), but the dose itself will be decreased since the filtration hardens the beam by selectively removing many lower energy photons.

Image Quality Factors The relationship between patient dosage and spatial resolution, noise (and hence contrast resolution), and slice thickness have been described earlier in this chapter and are based on Equation 8.9. This equation may be rewritten for the dose:

$$D \propto \frac{1}{w^3 \sigma^2 h}. \qquad (8.18)$$

In summary:

1. Doubling the pixel size (w) but keeping the standard deviation (σ) of the noise and the slice thickness (h) constant permits a reduction in dose by a factor of 8.
2. Permitting the standard deviation (σ) of the noise to be doubled while the pixel size (w) and the slice thickness are kept constant allows the dose to be reduced by a factor of 4.
3. Doubling the slice thickness with the pixel size (w) and the standard deviation (σ) of the noise held constant allows reduction in the dose by a factor of 2.

Dosage Measurements (Dosimetry)

Dosimeters Three basic measurement devices or dosimeters are employed in CT dosimetry: ionization chambers, thermoluminescent dosimeters (TLD), and film.

Ionization Chambers Ionization chambers rely on the production and measurement of ions by the radiation. They serve as a standard against which most other types of dosimeters are evaluated and calibrated. The advantages of ionization chambers include the following: a fairly constant sensitivity or energy response over a wide energy range, a linear response with dosage, application over a wide range of doses and dose rates, calibration stability over long periods of time, and convenience of use (with an immediate readout). Disadvantages include the relatively large dimensions (about a centimeter) in chambers of adequate sensitivity for lower dose levels (CT dose distributions may change dramatically over millimeters), and the need for performing a complete scan for each point to be measured since only one chamber can be used at a time.

Thermoluminescent Dosimeters TLDs consist of crystalline substances that trap electrons excited by the radiation at impurity trap sites. The crystalline substances are later heated, resulting in a release of the trapped electrons and emission of light as these electrons return to their ground state. The emitted light is measured and provides an estimate of an exposure or absorbed dose.

TLDs are the most widely used CT dosimeters. Lithium fluoride (LiF) is the most useful material, in the form of either loose powder or chips. Typical chip dimensions are $3 \times 3 \times 1$ mm.

A significant advantage of TLDs is that arrays of chips can be used to measure several dose profiles in a single scan, thus requiring relatively little scanner time. Disadvantages of TLDs include lack of immediate readout since the TLDs have to be processed, a variation in response with the relative orientation of the chips and the incident radiation, variations in sensitivity among nominally identical chips, and possible change in sensitivity of a particular chip with time, thus requiring recalibration after use. Also, the energy response of lithium fluoride is not as good as that of typical ionization chambers.

Film   Film may be used as a radiation measurement device. Narrow film strips can be inserted into holes in phantoms or attached to surfaces. Sheets of film may be wrapped around the surface of phantoms. The film darkening or density is measured with either a hand or computerized film densitometer.

Film offers the advantages of high spatial resolution, relatively little dependence on the angle of the film and incident radiation (Pentlow, 1981), and less difficulty in processing than with large numbers of TLDs. The films can be developed in automatic processors, provided strict control of conditions is maintained. A nearly spatially continuous response curve can be obtained with film. A significant disadvantage of film is its strong dependence on beam energy or quality. However, this is partly offset by the fact that the energy spectrum at different points in a scanned phantom or patient does not vary as much as might be expected (Pentlow, 1981).

Conditions and Techniques   An evaluation of the dose distribution should include measurements of the skin or surface dosages and dosages within the body or phantom. Appropriate measurements would be at four surface sites and the center, that is, the top, bottom, center, and both sides of a phantom, (McCullough and Payne, 1978; Pentlow, 1981). The surface measurements can be at 90° intervals. In CT units that only scan through 180°, the surface doses will vary dramatically. For these scanners the surface sites measured should include those corresponding to the maximum and minimum entrance and exit sites, respectively. Scanners having a rotation of exactly 360° or some integral multiple of 360° will have relatively little or no variation in surface dose.

TLD chips closely spaced along the thickness of the scan section (the Z direction) can be used to obtain a dose profile along the thickness of the scan. For example, 12 chips can be placed with the narrowest (typically 1 mm) dimension aligned along the Z direction (see Figure 8.12). The effect of a series of scans can be obtained by superimposing the single scan profiles (spaced at the appropriate distance between scans) and summing the profiles (the contributions from the separate scans). Figure 8.13 illustrates a summated total dose from multiple slices.

McCullough and Payne have previously suggested that any dose values should include the following minimum information; kVp, mA (either actual or "effective" if the tube is pulsed, i.e., the product of the actual mA and the duty cycle), total scan time (or the mAs), angular limits of the scan (scan angle), size and shape of the subject being scanned as well as the material of which it is composed, and the nature and quantity of any bolus of contrast. If variable filtrations are available, the one used should be described. McCullough and Payne also felt that, for comparisons, it would be useful to have the following additional information: slice thickness (the FWHM of the sensitivity profile of the slice at the isocenter), scan noise (in terms of its standard deviation expressed as a percent of the attenuation of water), and a measured estimate of the transverse resolution. When multiple scans are done, the table incrementation and the number of scans per study should be indicated.

Extensive dosage measurement data for different CT units are available from Pentlow (1981), from McCullough and Payne (1978), and from numerous other sources, including company brochures and specifications.

ACCURACY AND RELIABILITY OF CT NUMBERS

CT Numbers and Linear Attenuation Coefficients

Basic Relationship   The basic relationship between the CT number and the linear attenuation coefficient of a substance (Equation 2.20) is repeated here for convenience:

$$\text{CT number} = \frac{\mu_{\text{substance}} - \mu_{H_2O}}{\mu_{H_2O}} \times K.$$

Both $\mu_{\text{substance}}$ and μ_{H_2O} vary with the effective energy or kV of the x-ray beam at which the measurements are made.

For the original EMI CT unit (Mark I), the effective energy of a 120-kVp beam after passing through 27 cm of water was 73 keV, and μ_{H_2O} at this energy has a value of .19 cm^{-1} (Zatz, 1981). K was given the value of 500 EMI or old Hounsfield units.

Contrast Scale   Since the CT number scale is not the same for all scanners, it is useful to determine the contrast scale (the change in μ per CT number). This permits the CT number standard deviation to be expressed in a form independent of a particular scanner. Equation 2.20 may be rewritten as

$$\text{CT number} = \mu_{\text{substance}} \frac{K}{\mu_{\text{H}_2\text{O}}} - K. \quad (8.19)$$

The relationship between the change in μ and a change in the CT number (ΔCT) can be written as

$$\Delta\mu = (\Delta\text{CT}) \frac{\mu_{\text{H}_2\text{O}}}{K}. \quad (8.20)$$

If (ΔCT) is taken equal to 1, then the change in μ per CT number is

$$\frac{\Delta\mu}{\text{CT number}} = \frac{\mu_{\text{H}_2\text{O}}}{K}. \quad (8.21)$$

This may be expressed as a percent:

$$\frac{\% \mu}{\text{CT number}} = \frac{\mu_{\text{H}_2\text{O}}}{K} \times 100. \quad (8.22)$$

For EMI (old Hounsfield) units, $K = 500$, and

$$\frac{\% \mu}{\text{CT number}} = .2\% \ \mu_{\text{H}_2\text{O}}. \quad (8.23)$$

For new Hounsfield units, $K = 1{,}000$, and

$$\frac{\% \mu}{\text{CT number}} = .1\% \ \mu_{\text{H}_2\text{O}}. \quad (8.24)$$

Therefore, a change of 1 CT number corresponds to a change of .2% of the linear attenuation coefficient of a material compared to that of water for EMI units (old Housnfield units); 100 CT numbers will require a 20% change in μ relative to that of water. For new Hounsfield units, a change of 1 CT number corresponds to a .1% change in μ relative to that of water; 100 CT numbers require a 10% change in μ relative to that of water.

Basic Definitions

Accuracy of CT Numbers Accuracy is an indication of how well the measured value of a CT number conforms to the "true" value, which corresponds to the linear attenuation coefficient of a voxel. Accuracy depends upon a number of nonrandom systematic errors. These systematic errors are, at least in principle, capable of being corrected.

Precision of CT Numbers Precision indicates the capability to reproduce the same CT value in repeated measurements. Precision refers to statistical or random variations in the CT values, in contrast to systematic errors, which are responsible for errors in accuracy. Precision is an indication of how much a single measurement of the CT number of a single voxel of a substance, such as water, might be expected to differ from the average of a large set of measurements of the same voxel of water. If enough measurements are performed, statistical or random errors tend to cancel out, leaving only the systematic errors.

Accuracy and precision are both used in describing measurements to indicate the reliability with which the values are determined.

Linearity of CT Numbers Linearity of CT values exists when the relation between CT numbers and linear attenuation values is linear at a particular effective beam energy. The presence of linearity indicates that subject contrast is constant over the range of CT numbers of interest.

Spatial Uniformity Spatial uniformity indicates the capability of the scanner to measure the

Table 8.5. Factors affecting the reliability of CT value measurements

Factors affecting the CT value of water and the contrast scale
    Temporal drift of contrast scale
    kVp
    Beam filtration
    Patient (subject) parameters
      Size
      Shape
      Composition
    Temperature drift
    Contrast enhancement
Artifacts
    Beam hardening with poor (or no) polychromatic corrections
    High Z transitions
    Patient-related
      High densities (contrast, metal)
      Motion
      Centering
Statistical or random noise

same CT number of an object regardless of its position within the scan section. For a water phantom, the mean value of a group of adjacent voxels may differ, depending or whether the region measured is in the center or the periphery of the phantom.

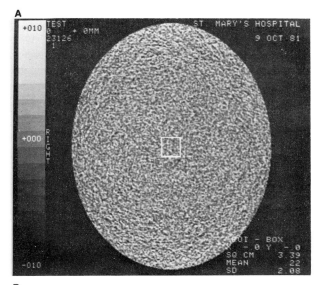

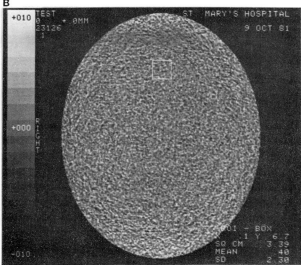

Figure 8.14. CT calibration scans of a water phantom. Measurement in (A) the center ($X = 0$, $Y = 0$) and (B) the periphery ($X = 1$, $Y = 6.7$) of the phantom. The area included in both measurements is 3.39 cm². The center measurement has a mean of .22 and a standard deviation of 2.08. The peripheral measurement has a mean of .40 and a standard deviation of 2.30. The close approximation of both mean measurements to the true value of zero for water indicates the accuracy of the measurements. The small standard deviations indicate a relatively high precision. The approximation of the mean measurements in the center and periphery indicates good spatial uniformity.

Figure 8.14 illustrates accuracy, precision, and spatial uniformity for measurements on a water phantom.

Factors Affecting the Reliability of CT Numbers

There are a number of different factors that determine the reliability of measured CT values. Table 8.5, modified from the listing by McCullough (1981), outlines these factors.

CT PHANTOMS

A phantom is a device designed and constructed to serve as a test object for the evaluation of one or more performance parameters of an imaging system. A number of different phantoms have been developed to evaluate the performance of CT scanners. Bergstrom (1981) has divided CT phantoms into five categories:

1. Composite phantoms, constructed for the evaluation of several different parameters of performance
2. Phantoms designed for the evaluation of a single performance parameter
3. Quality assurance phantoms
4. Dose phantoms
5. True or simulated (anthropomorphic) anatomical phantoms.

A composite phantom is made of several different sections or structures which enable the separate evaluation of each different parameter. Such phantoms have been constructed by the American Association of Physicists in Medicine (AAPM) and the Bureau of Radiological Health. The AAPM composite phantom has five sections. These permit the determination of contrast resolution, spatial resolution, contrast scale and linearity, slice thickness, and the CT value of water as well as a noise standard deviation.

Phantoms have been built to evaluate one specific parameter for scientific purposes. Examples of such phantoms include the slice thickness phantom of Brooks and Di Chiro (1977) and the phantom of Duerinckx and Macovski (1978) to evaluate beam hardening artifacts.

A General Electric Gray/White Phantom Mod III, designed to examine the capability of a CT system to image low contrast objects, is shown in Figure 8.15. This phantom is called a gray/white matter phantom because its contrast levels (.2–3%) include

GE GRAY/WHITE PHANTOM MOD III

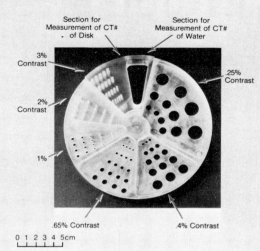

PHANTOM DESIGN

The GE Gray/White Phantom is constructed of a polystyrene disk. Each sector in this disk contains a pattern of holes. In the version displayed at the left, the holes are separated by their diameters in all sectors except the two largest sectors. Each sector has a different thickness. The smaller the sector the thicker it is.

With the disk immersed in water and centered in the scan plane, the partial volume effect will produce a CT number difference for a given sector hole given approximately by

$$CT_d \times t/z$$

Where CT_d is the CT number of the material of the disk, z is the slice thickness and t is the thickness of the sector. The ranges of sector thickness displayed at the left accurately reproduce contrast differences from .25% to 3%.

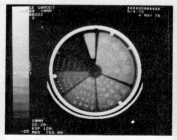 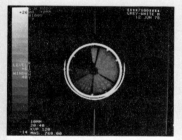

The above scans were performed at a dose of 6.45 Rad measured from TLD's placed on the phantom.* The 8800 scan is reconstructed on .8mm pixels and the 7800 scan is reconstructed on 1.3mm pixels. The detectability of low contrast objects from these types of images can be determined reproducibly by a single observer or the consensus of a group of observers.

GENERAL

The phantom described above is designed to examine the capability of a CT System to image low contrast objects. Anatomically we can think of gray/white matter differentiation, detection of metastases in the liver, and lesions of the adrenal glands as a few of the many areas which require imaging of low contrast objects of small spatial dimensions. The CT System that can image these types of pathology with the lowest dose will have the greatest value to the medical community and their patients.

The study of the detectability of low contrast objects is not new and its extension to computed tomography is only natural.

Measurements made under clinical conditions on the GE Gray/White Phantom MOD III show detectability of 5mm at .39% contrast at a dose of about 6 Rads for both the CT/T 7800 and 8800 Systems.*

Measurements of this type provide a quantitative way of stating the image performance of a scanner and a definitive means of comparing scanner performance.

*Dose value furnished by Gerald Cohen, Ph.D., Alleghany General Hospital.

Figure 8.15. Phantom design and description of the General Electric Gray/White Phantom Mod III. This phantom is designed to examine the capability of a CT system to image low contrast objects. (Courtesy of General Electric Medical Systems.)

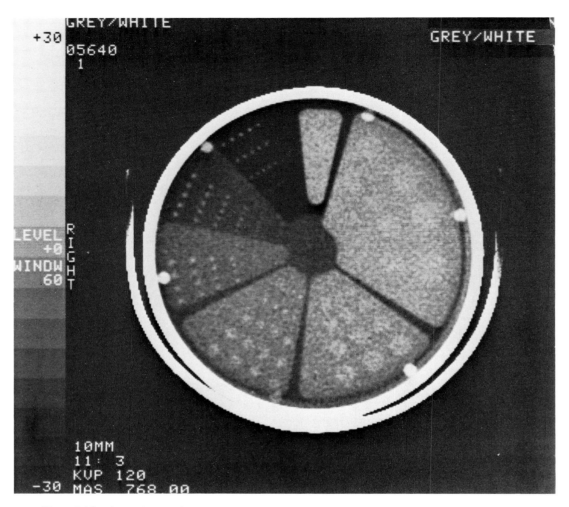

Figure 8.16. A scan image of the General Electric Gray/White Phantom Mod III. (Courtesy of General Electric Medical Systems.)

the difference between gray and white matter of the human brain (.6–1%). This phantom has been described by Cohen and DiBianca (1979). In this phantom the different contrasts are achieved with a partial volume effect. If the material in the phantom only occupies a fifth of the slice thickness, the contrast will only be about a fifth of the contrast. A separate scan image of this phantom is shown in Figure 8.16 between the material and water.

Quality assurance phantoms are usually simple phantoms with features similar to the contrast scale/linearity section of the AAPM phantom. They are usually produced by the equipment manufacturer.

Dose phantoms may or may not be the same as the performance evaluation phantoms. One model is simply a polystyrene or Perspex block in which are drilled holes to accommodate TLDs.

True or simulated (anthropomorphic) anatomical phantoms have been used to provide a simulation of patient scanning. However, the nature of the phantom does not lend itself to a rigorous mathematical evaluation.

REFERENCES AND SUGGESTED READINGS

Image Clarity (Visibility) in Radiography

Christensen, E. E., Curry, T. S., and Dowdey, J. E. The radiographic image. In An Introduction to the Physics of Diagnostic Radiology, 2nd ed., Chap. 13, pp. 161–184. Lea & Febiger, Philadelphia, 1978.

Morgan, R. H. The frequency response function. A valuable means of expressing the information recording capability of diagnostic x-ray systems. American Journal of Roentgenology 88:175–186, 1962.

Morgan, R. H., Bates, L. M., Rao, U. V. G., and Marinaro, A. The frequency response characteristics of x-ray films and screens. American Journal of Roentgenology 92:426–440, 1964.

Rao, G. U. V., Beachley, M. O., Bosch, H. A., Kan, P. T. The relevance of image analysis in clinical radiography. (Scientific exhibit shown at the 81st annual meeting of the American Roentgen Ray Society, San Francisco, March 23–27, 1981, and awarded the Silver Medal of the Society).

Rossman, K. Point spread-function, line spread-function, and modulation transfer function. Tools for the study of imaging systems. Radiology 93:257–272, 1969a.

Rossman, K. Image quality. Radiological Clinics of North America 7:419–433, 1969b.

Seeman, H. Physical factors which determine roentgenographic contrast. American Journal of Roentgenology 80:112–116, 1958.

Sprawls, P. Image blur and resolution. In The Physical Principles of Diagnostic Radiology. Chap. 15, pp. 193–217. University Park Press, Baltimore, 1977.

Spatial Resolution in Computed Tomography

Alvarez, R. E., and Stonestrom, J. P. Optimal processing of computed tomography images using experimentally measured noise properties. Journal of Computer Assisted Tomography 3:77–84, 1979.

Axelsson, B. An investigation of the slice geometry of the EMI head scanner. Journal of Computer Assisted Tomography 1:187–190, 1977.

Bassano, D. A., Chamberlain, C. C., Mozley, J. M., and Kieffer, S. A. Physical, performance, and dosimetric characteristics of the Δ-scan 50 whole-body/brain scanner. Radiology 123:455–462, 1977.

Bergstrom, M. Performance evaluation of scanners. In T. H. Newton and D. G. Potts (eds.), Radiology of the Skull and Brain: Technical Aspects of Computed Tomography, Vol. 5, Chap. 123, Part XVII, pp. 4212–4227. C. V. Mosby, St. Louis, 1981.

Blumenfeld, S. M., and Glover, G. Spatial resolution in computed tomography. In T. H. Newton and D. G. Potts (eds.), Radiology of the Skull and Brain: Technical Aspects of Computed Tomography, Vol. 5, Chap. 112, Part XVI, pp. 3918–3940. C. V. Mosby, St. Louis, 1981.

Bracewell, R. N. Correction for collimator width (restoration) in reconstructive x-ray tomography. Journal of Computer Assisted Tomography 1:6–15, 1977.

Brooks, R. A., and Di Chiro, G. Slice geometry in computer assisted tomography. Journal of Computer Assisted Tomography 1:191–199, 1977.

Cohen, G. Contrast-detail-dose analysis of six different computed tomographic scanners. Journal of Computer Assisted Tomography 3:197–203, 1979.

Cohen, G., and DiBianca, F. A. The use of contrast-detail-dose evaluation of image quality in a computed tomographic scanner. Journal of Computer Assisted Tomography 3:189–195, 1979.

General Electric Company. CT/T technology continuum. Technical performance of the CT/T system. General Electric Publication No. 4870.

Glover, G. H., and Eisner, R. L. Theoretical resolution of computed tomography systems. Journal of Computer Assisted Tomography 3:85–91, 1979.

Hilal, S. K., and Trokel, S. L. Computerized tomography of the orbit using thin sections. Seminars in Roentgenology 12:137–147, 1977.

Hounsfield, G. N. Potential uses of more accurate CT absorption values by filtering. American Journal of Roentgenology 131:103–106, 1976.

Hounsfield, G. N. Picture quality of computed tomography. American Journal of Roentgenology 127:3–9, 1976.

Joseph, P. M., Spital, R. D., and Stockham, C. D. The effects of sampling on CT images. Computerized Tomography 4:189–206, 1980.

Judy, P. F. The line spread function and modulation transfer function of a computed tomographic scanner. Medical Physics 3:233–236, 1976.

MacIntyre, W. J., Alfidi, R. J., Haaga, J., Chernak, E., and Meany, T. F. Comparative modulation transfer functions of the EMI and Delta scanners. Radiology 120:189–191, 1976.

Margulis, A. R., Boyd, D. P., and Korobkin, M. T. Comparison of bimodal (translate-rotate) and pure rotary body CT scanners. In P. Gerhardt and E. van Kaick (eds.), Total Body Computerized Tomography. International Symposium, Heidelberg, 1977, pp. 10–15. Georg Thieme, Stuttgart, 1979.

McCullough, E. C., Payne, J. T., Baker, H. L., Hattery, R. R., Sheedy, P. F., Stephens, D. H., and Gedgaudas, E. Performance evaluation and quality assurance of computed tomography scanners, with illustrations from the EMI, ACTA, and Delta scanners. Radiology 120:173–178, 1976.

Ommaya, A. K., Murray, G., Ambrose, J., Richardson, A., and Hounsfield, G. Computerized axial tomography: Estimation of spatial and density resolution capability. British Journal of Radiology 49:604–611, 1976.

Osborn, A. G., and Wing, S. D. Thin section computed tomography in the evaluation of third ventricle colloid cysts. Radiology 124:257–258, 1977.

Ramachandran, G. N., and Lakshminarayanan, A. V. Three-dimensional reconstruction from radiographs and electron micrographs: Application of convolutions instead of Fourier transforms. Proceedings of the National Academy of Sciences 68:2236–2240, 1971.

Robbins, A. H., Pugatch, R. D., Gerzof, S. G., Spira, R., Rankin, S. C., and Gale, D. R. An assessment of the role of scan speed in perceived image quality of body computed tomography. Radiology 139:139–146, 1981.

Shepp, L. A., and Logan, B. F. The Fourier reconstruction of a head section. I.E.E.E. Transactions on Nuclear Science NS-21(3):21–43, 1974.

Tanaka, E., and Iinuma, T. A. Correction functions and statistical noises in transverse section picture reconstruction. Computers in Biology and Medicine 6:295–306, 1976.

Technicare. Corporation Technical supplement. The Delta Scan 2000 series of computed tomography scanners, 1978.

Wagner, L. K., and Cohen, G. Energy dependence of contrast-detail-dose and object-detectability-dose curves for CT scanners. Journal of Computer Assisted Tomography 6:378–382, 1982.

Weinstein, M. A., Berlin, A. J., and Duchesneau, P. M.

High resolution computed tomography of the orbit with the Ohio Nuclear delta head scanner. Radiology 127:175–177, 1976.

Zatz, L. M. Image quality in cranial computed tomography. Journal of Computer Assisted Tomography 2:336–340, 1978.

Zatz, L. M. Basic principles of computed tomography scanning, In T. H. Newton and D. G. Potts (eds.), Radiology of the Skull and Brain: Technical Aspects of Computed Tomography, Vol. 5, Chap. 109, Part XVI, pp. 3853–3876. C. V. Mosby, St. Louis, 1981.

Contrast Resolution and Noise in Computed Tomography

Alvarez, R. E., and Stonestrom, J. P. Optimal processing of computed tomography images using experimentally measured noise properties. Journal of Computer Assisted Tomography 3:77–84, 1979.

Barrett, H. H., Gordon, S. K., and Hershel, R. S. Statistical limitations in transaxial tomography. Computers in Biology and Medicine 6:307–323, 1976.

Bassano, D. A., Chamberlain, C. C., Mozley, J. M., and Kieffer, S. A. Physical, performance, and dosimetric characteristics of the Δ-scan 50 whole-body/brain scanner. Radiology 123:455–462, 1977.

Bergstrom, M. Performance evaluation of scanners. In T. H. Newton and D. G. Potts (eds.), Radiology of the Skull and Brain: Technical Aspects of Computed Tomography, Vol. 5, Chap. 123, Part XVII, pp. 4212–4227. C. V. Mosby, St. Louis, 1981.

Brooks, R. A., and Di Chiro, G. Statistical limitations in x-ray reconstructive tomography. Medical Physics 3:237–240, 1976.

Chesler, D. A., Riederer, S. J., and Pelc, N. J. Noise due to photon counting statistics in computed x-ray tomography. Journal of Computer Assisted Tomography 1:64–74, 1977.

Chew, E., Weiss, G. H., Brooks, R. A., and Di Chiro, G. Effect of CT noise on detectability of test objects. American Journal of Roentgenology 131:681–685, 1978.

Cohen, G. Contrast-detail-dose analysis of six different computed tomographic scanners. Journal of Computer Assisted Tomography 3:197–203, 1979.

Cohen, G., and DiBianca, F. A. The use of contrast-detail-dose evaluation of image quality in a computed tomographic scanner. Journal of Computer Assisted Tomography 3:189–195, 1979.

Duerinckx, A. J., and Macovski, A. Nonlinear polychromatic and noise artifacts in x-ray computed tomography images. Journal of Computer Assisted Tomography 3:519–526, 1979.

Fullerton, G. D., and White, D. R. Anthropomorphic test objects for CT scanners. Radiology 133:217–222, 1979.

General Electric Company. CT/T technology continuum. Technical performance of the CT/T system. General Electric Publication No. 4870.

Hanson, K. M.: Noise and contrast discrimination in computed tomography. In T. H. Newton and D. G. Potts (eds.), Radiology of the Skull and Brain: Technical Aspects of Computed Tomography, Vol. 5, Chap. 113, Part XVI, pp. 3941–3955. C. V. Mosby, St. Louis, 1981.

Hanson, K. M. On the optimality of the filtered back projection algorithm. Journal of Computer Assisted Tomography 4:361–363, 1980.

Hilal, S. K., and Trokel, S. L. Computerized tomography of the orbit using thin sections. Seminars in Roentgenology 12:137–147, 1977.

Hounsfield, G. N. Potential uses of more accurate CT absorption values by filtering. American Journal of Roentgenology 131:103–106, 1976.

Hounsfield, G. N. Picture quality of computed tomography. American Journal of Roentgenology 127:3–9, 1976.

Joseph, P. M. Artifacts in computed tomography. In T. H. Newton and D. G. Potts (eds.), Radiology of the Skull and Brain: Technical Aspects of Computed Tomography, Vol. 5. Chap. 114, Part XVI, pp. 3956–3992. C. V. Mosby, St. Louis, 1981.

Joseph, P. M., Hilal, S. K., Schulz, R. A., and Kelcz, F. Clinical and experimental investigation of a smoothed CT reconstruction algorithm. Radiology 134:507–516, 1980.

Joseph, P. M., Spital, R. D., and Stockham, C. D. The effects of sampling on CT images. Computerized Tomography 4:189–206, 1980.

Koehler, P. R., Anderson, R. E., and Baxter, B. The effect of computed tomography viewer controls on anatomical measurements. Radiology 130:189–194, 1979.

McCullough, E. C. Factors affecting the use of quantitative information from a CT scanner. Radiology 124:99–107, 1977.

McCullough, E. C., Payne, J. T., Baker, H. L., Hattery, R. R., Sheedy, P. F., Stephens, D. H., and Gedgaudas, E. Performance evaluation and quality assurance of computed tomography scanners, with illustrations from the EMI, ACTA, and Delta scanners. Radiology 120:173–178, 1976.

Ommaya, A. K., Murray, G., Ambrose, J., Richardson, A., and Hounsfield, G. Computerized axial tomography: Estimation of spatial and density resolution capability. British Journal of Radiology 49:604–611, 1976.

Osborn, A. G., and Wing, S. D. Thin section computed tomography in the evaluation of third ventricular colloid cysts. Radiology 124:257–258, 1977.

Robbins, A. H., Pugatch, R. D., Gerzof, S. G., Rankin, S. C., and Gale, D. R. An assessment of the role of scan speed in perceived image quality of body computed tomography. Radiology 139:139–146, 1981.

Tanaka, E., and Iinuma, T. A. Correction functions and statistical noises in transverse section picture reconstruction. Computers in Biology and Medicine 6:295–306, 1976.

Technicare Corporation. Technical supplement. The Delta Scan 2000 series of computed tomography scanners, 1978.

Tretiak, O. J. Noise limitations in x-ray computed tomography. Journal of Computer Assisted Tomography 2:477–480, 1978.

Wagner, L. K., and Cohen, G. Energy dependence of contrast-detail-dose and object-detectability-dose curves for CT scanners. Journal of Computer Assisted Tomography 6:378–382, 1982.

Zatz, L. M. Image quality in cranial computed tomography.

Journal of Computer Assisted Tomography 2:336–340, 1978.

Zatz, L. M. Basic principles of computed tomography scanning. *In* T. H. Newton and D. G. Potts (eds.), Radiology of the Skull and Brain: Technical Aspects of Computed Tomography, Vol. 5, Chap. 109, Part XVI, pp. 3853–3876. C. V. Mosby, St. Louis, 1981.

Patient Dosage in Computed Tomography

Balter, S. A philosophy of "dose" specification for computed tomography. Medicamundi 22:11–12, 1977.

Bassano, D. A., Chamberlain, C. C., Mozley, J. M., and Kieffer, S. A. Physical, performance, and dosimetric characteristics of the Delta Scan 50 whole-body/brain scanner. Radiology 123:455–462, 1977.

Bhave, D. G., Kelsey, C. A., Burstein, J., and Brogdon, B. G. Scattered radiation doses to infants and children during EMI head scans. Radiology 124:379–380, 1977.

Brasch, R. C., Boyd, D. P., and Gooding, C. A. Computed tomographic scanning in children: Comparison of radiation dose and resolving power of commercial CT scanners. American Journal of Roentgenology 131:95–101, 1978.

Cohen, G. Contrast-detail-dose analysis of six different computed tomographic scanners. Journal of Computer Assisted Tomography 3:197–203, 1979.

Cohen, G., and DiBianca, F. A. The use of contrast-detail-dose evaluation of image quality in a computed tomographic scanner. Journal of Computer Assisted Tomography 3:189–195, 1979.

Dixon, R. L., and Ekstrand, K. E. A film dosimetry system for use in computed tomography. Radiology 127:255–258, 1978.

General Electric Company. CT/T technology continuum. Technical performance of the CT/T system. General Electric Publication No. 4870.

General Electric Company. CT/T technology continuum update. The significance of dose and sensitivity profiles. General Electric Publication No. 4998, 1979.

Gordon, R. Dose reduction in computerized tomography. Guest editorial. Investigative Radiology 11:508–517, 1976.

Gross, G. P., and McCullough, E. C. Radiation protection requirements for a whole-body CT scanner. Radiology 122:825–826, 1977.

Hobday, P., and Parker, R. P. Radiation exposure to the patient in computerized tomography. British Journal of Radiology 51:925–926, 1978.

Isherwood, I., Young, I. M., Bowker, K. W., and Brumall, G. K. Radiation dose to the eyes of the patient during neuroradiological investigations. Neuroradiology 10:137–141, 1975.

Koch, H., Freundlich, D., Zaklad, H., and Koch, B. Low dose CT imaging. *In* P. Gerhardt and E. van Kaick (eds.), Total Body Computerized Tomography. International Symposium, Heidelberg, 1977, pp. 60–65. Georg Thieme, Stuttgart, 1979.

Krauss, O., and Schuhmacher, H. Absorbed dose to the patient by computerized whole body x-ray. *In* P. Gerhardt and E. van Kaick (eds.), Total Body Computerized Tomography. International Symposium, Heidelberg, 1977, pp. 52–56. Georg Thieme, Stuttgart, 1979.

Linke, G., Pauli, K., and Pfeiler, M. Exposure of the patient to radiation in computerized axial tomography. Electromedica 1/76, pp. 15–18.

McCullough, E. C., and Payne, J. T. Patient dosage in computed tomography. Radiology 129:457–463, 1978.

McCullough. E. C. Payne, J. T., Baker, H. L., Hattery, R. R., Sheedy, P. F., Stephens, D. H., and Gedgaudus, E. Performance evaluation and quality assurance of computed tomography scanners, with illustrations from the EMI, ACTA, and Delta scanners. Radiology 120:173–188, 1976.

Pentlow, K. S. Dosimetry in computed tomography. *In* T. H. Newton and D. G. Potts (eds.), Radiology of the Skull and Brain: Technical Aspects of Computed Tomography, Vol. 5, Chap. 124, Part XVII, pp. 4228–4258. C. V. Mosby, St. Louis, 1981.

Perry, B. J., and Bridges, C. Computerized transverse axial scanning (tomography): Part 3. Radiation dose considerations. British Journal of Radiology 46:1048–1051, 1973.

Shrivastava, P. N., Lynn, S. L., and Ting, J. Y. Exposures to patient and personnel in computed axial tomography. Radiology 125:411–415, 1977.

Trefler, M., and Haughton, V. M. Patient dose and image quality in computed tomography. American Journal of Roentgenology 137:25–27, 1981.

Villafana, T., Scouras, J., Kirkland, L., and McElroy, N. Health physics aspects of the EMI computerized tomography brain scanner. Health Physics 34:71–82, 1978.

Wall, B. F., Green, D. A. C., and Veerappan, R. The radiation dose to patients from EMI and body scanners. British Journal of Radiology 122:699–702, 1977.

Accuracy and Reliability of CT Numbers

Bergstrom, M. Performance evaluation of scanners. *In* T. H. Newton and D. G. Potts (eds.), Radiology of the Skull and Brain: Technical Aspects of Computed Tomography, Vol. 5, Chap. 123, Part XVII, pp. 4212–4227. C. V. Mosby, St. Louis, 1981.

Bydder, G., and Kreel, L. The temperature dependence of computed tomography attenuation values. Journal of Computer Assisted Tomography 3:506–510, 1979.

McCullough, E. C. Potentials of computed tomography in radiation therapy treatment planning. Radiology 129:765–768, 1978.

McCullough, E. C. Computed tomography in radiation therapy treatment planning. *In* T. H. Newton and D. G. Potts (eds.), Radiology of the Skull and Brain: Technical Aspects of Computed Tomography, Vol. 5, Chap. 127, Part XVIII, pp. 4301–4311. C. V. Mosby, St. Louis, 1981.

McDavid, W. D., Waggener, R. G., Sank, V. J., Dennis, M. J., and Payne, W. H. Correlating computed tomographic numbers with physical properties and operating kilovoltage. Radiology 123:761–762, 1977.

Phelps, M. E., Gado, M. H., and Hoffman, E. J. Correlation of effective atomic number and electron density with attenuation coefficients measured with polychromatic x-rays. Radiology 117:585–588, 1975.

Phelps, M. D., Hoffman, E. J., and Ter-Pogossian, M. M. Attenuation coefficients of various body tissues, fluids, and lesions at photon energies of 18 to 136 keV. Radiology 117:573–583, 1975.

Pullan, B. R., Ritchings, R. T., and Isherwood, I. Accuracy and meaning of computed tomography attenuation values. *In* T. H. Newton and D. G. Potts (eds.), Radiology of the Skull and Brain: Technical Aspects of Computed Tomography, Vol. 5, Chap. 111, Part XVI, pp. 3904–3917. C. V. Mosby, St. Louis, 1981.

Rao, P. S., and Gregg, E. C. Attenuation of monoenergetic gamma rays in tissues. American Journal of Roentgenology 123:631–637, 1975.

Thaler, H. T., Rottenberg, D. A., Pentlow, K. S., and Allen, J. C. A method of correcting for linear drift in computed tomography brain scans. Journal of Computer Assisted Tomography 3:251–255, 1979.

Wittenberg, J., Maturi, R. A., Ferrucci, J. T., and Margolies, M. N. Computerized tomography of in vitro abdominal organs—Effect of preservation methods on attenuation coefficient. Computerized Tomography 1:95–101, 1977.

Zatz, L. M. Basic principles of computed tomography scanning. *In* T. H. Newton and D. G. Potts (eds.), Radiology of the Skull and Brain: Technical Aspects of Computed Tomography, Vol. 5, Chap. 109, Part XVI, pp. 3853–3876. C. V. Mosby, St. Louis, 1981.

Zatz, L. M., and Alvarez, R. E. An inaccuracy in computed tomography: The energy dependence of CT values. Radiology 124:91–97, 1977.

CT Phantoms

Bassano, D. A., Chamberlain, C. C., Mozley, J. M., and Kieffer, S. A. Physical performance and dosimetric characteristics of the Δ-Scan 50 whole-body/brain scanner. Radiology 123:455–462, 1977.

Bergstrom, M. Performance evaluation of scanners. *In* T. H. Newton and D. G. Potts (eds.), Radiology of the Skull and Brain: Technical Aspects of Computed Tomography, Vol. 5, Chap. 123, Part XVII, pp. 4212–4227. C. V. Mosby, St. Louis, 1981.

Brooks, R. A. and Di Chiro, G. Slice geometry in computer assisted tomography. Journal of Computer Assisted Tomography 1:191–199, 1977.

Chew, E., Weiss, G. H., Brooks, R. A., and Di Chiro, G. Effect of CT noise on detectability of test objects. American Journal of Roentgenology 131:681–685, 1978.

Cohen, G., and DiBianca, F. A. The use of contrast-detail-dose evaluation of image quality in a computed tomography scanner. Journal of Computer Assisted Tomography 3:189–195, 1979.

Duerinckx, A. J., and Macovski, A. Polychromatic streak artifacts in computed tomography images. Journal of Computer Assisted Tomography 2:481–487, 1978.

Fullerton, G. D., and White, D. R. Anthropomorphic test objects for CT scanners. Radiology 133:217–222, 1979.

Joseph, P. M., Hilal, S. K., Schulz, R. A., and Kelz, F. Clinical and experimental investigation of a smoothed CT reconstruction algorithm. Radiology 134:507–516, 1980.

McCullough, E. C., Payne, J. T., Baker, H. L., Hattery, R. R., Sheedy, P. F., Stephens, D. H., and Gedgaudas, E. Performance evaluation and quality assurance of computed tomography scanners, with illustrations from the EMI, ACTA, and Delta scanners. Radiology 120:173–188, 1976.

Zatz, L. M. Image quality in cranial computed tomography. Journal of Computer Tomography 2:336–346, 1978.

CHAPTER 9
FURTHER APPLICATIONS OF COMPUTED TOMOGRAPHY AND OTHER TOMOGRAPHIC TECHNIQUES

FURTHER APPLICATIONS OF COMPUTED TOMOGRAPHY

Computed Radiography
  Principles and System Design
  Clinical Applications
  Comparison of Computed Radiography and Conventional Radiography
Multiplanar Reconstruction (Reformatted Images in Nontransverse Planes)
Dynamic Computed Tomography
Applications of Computed Tomography in Radiation Therapy
High Resolution Computed Tomography
Gated Scanning
Dual Energy Scanning

OTHER TOMOGRAPHIC TECHNIQUES

Ultrafast Transmission Scanning
  Dynamic Spatial Reconstructor
  Scanning Electron Beam Systems
Emission Computed Tomography
  General Description
  Gamma Ray Emission Computed Tomography
  Positron Emission Computed Tomography
Ultrasound
  Historical Background
  General Principles
  Imaging Techniques
Nuclear Magnetic Resonance Imaging
  Historical Background
  Basic Principles of NMR
  Fundamental Parameters of NMR
  Techniques of Imaging with NMR
  Biological Effects
Microwave Computed Tomography

REFERENCES AND SUGGESTED READINGS

The first part of this chapter discusses additional applications of computed tomography, including a number of refinements and modifications of the basic techniques described earlier. These include computed radiography, multiplanar reconstruction, dynamic CT, applications of CT in radiation therapy, high resolution CT, gated CT, and dual energy scanning. The fundamental concepts are stressed in each instance. The remainder of the chapter deals with other tomographic imaging techniques. The unifying feature of these techniques is that each is used to produce a tomographic or sectional image. The nature of the physical interaction ultimately responsible for producing image information is quite different for these different tomographic techniques. The physical basis of each technique and the physical parameter to be measured in each case are discussed with emphasis on fundamental concepts. Topics discussed include ultrafast transmission scanning, emission CT, ultrasound, nuclear magnetic resonance, and microwave CT.

FURTHER APPLICATIONS OF COMPUTED TOMOGRAPHY

Computed Radiography

Principles and System Design Computed radiography (also called computed digital radiography or digital computed radiography) is a technique for obtaining a radiograph-like image by moving a patient through a CT gantry. As the bed on which the patient lies is translated through the gantry at constant speed, the x-ray tube is activated or pulsed, and the detector array measures the x-ray beam transmitted through the patient. The radiographic image obtained with this method resembles a conventional radiograph and has been called a scout view (General Electric), indicating its initial primary application as a localization technique prior to performing CT.

The scout view or computed radiograph performed with the patient positioned on the CT bed permits accurate localization and orientation of the CT scanning slices for an optimal and efficient examination. With clinical usage, computed radiography has emerged as an effective diagnostic imaging technique in its own right.

The technique of digital computed radiography, as illustrated in Figure 9.1 by a third generation rotating tube and detector array, is performed in the following manner. With the x-ray tube fixed in a stationary position, the patient is translated on the bed through the CT gantry at constant speed (e.g., 6 cm/s) while the highly collimated fan beam of x-rays passes through the patient. The stationary x-ray tube is aligned prior to scanning for either a frontal or a lateral view. It may also be rotated 8° laterally from an anteroposterior position for stereo views. In a rotating detector system, the entire detector array is always aligned opposite to the x-ray tube and is stationary when the tube is fixed. In a fixed detector system, a portion of the detector system opposite the fixed x-ray tube is used.

When the x-ray tube is pulsed, each detector element intercepts a portion of the transmitted x-ray fan beam. The data in each detector element are recorded in a signal channel for each individual detector element. Signal data are recorded in all the detector elements for a single pulse (or for a specified measurement time, for a continuously operating tube). Each pulse thus yields one line or profile of x-ray information, that is, one line of information across the patient. Multiple x-ray pulses occur during patient translation through the gantry, each resulting in a new set of x-ray data or an x-ray profile. As the patient is translated through the gantry, a longitudinally contiguous set of x-ray profiles is generated. The information is digitized and processed as it is collected. At the end of the translation and data processing, the image is displayed. Spatial efficiency may be improved by collimating the fan beam to a slice thickness of 1.5 mm and either sampling at 1.5-mm increments or taking overlapping samples at .75-mm intervals.

Computed radiography is usually performed with either third generation units (rotating tube and detectors) employing pulsed radiation, as shown in Figure 9.1, or with fourth generation units (rotating tube and stationary detectors) employing continuous radiation. In principle, computed radiography can also be performed with first and second generation units (translational-rotational systems). However, because of the relatively fewer detector elements that are available in translational-rotational systems to obtain a profile, the detector or detectors must be translated across the patient for each data line or profile. This would involve a proportional increase in the total time required to obtained a computed radiograph.

Because the image information is converted into and stored in digital form, it can be processed and manipulated with digital technique. This allows digital processing of the image as with CT sections.

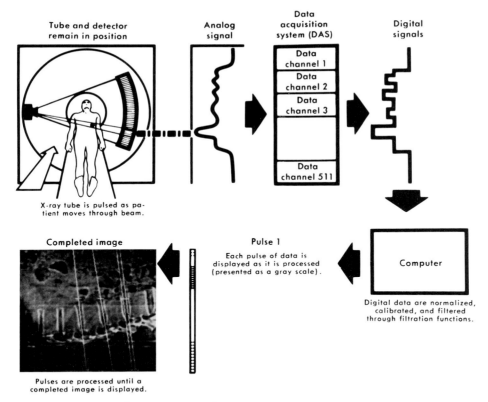

Figure 9.1. Diagram of the CT scanner, demonstrating the essential system components and the sequence of data acquisition and data modifications required to form an electronic digital image. (Reproduced by permission from W. D. Foley et al. Digital radiography of the chest using a computed tomography instrument. Radiology 133:231–234, 1979.)

There are several significant advantages of digital computed radiography. The use of the very efficient high pressure xenon or scintillation crystal detectors enables a low patient dose (e.g., an incident skin dose of 100 mrad for a pulsed output scanner at maximum tube output; Foley and DiBianca, 1981). The thin slit collimation of the detector results in rejection of scatter radiation, thus improving image contrast. In particular, there is good low contrast sensitivity for large objects. The x-ray detectors, particularly high pressure xenon cells, have a relatively wide dynamic range (the range of x-ray intensities over which the detectors are linear in their response).

Finally, the image can be processed and modified with digital techniques. This permits the use of edge enhancement and also allows direct view manipulation of the image on the display monitor.

The principal disadvantages are the relatively poor high contrast spatial resolutions and the long exposure or image formation time. The spatial resolution for digital computed radiography is about .5 line pairs per mm for high contrast detail. The image formation time for digital computed radiography is about 5–7 s, compared to times of significantly less than 1 s for conventional radiography.

Computed radiography is a specific example of or a particular approach to a more general group of imaging techniques that fall under the heading of scanned projection radiography. The basis of scanned projection radiography is the employment of a detector system that views only a small part of the patient at any point in time. The detector system scans the patient over the region of interest by mechanically translating either the patient or the x-ray source and detector system. Computed radiography thus represents an approach to scanned projection radiography in which the x-ray tube and detector system in the gantry of a CT unit are used, and in which the patient is translated through the gantry with the x-ray tube and detectors fixed in position. Other approaches to scanned projection radiography which do not use CT systems include the employment of a

Further Applications   215

pencil beam scanner with a scintillating screen that is scanned in a line-by-line fashion with an array of light-sensitive detectors.

Because of the slitlike nature of the detector apertures used, computed radiography may also be considered as a kind of slit beam radiography, in distinction to the large area beam radiography of conventional radiography.

The digital nature of the computed radiograph is shared with other digital imaging systems such as digital subtraction fluoroscopy or angiography. The latter techniques differ in the detector or receptor system and the method of data acquisition.

Clinical Applications Because a computed radiograph is performed with a patient lying on the CT table, specific planes or sections can be selected in reference to the computed radiograph and then related to a table index scale at the image margin (Figure 9.2). The operator may then position the table by computer control through the operator console, so that computed tomograms are obtained at the selected sections. In addition, the correct alignment of angled sections can be determined from a lateral projection (Figure 9.3). This expedites the performance of CT examination, permitting the selection of the optimal scanning sections through the correct region of interest. The inefficiency of scanning too many body sections can be avoided, thus reducing radiation exposure and x-ray tube use. The efficiency and time requirements for the examination can be improved, allowing better patient throughput.

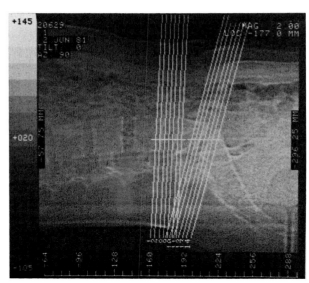

Figure 9.3. Selection of levels for CT scans with appropriate angulation for gantry tilt for optimal orientation relative to the disk space.

Without computed radiography, localization techniques for CT have been a great deal more cumbersome. For example, a preliminary radiograph might be performed with localization markers attached to the patient. After selection of the desired scan sections the patient would then be moved to the CT gantry. This technique is more inefficient and time-consuming, less accurate, and necessitates a separate radiograph with a higher radiation exposure than a comparable computed radiograph. Another less accurate localization technique that has been employed is the use of an external laser beam to reference external or topographical landmarks in the CT gantry. In contrast, CT permits localization on the basis of internal structures or organs.

Some other clinical examples of computed radiography are illustrated in Figures 9.4–9.6.

In batch image reconstruction, the image data for multiple sequential scans are stored in the computer memory during scanning. Reconstruction and display can be done during but mostly after the scanning. A computed radiograph can be used to localize the region of interest. Thus an entire scan sequence can be performed without monitoring individual scans but with the assurance that the region of interest has been included in the scan sequence. The time for such a study would then be limited only by the time necessitated for patient positioning, performance of

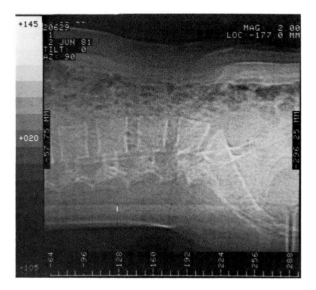

Figure 9.2. Computed radiograph of the lumbosacral spine, lateral view. The numbers at the bottom of the image indicate the position in centimeters along the table.

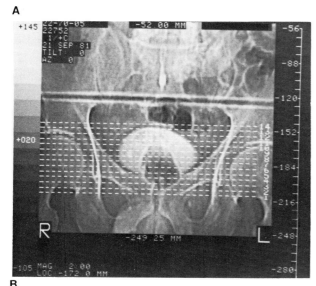

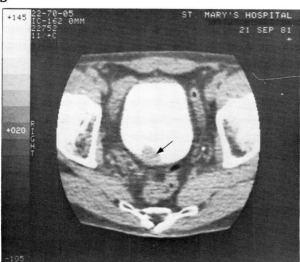

Figure 9.4. *A*, Computed radiograph illustrating the contrast-filled bladder and showing the levels of selected transverse scans through the bladder. *B*, One transverse CT scan through the bladder illustrating a tumor (arrow).

the computed radiograph, selection of appropriate scan sections, scanning time, table incrementation, and tube cooling. It may still be appropriate to have the patient remain in the department until after the individual scans have been examined in the event that any additional scans are necessary.

Computed angiotomography, or dynamic scanning, consists of obtaining multiple scans in rapid sequence during and following injection of a bolus of contrast material. The scans may be performed at the same or contiguous levels. Batch image recon-

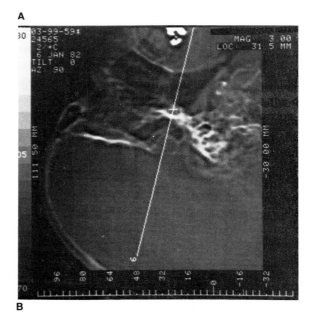

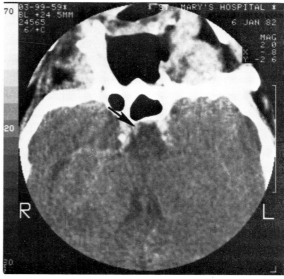

Figure 9.5. Coronal imaging of the sella turcica. *A*, Magnified computed radiograph of the head illustrating selection of an appropriately oriented section through the sella turcica. *B*, The corresponding coronal CT section shows a small pituitary (arrow) in an otherwise "empty" sella. The image has been inverted relative to its display on the monitor for a more appropriate anatomical presentation.

Further Applications 217

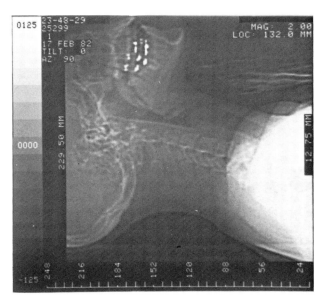

Figure 9.6. Computed radiograph showing a lateral view of the cervical spine.

may, for example, increase the perceptivity of low contrast lesions such as some lung tumors. Its clinical efficacy is, however, offset by the relatively poorer spatial resolution, long image formation time, and the relatively high equipment cost.

Comparison of Computed Radiography and Conventional Radiography A comparison of computed radiography and conventional radiography (standard film-screen radiography) has been discussed and analyzed in some detail by Cohen et al. (1979) and by Foley and DiBianca (1981).

Contrast Resolution In conventional radiography, the ratio of the scatter to the primary radiation is of the order of 70–100%. In computed radiography, the scatter-to-primary ratio on a General Electric CT/T 8800 system is about 4–5% (Foley and DiBianca, 1981). Since scatter is one of the primary limitations to contrast resolution, this reduced scatter-to-primary radiation ratio permits a significant improvement in contrast. In computed radiography, the out-of-plane scattered radiation (the scattered radiation that is deflected out of the section being irradiated by the primary beam) is rejected since it is not incident on the detectors. Because this is the major portion of scattered radiation, its rejection is the primary reason for the significantly improved scatter-to-primary radiation for slit beam compared to wide area radiography. In-plane scattered radiation (scattered radiation that remains in the section of the primary beam) will fall on the detectors but may not be recorded because of detector collimation.

The greatly improved efficiency of CT detector systems in capturing and detecting incident radiation (about 50–90%), compared to even the relatively efficient rare earth film-screen combinations of conventional radiography, permits a significant noise reduction per equivalent dose and a further increase in contrast resolution.

Dynamic Range The dynamic range of a computed radiographic display is an indication of the range of signal strengths that may be accurately recorded and displayed. This is equivalent to the latitude of a film-screen combination in conventional radiography. The dynamic range in computed radiography is of the order of 10,000:1, compared to about 100:1 for conventional radiography (Foley and DiBianca, 1981). The wider dynamic range is the result of an electronic rather than a film recording system. This increases the range of tissue densities that can be recorded and displayed.

Spatial Resolution Conventional radiographic film screen combinations permit spatial resolution in the range of 3–8 line pairs per mm. This is determined by the screen thickness.

For the General Electric CT/T 8800, the spatial resolution of a computed radiograph is about .5 line pairs per mm. For this system the spatial resolution in the plane of the fan beam is determined by the detector aperture in the field of view (.74 mm) and the sampling distance between detectors projected to the center of the field of view (.83 mm). In the longitudinal plane the spatial resolution is determined by the width of the collimated fan beam (1.5 mm) and the sampling distance (either samples at 1.5-mm intervals or overlapped samples at .75-mm intervals). The poorer spatial resolution is reflected in the poorer detail of bone trabeculae, lung markings and small nodules, and opacified renal calyces.

Temporal Resolution The time required to perform a computed radiograph is typically 5–10 s, considerably longer than the subsecond exposure times of conventional radiography. The local temporal resolution or time to collect data from several contiguous scan lines is faster, of the order of 50 ms. The poorer temporal resolution of computed radiography limits its applications in areas where patient motion is a problem or where rapid sequential radiographs are required.

Image Manipulation The digital nature of a computed radiograph permits manipulation to modify the image in order to enhance useful information relative to noise. Such techniques are not available in any practical fashion with conventional radiography.

Multiplanar Reconstruction (Reformatted Images in Nontransverse Planes)

One of the most important limitations of CT has been the constraint on the orientation of the body cross-sections that can be imaged. The usual scans are axial or transverse, that is, perpendicular to the long axis of the body. Coronal sections of the head as well as nontransverse sections of the limbs in adults and of the body in infants may be obtained by appropriate patient positioning within the gantry. However, the necessary positioning is often awkward and frequently uncomfortable for the patients, thus further limiting the capability of imaging nontransverse sections.

To obtain images of sections perpendicular to the original transverse scans (i.e., sagittal, coronal, or oblique) while circumventing the limitations and difficulties of direct nonaxial scanning, an indirect approach has been developed. The direct scanning in the CT gantry is still performed for transverse sections. A multiplanar reconstruction is then performed, reformatting the series of original transverse scan sections into new sets of body sections corresponding to nonaxial or nontransverse planes. Initially, the reformatted image sections were limited to planes perpendicular to the original transverse sections: coronal, sagittal, or oblique. Further refinements have expanded the technique to include image sections at any arbitrary, nonperpendicular orientation to the original transverse sections.

In the original pioneering work in this field by William V. Glenn, Jr., et al. (1975), the reconstruction technique involved taking overlapping thick (8 mm) CT sections and then constructing a larger number of thinner (2 mm) nonoverlapped sections. This process of making thin transverse sections from thicker overlapped sections is called deconvolution. Each voxel in a thick section, typically measuring 8 × 1.5 × 1.5 mm, is divided into smaller voxels measuring 2 × 1.5 × 1.5 mm. These smaller, more cubic voxels are then used as the basic picture elements in reconstructing sagittal and coronal sections. That is, the smaller cubelike voxels are the basic building blocks or picture elements in vertically oriented image planes perpendicular to the original transverse scans. The use of multiple overlapping scans results, however, in each smaller element of tissue residing within several different scan sections, thus significantly increasing the radiation dose to that tissue element.

An alternative approach involves the use of multiple contiguous but not overlapping transverse sections. By selecting out of each transverse section all the elements or voxels in the same corresponding or contiguous row from one transverse or axial section to the next, a coronal section is reconstructed. Similarly, by selecting all the elements or voxels in successive corresponding columns from the transverse sections, a sagittal section is reconstructed. This is illustrated in Figure 9.7. Using this approach, the spatial resolution along the direction of the body axis, perpendicular to the original transverse scans, can be no better than the thickness or depth of the transverse scans. This resolution may be improved by employing thinner sections of 5 or even 1.5 mm. The use of thinner sections, however, entails a greater radiation dose, since approximately the same number of photons must be used in each thin section as in a single thick section to avoid increasing the statistical noise in a section. Also, more scans are required to cover a fixed thickness of the body, necessitating both a longer scanning time and a longer reconstruction time to obtain the multiplanar images. The reformatted images have been useful in a variety of clinical situations, as illustrated in Figures 9.8–9.14. Generally, coronal images of the head, when appropriate, may be obtained by direct scanning in the coronal plane. The direct coronal scans are of superior image quality compared to the coronal images obtained by reformatting original transverse scans.

Dynamic Computed Tomography

Dynamic computed tomography, or rapid sequence CT scanning, is a method of obtaining dynamic physiological or functional information in addition to the usual static anatomical information about tissue cross-sections. In particular, dynamic CT allows investigation of vascular blood flow and tissue perfusion. Multiple fast CT scans, varying from approximately 1–5 s, are performed in rapid sequence for a specific cross-section. That is, the patient table is not moved between scans, so that the same tissue cross-section is repeatedly scanned, with a short interscan delay typically of about 1 or 2 s.

To achieve dynamic CT imaging, the following requirements must be met: the computer must have sufficient memory to store the large quantity of raw data from all of the images obtained (typically 6–16)

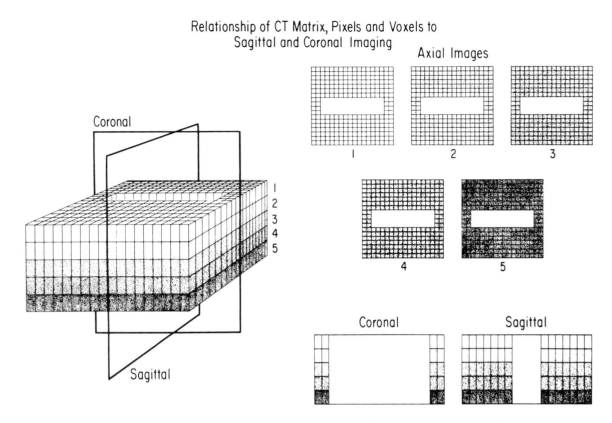

Figure 9.7. Multiplanar reconstruction. Selection of voxels in corresponding rows or columns of adjacent axial sections allows formation of coronal or sagittal sections.

in a single dynamic sequence; the scanning apparatus must have the mechanical capability of performing successive fast scans (1–5 s) in a rapid sequence (about 1 or 2 s between the termination of one scan and the initiation of the following scan); the x-ray tube must be capable of sustaining the heat load generated by the total number of scans in the sequence, with little cooldown period between the successive scans.

To increase the rapidity of the scanning sequence, a short interscan time is essential. This necessitates the capability of rapid bidirectional scanning; that is, a clockwise-counterclockwise-clockwise sequence of the tube (fourth generation) or tube and detector array (third generation) motion can be performed without a significant delay in reversing the direction of rotation.

Another technique for rapid image acquisition involves limiting the number of views per image and having images that are overlapping in time, so that consecutive temporal images have views in common. This may be facilitated by overscanning, that is, scanning more than 360° in a single rotational motion so that more views are available as the tube (or tube and detector array) is rotated in either the clockwise or counterclockwise direction.

As an example, the Picker Synerdyne can be programmed to obtain three images in 402° of data acquisition in 1.7 s. Following an interscan delay of less than 1 s, another three images may be obtained by scanning through 402° in the opposite direction during 1.7 s. Successive images will share views with other images obtained during the same scan.

An important application of this technique is the improved identification and delineation of vascular structures, also referred to as computed angiotomography. The transient dense opacification of vessels after an intravenous bolus injection of contrast can be followed in time by rapid sequence fast scans. This not only permits the identification of a normal vascular structure, but also allows detailed examination of intravascular disease. This includes assessment of the patency of a coronary artery bypass graft, delineation of intracardiac masses (mural thrombi,

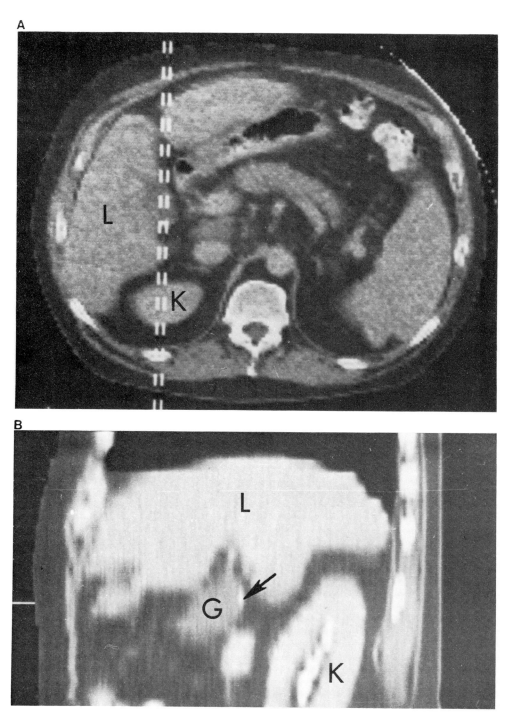

Figure 9.8. *A*, Transverse CT section of the upper abdomen indicating the location of a sagittal plane through the right kidney (*K*) and liver (*L*) to be reconstructed from adjacent transverse scans. *B*, The reformatted image of the sagittal section demonstrates the right kidney, liver, gallbladder (*G*), and a gallstone (arrow). The white line on the reader's left indicates the level of the transverse section shown in *A*.

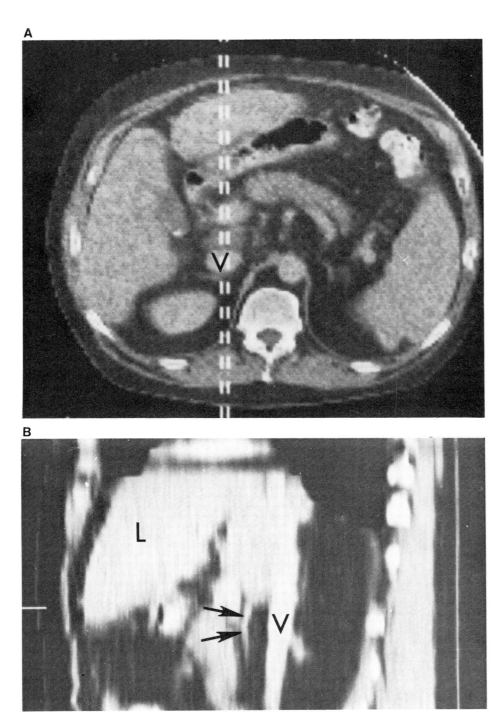

Figure 9.9. *A*, A new sagittal plane has been selected for reconstruction through the inferior vena cava (*V*). *B*, Sagittal section illustrating the opacified inferior vena cava, liver (*L*), and right adrenal gland (arrows).

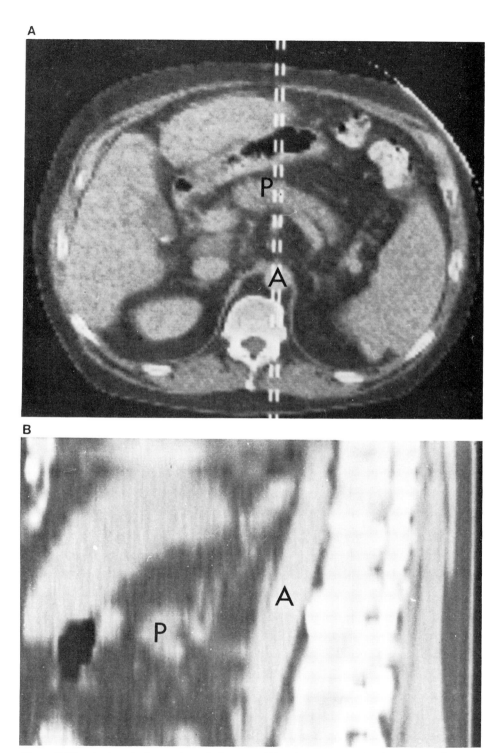

Figure 9.10. *A*, A sagittal scan through the aorta (*A*) and pancreas (*P*) has been selected. *B*, The corresponding reconstructed sagittal section.

Further Applications 223

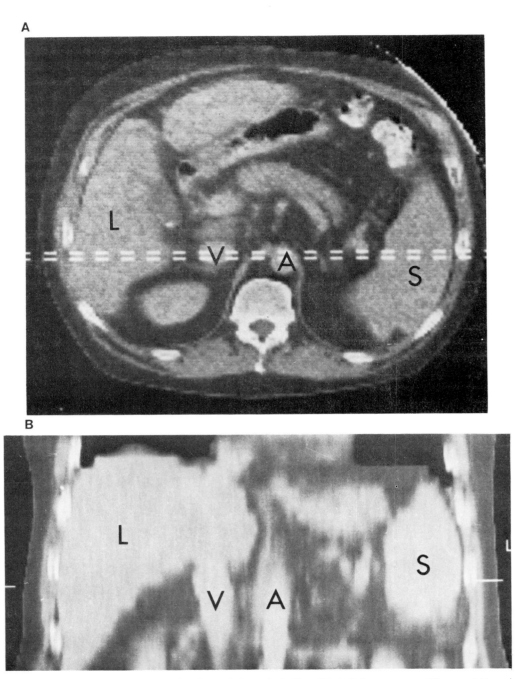

Figure 9.11. A, A coronal scan is to be obtained through the liver (L), inferior vena cava (V), aorta (A), and spleen (S). B, The reformatted coronal scan is illustrated. The white lines on the sides indicate the level of the section in A.

myxomas, and other primary or secondary tumors), the internal flap in aortic dissections, and thrombi within larger systemic and pulmonary vessels.

Another particularly significant general area of investigation is the study of blood flow to and tissue perfusion within an organ. A great deal of work has been performed in perfusion studies, especially in the brain and the kidneys. Most frequently, multiple rapid sequence scans are obtained following injection of the intravenous bolus, and the successive images

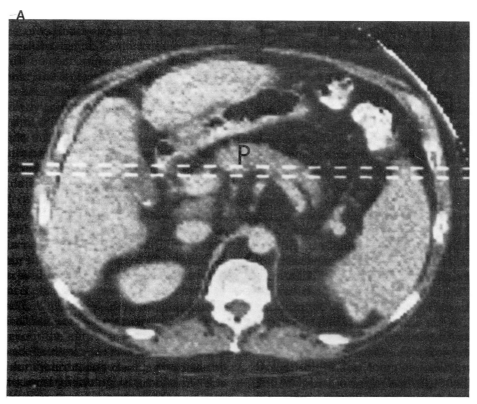

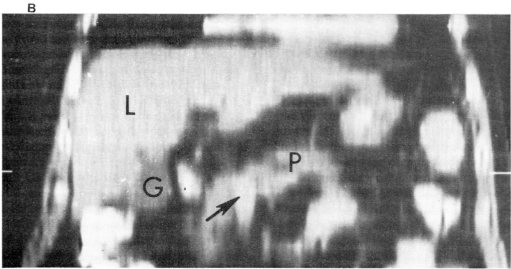

Figure 9.12. *A*, A coronal scan is to be selected at the level of the pancreas. *B*, The coronal scan shows the liver (*L*), gallbladder (*G*), pancreas (*P*), and superior mesenteric vein (arrow).

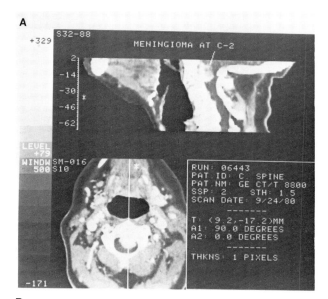

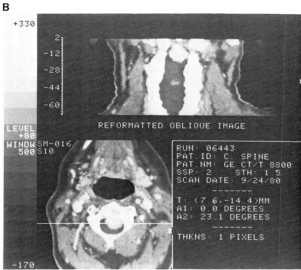

Figure 9.13. *A*, Superiorly, a sagittal image that has been reformatted from a series of transverse scans illustrating a meningioma at the level of C2; inferiorly, one of the transverse sections used in the reformatting as well as appropriate patient and scan information. *B*, A reformatted oblique image oriented along the spinal column and illustrating the meningioma. (Courtesy of General Electric Medical Systems.)

are displayed side by side, allowing direct visual assessment of gross changes in the tissue density (Figures 9.15 and 9.16). More precise identification of density changes (time-density curves) can be obtained by positioning cursor boxes of arbitrary area at different locations within the tissue cross-section and mapping the quantitative changes of the CT density of the tissue enclosed within each cursor box as a function of time (Figures 9.17 and 9.18).

Comparison of the two cerebral hemispheres permits diagnosis of ischemia by a more slowly rising perfusion curve with a depressed peak. Infarction may also be identified and distinguished from ischemia by the presence of an essentially flat perfusion curve with time (Figure 9.19). Several patterns associated with brain tumors have also been described. In the kidneys, decreased perfusion of one kidney early after injection may indicate renal arterial stenosis.

Estimates of cerebral blood flow may also be made relying on classical principles of indicator dilution analysis, which is the estimation of the volume of body compartments such as the vascular system by the dilution of a fixed amount of an indicator substance added to the compartment. This is relatively easier to do in the brain than elsewhere in the body, since the contrast does not normally enter the extravascular space in the intact brain.

Another approach to the study of blood flow by dynamic CT uses inhaled stable (nonradioactive or nondecaying) xenon. The rate of perfusion of tissue by xenon during inhalation and its washout after inhalation is stopped are dependent on blood flow and xenon solubility within the tissue. The xenon inhalation method may also be used in the study of regional lung ventilation.

An alternative use of great practical value for rapid sequence CT scanning is the rapid acquisition of serial, spatially adjacent axial cross-sections. This requires the capability for fast and accurate table incrementation during the study; a minimum of about a 2-s interscan time interval is usually needed. This rapid acquisition of multiple scans may allow an examination to be completed in a few minutes, minimizing patient time on the scanning bed. Rapid sequence scanning minimizes the possibility of patient motion between scans; in fact, several adjacent scans may be obtained during a single breath holding. This results in more accurate registration of the slices for any subsequent image reformatting in nonaxial planes.

In CT systems not equipped for dynamic scanning, some limited information concerning better opacification and identification of vascular structures may be obtained by scanning during or immediately following bolus injection of contrast (for example, 10–20 ml of intravenous contrast) at a particular level. A series of such scans can be performed, with a bolus injection occurring during or immediately preceding each scan. This is useful in distinguishing

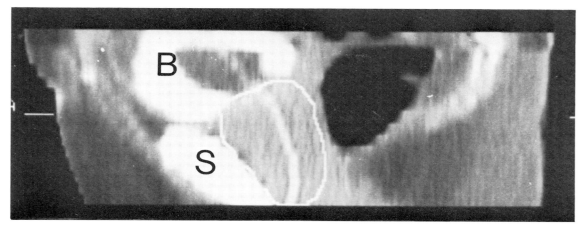

Figure 9.14. A reformatted sagittal image of the prostate gland, outlined by a trace. The bladder (*B*) and symphysis (*S*) are indicated. Contrast is seen in the urethra. Defect at the bladder base is water in a Foley catheter balloon.

between vascular and nonvascular structures, especially in the mediastinum (Figure 9.20).

Applications of Computed Tomography in Radiation Therapy

The significance of CT in planning portals for radiation therapy was appreciated from its inception. Traditionally, radiation portals have been designed on the basis of clinical evaluation, conventional radiographic studies, and radionuclide and ultrasound images, followed by simulation and computation of a treatment plan. Soon after the introduction of CT, this approach was frequently altered to include the findings of CT in the initial planning, in much the same way as conventional radiographic studies, or as a final modification. CT was recognized as a valuable approach for the follow-up evaluation of the response of the tumor to therapy.

An even more significant application of CT in radiation therapy involves planning portals directly

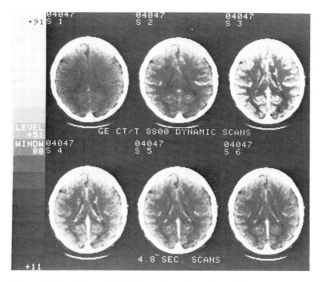

Figure 9.15. Dynamic CT scanning. A series of six scans in temporal sequence, each of 4.8 s duration, at the level of the bodies of the lateral ventricles, following a bolus of intravenous contrast. Perfusion can be identified as the contrast transmits through the brain. (Courtesy of General Electric Medical Systems.)

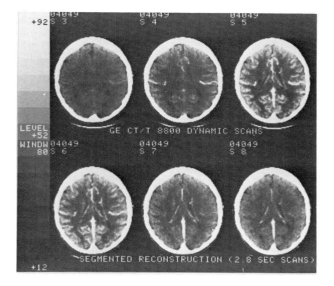

Figure 9.16. Dynamic CT scanning. A series of six scans in temporal sequence after a bolus of intravenous contrast. Each scan is reconstructed on the basis of 2.8 s of scan data. This allows more rapid accumulation of images and perfusion data.

Further Applications

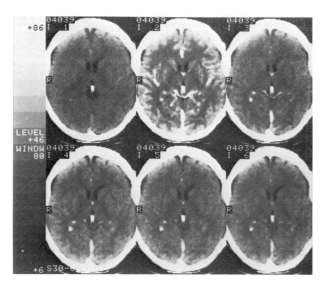

Figure 9.17. Dynamic CT scanning. Six consecutive scans, each of 4.8 s duration, at the level of the anterior horns of the lateral ventricle after a bolus of intravenous contrast.

from the CT images. CT provides information about the tumor location and size, its relationship to internal organs and structures, the patient's contours, and tissue composition, all of which affect the dose distribution. One method of directly using this information involves the magnification of a scan to lifesize proportions. The patient contours, tumor volume, and heterogeneities are traced. The different shapes

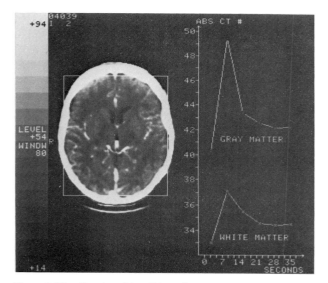

Figure 9.18. Graphs of the CT numbers in gray matter and white matter as a function of time following the bolus for the sequence of scans from Figure 9.17.

are entered into a treatment planning system along with appropriate electron density values or associated Compton linear attenuation coefficients. In another approach, the CT image is transferred to a floppy disk and displayed on a diagnostic display console (DDC) that is independent of the main computer and capable of displaying images from a floppy disk. The external body contour and the tumor contours are then traced with a cursor or light pen on the image as it is displayed on the independent DDC. A disk reader in the DDC transfers the data to a radiation therapy planning system such as the older EMI RAD-8 or Artronix PC-12 or the newer AECL (Atomic Energy of Canada, Limited) Theraplan or the ATC treatment planning system. Quantitative CT density information, which incorporates a general map of electron density, is included with the scan, and this allows for tissue heterogeneity corrections.

In megavoltage beam therapy (^{60}Co through 25 MV x-rays), the Compton effect or scattering is by far the dominant mode of interaction between the x-ray beam and the irradiated tissues up to about 10 MV. At higher energies, the process of pair production becomes increasingly important. Compton scattering depends primarily on the electron density (e/cm^3). The shapes of the isodose curves are therefore determined to a great extent by the electron density of the irradiated tissue.

For therapy planning purposes, the linear attenuation coefficient may be assumed as a first approximation to be equal to the Compton linear attenuation coefficient. Equation 2.14 may then be written as

$$\text{CT number} = \frac{\mu_e - \mu_{H_2O}}{\mu_{H_2O}} \times K, \tag{9.1}$$

when the linear attenuation coefficient for an arbitrary tissue μ_e (other than bone) and water μ_{H_2O} are determined entirely by the Compton effect. Equation 9.1 may be solved for the ratio μ_e/μ_{H_2O}, giving

$$\frac{\mu_e}{\mu_{H_2O}} = \frac{\text{CT number} + K}{K}, \tag{9.2}$$

where K is equal to 500 or 1,000, depending on whether old or new Hounsfield units are used. Since

$$\mu_e \propto N_e, \tag{9.3}$$

where N_e is equal to the electron density of an arbitrary tissue, then

$$\frac{N_e}{N_{H_2O}} = \frac{\mu_e}{\mu_{H_2O}} = \frac{\text{CT number} + K}{K}. \tag{9.4}$$

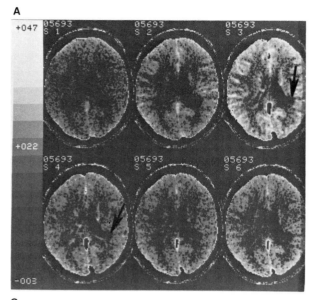
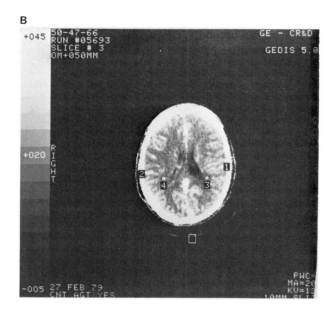
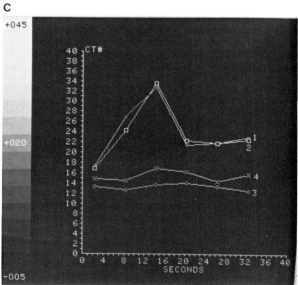

Figure 9.19. Cerebral infarction. A, Nonperfusion of the paraventricular white matter near the left atrium (arrow). When the contralateral normal white matter curve is compared to that of the infarction, one notes the disappearance of the small elevation of the perfusion curve in the infarcted area. This is an infarction in deep left parietal white matter near the atrium. B, Selection of four areas whose perfusion curves will be examined. C, Curve 3 represents the abnormal white matter perfusion curve. Curve 4 is the contralateral (right) normal control area. Curves 1 and 2 represent normal temporal cortical curves. (Reproduced by permission from E. R. Heinz et al. Dynamic computed tomography study of the brain. Journal of Computer Assisted Tomography 3:641–649, 1979.)

Thus, a reasonably accurate estimate of the electron densities of different soft tissues may be obtained from the CT numbers. Unfortunately, the electron density of tumors may be quite similar or identical (isodense) to that of normal tissues. Intravenous contrast enhancement may result in uneven changes in the CT numbers, thus permitting a separation of tumor from normal tissue. This separation may then be traced as a tumor boundary, It may be appropriate to perform a scan of a particular section before and after intravenous contrast enhancement. The border between tumor and normal tissue may be identified better in the enhanced section. This border can then be traced on the unenhanced section where the tumor and normal tissue are isodense, using the enhanced section as a guide. Thus, the electron density information used in therapy planning will not be falsely elevated because of intravenous contrast enhancement.

The accurate delineation of tumor borders by this method permits better planning of therapy, to deliver an optimal tumor dose while limiting the irradiation of noninvolved tissues, including vital and often radiation-sensitive organs. However, to accomplish this the array of CT numbers composing a scan

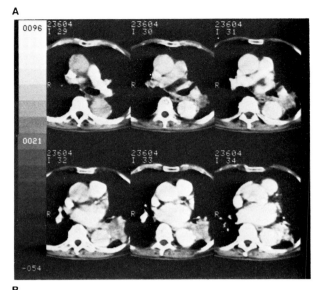

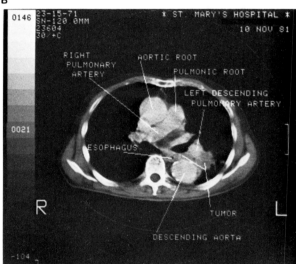

Figure 9.20. A patient with a mediastinal mass. A, Six spatially sequential scans in the thorax, each performed immediately after a bolus of intravenous contrast, which allow vascular and nonvascular structures to be distinguished. B, The different normal structures and tumor are indicated for the second scan in the sequence.

has to be converted to an array of attenuation coefficients or electron densities using Equation 9.2 or 9.4. This usually entails significant computer effort. Whether or not such an effort is worthwhile has been the subject of several debates. For example, McCullough (1978) has described the limitations in the use of CT numbers in planning megavoltage beam therapy. These include the following: 1) inhomogeneity corrections are really useful only in a small number of therapy plans; 2) there is a lack of sensitivity for various correction schemes for megavoltage photon beam therapy (as documented by Geise and McCullough, 1977); 3) there is an inherent inaccuracy in correction schemes; 4) determinations of electron density in vivo are inaccurate; and 5) there is a relatively narrow range of CT numbers and electron densities for most soft tissues (the greatest difference is usually the approximately 9% difference between fat and nonfatty soft tissues).

McCullough (1978) listed several technical factors that limit the accuracy of in vivo determination of electron densities. These include: (1) variation in CT number of H_2O and contrast scale with kVp, size and shape of the patient, and composition of the patient; 2) artifactual behavior related to poor (or no) polychromatic corrections, the algorithm frequency response, uniform imaging of complex subjects, machine performance and variations in patient bolusing (intravenous contrast enhancement), centering, or movement; and 3) scan (photon) noise.

Prasad and others (1979) have attempted pixel-by-pixel corrections for tissue inhomogeneities with a CT-interfaced treatment planning system. The CT number associated with each pixel was converted into a physical density. The resulting data were compared with dose measurements performed in a phantom. This showed that the pixel calculations resulted in an overestimate of the dose by 5–7% in locations adjoining the lung. The overestimate was felt to be due to the fact that the loss of scatter at greater depths is reflected in the measured values but not in the computed values. This happened because the loss of scatter was not taken into account by the algorithm, which would have to be improved. However, there were several advantages cited. Using pixel calculations from CT, it is not necessary to outline the various inhomogeneities or to assign appropriate physical or electron densities. After generating and storing a table correlating CT numbers and electron densities for routine scans, the system automatically converts CT numbers to densities for dose calculations at megavoltage energies. This can be helpful in radiation therapy planning, in which assignment of densities may present a problem since such density values are usually not available and can vary significantly between patients.

In spite of the above controversies, radiotherapy treatment planning programs are now being directly incorporated within or interfaced to many CT units. Typically, a trackball-controlled cursor or possibly a light pen is used to trace the external patient outline for the CT slices. Alternatively, this is done auto-

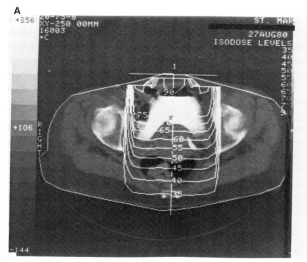

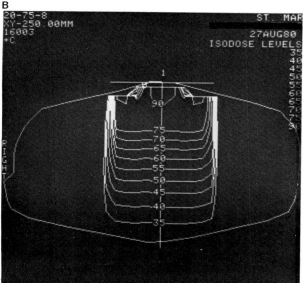

Figure 9.21. Radiation therapy plan using a single portal, showing (A) soft tissue structures with contrast in the bladder, and (B) superimposed over a body contour. Contrast is useful to define the bladder boundaries; however, final portals may be planned on unenhanced sections so that contrast does not falsely alter the electron density information.

matically under the control of the computer. The tumor or target is also outlined using a trackball or similar approach. Structures for inhomogeneity correction or for relative sparing are also outlined.

Information about the different megavoltage beams that are employed by the therapist (e.g., beam energy, cobalt or linear accelerator, source wedges) is incorporated into the computer software. An appropriate therapeutic approach is then selected, for example, skin-surface-dose (SSD) or rotational iso-centric therapy. The therapy planner may then create a therapy plan by selecting particular radiation beams and positioning them in appropriate physical relationships to tumor and normal tissues. The isodose levels of a therapy plan can be displayed superimposed over the tissue cross-section, or over the external contour only of the section, permitting evaluation of the adequacy of a plan. If a particular beam pattern does not deliver adequate tumor irradiation or does not permit appropriate sparing of a vital organ, one or more of the beams can be easily repositioned and a new plan devised. This plan can be revised repeatedly until a satisfactory or optimal dose plan is achieved and displayed on the console. Figures 9.21 and 9.22 illustrate therapy plans performed on a CT unit.

In addition to generating or calling up appropriate isodose curves corresponding to a particular plan, a trackball-controlled cursor is usually available to display the dose at any point. The completed treatment plan may also be viewed in sagittal or coronal planes, with an appropriate display of the beam data.

By combining the localization images and the computerized plan, the patient bed can be positioned so that a crosshair laser targets or indicates the treatment beam boundaries directly on the patient (Pfizer PZ-SIM). After the targets have been determined, all therapy beam coordinates are accurately marked on the skin prior to treatment.

In addition to planning external beam radiation, CT is used in planning interstitial or intracavitary

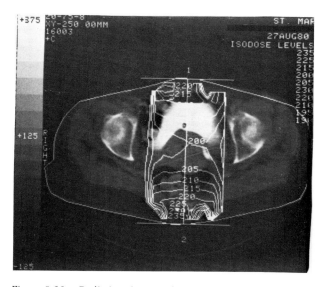

Figure 9.22. Radiation therapy plan using two portals. Contrast is present to define the bladder.

Further Applications

radiation therapy, in which radioactive seeds are implanted within the interstitium of an organ or within a cavity. Figure 9.23 illustrates volumetric determination of the prostate gland for accurate dosimetry planning prior to placement of iodine-125 radioactive seeds. Gold-198 has also been employed. The width of the gland is determined on a transverse scan. An approximation of the depth (anterior-posterior dimension) and the length of the gland can be obtained as well from the transverse scans; the length is determined from the number of successive transverse scans on which the gland appears. However, the depth and length of the gland can be more accurately determined by direct measurement from a sagittal reconstruction, as shown in Figure 9.24. The adequacy of seed implantation can be assessed by a postimplantation scan, as illustrated in Figure 9.25. Isodose curves of interstitial implants may be superimposed on the CT images as well.

Intracavitary placement, using a Fletcher type of applicator, of radium or cesium-137 sources for cervical carcinoma may also be assessed by CT to evaluate placement of the sources. Isodose curves can be computed, and the radiation dose to particular structures or specific anatomical landmarks can be estimated. In particular, the dose to the so-called point A (located 2 cm superior and 2 cm lateral to the external cervical os) and point B (located 2 cm superior and 5 cm lateral to the external cervical os) may be com-

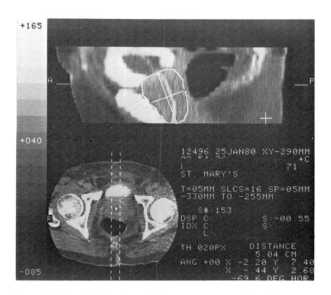

Figure 9.24. The borders of the prostate are outlined by a trace in a sagittal reconstruction of the gland. The length of the gland along its true longitudinal axis is indicated. The depth of the gland, measured perpendicular to the long axis, is also indicated. (Reproduced by permission from C. L. Morgan et al. Computed tomography in the evaluation, staging, and therapy of carcinoma of the bladder and prostate. Radiology 140:751–761, 1981.)

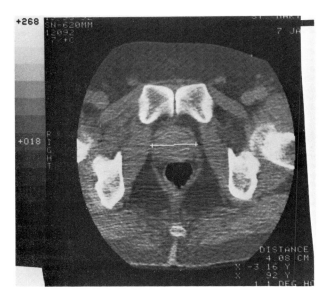

Figure 9.23. A measurement of the transverse dimension of the prostate. Anteroposterior and longitudinal measurements can also be estimated from CT scans.

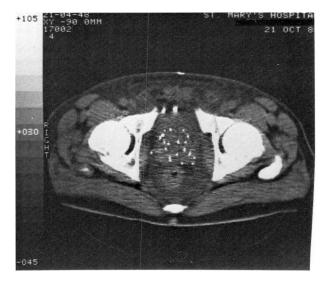

Figure 9.25. CT scans illustrating the placement of radioactive iodine-125 seeds that have been implanted in the prostate for therapy. (Reproduced by permission from C. L. Morgan et al. Computed tomography in the evaluation, staging, and therapy of carcinoma of the bladder and prostate. Radiology 140:751–761, 1981.)

puted from the scans. CT also permits a more accurate computation of the dose to the pelvic bones.

CT also is extremely valuable in staging the extent of disease in tumor patients prior to selection of those patients who might benefit from external beam radiation or interstitial or intracavitary implants.

High Resolution Computed Tomography

Higher spatial resolution in CT images provides significantly improved anatomical detail in certain regions, in particular the spine and temporal bone. Small anatomical structures, such as the semicircular canals in the temporal bone, require resolution of less than .6 mm for adequate detail. A pixel size of .8–1.0 mm may not provide adequate spatial resolution for small anatomical structures in a tissue slice. To avoid this problem, it is desirable to use smaller pixels (e.g., about 0.25 mm), to reconstruct scan data. Also, to ensure improved spatial resolution, the slice thickness should be reduced. Thin (approximately 5 mm) or ultrathin (approximately 1.5 mm) sections should be employed. Typically, sections approximately 5 mm will suffice in the spine, but good spatial resolution in the temporal bone necessitates the use of ultrathin sections of 1–2 mm. Thus, the size of a representative voxel may be reduced from a routine volume of about $10 \times 1 \times 1$ mm to a much smaller $1.5 \times .25 \times .25$ mm.

Several approaches have been devised to provide images with increased spatial resolution. These have been described by Blumenfeld and Glover (1981). In translational-rotational units, the detector apertures have been reduced and the spatial sampling frequency increased over a smaller region of interest. If the region of interest comprises only a short portion of the total translation, a "target scan" of the selected region of interest is obtained. Artifacts are reduced, and the accuracy of CT numbers is maintained by measurements outside this target area, which are taken at a lower spatial frequency. Alternatively, the translation may be limited to just the projected dimension of the target, so that no measurements are taken outside the target area. The appearance of the image when either of these approaches is used may be improved further by the use of special reconstruction algorithms.

A reduced field of view may also be reconstructed in purely rotational systems. Commercial systems may offer a choice of several different standard field sizes. For example, the General Electric CT/T 8800 provides a 42-cm large body, a 35-cm small body, and a 25-cm infant size. Each of these corresponds to successively better spatial resolutions. However, if a small field of view is reconstructed within a large object, bothersome artifacts may occur.

Another technique that has been employed in third generation scanners is a radial shift of the tube and detectors relative to the center of the field of view. This has been described in Chapter 3. This approach permits full utilization of all the detectors in the array regardless of the size of the object being imaged. For smaller objects this effectively decreases the effective ray spacing in the object. The ray spacing at the detector array is simply the distance between the centers of the detector elements. This spacing decreases as one traces the rays back to the tube. For smaller objects the tube may be moved closer to the object, so that the effective ray spacing is decreased, thus increasing spatial resolution.

The process of target reconstruction permits the achievement of higher spatial resolution by selecting a small region of interest (target) within the larger area scanned, which is then reconstructed again from the raw data. The convolution kernel of the target reconstruction algorithm is extended in its spatial frequency response to match a new, smaller pixel size. As an example, the General Electric CT/T REVIEW may reconstruct the target on pixels as small as .25 mm.

Different algorithms may be employed in the target reconstruction. Each of these involves the use of a particular convolution filter. Each filter offers a different compromise or tradeoff between noise and spatial resolution. One algorithm may maximize spatial resolution, but with a concomitant increase in noise and decrease in contrast discrimination. Another algorithm may try to reduce noise, sacrificing some spatial resolution. Since each uses the initial raw data, both types of target reconstruction can be performed without any additional patient exposure.

Examples of high resolution CT images are illustrated in Figures 9.26–9.31.

Another form of data manipulation involves the application of a special mathematical filter to enhance the edges of structures ("sharpen up" the picture). Edge enhancement may be applied to the target reconstruction or to the original standard image. More accurate attempts to correct beam hardening associated with the relatively larger amounts of bone in the temporal areas and spine may further improve the image quality and resolution.

A useful technique when displaying bony structures is the extension of the range of CT numbers. The extended CT scale has been described already

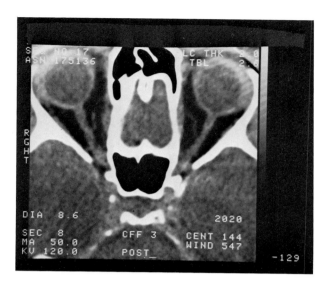

Figure 9.26. High resolution transverse section through the orbits. (Courtesy of Technicare Corporation.)

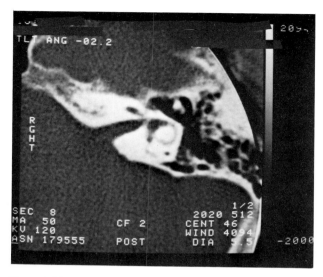

Figure 9.28. High resolution section transverse section through the temporal bone illustrating internal auditory canal, middle ear, and mastoids. (Courtesy of Technicare Corporation.)

in detail in Chapter 6. The use of an extended CT scale and reconstructed target scans permits a significant improvement in the imaging of small bone detail, as in the middle ear. An example of the use of a target scan and extended scale is shown in Figure 9.32.

Gated Scanning

Satisfactory imaging of the rapidly moving myocardium cannot be performed unless the time of scanning or image formation is significantly less than the typical 800- to 1,000-ms cardiac cycle. Data gathering would have to be confined to a small fraction of the CT scanning cycle. The small amount of information accumulated in this brief interval results in the reconstruction of images of relative poor quality. The problem is one of obtaining sufficient data for discrete short intervals of the cardiac cycle to permit reconstruction of an image of reasonable quality

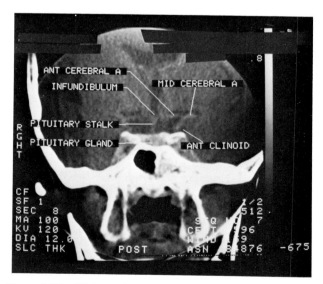

Figure 9.27. High resolution coronal head section at the level of the pituitary gland. (Courtesy of Technicare Corporation.)

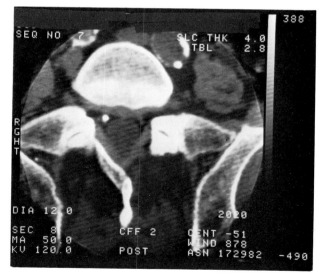

Figure 9.29. High resolution transverse section through the lower lumbar spine. (Courtesy of Technicare Corporation.)

234   Basic Principles of Computed Tomography

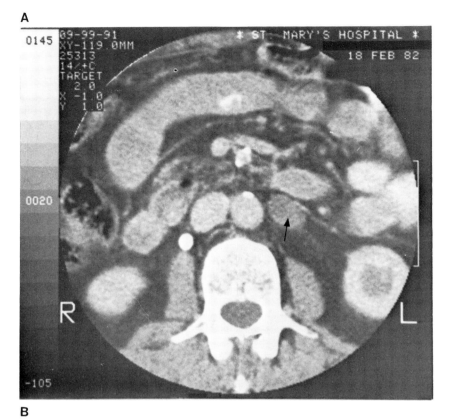
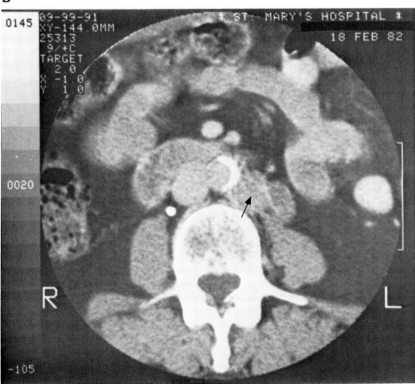

Figure 9.30. High resolution scans illustrating (A) dilated left ureter (arrow), and (B) at a more caudad level the enlarged paraaortic nodes (arrow) responsible for the obstruction.

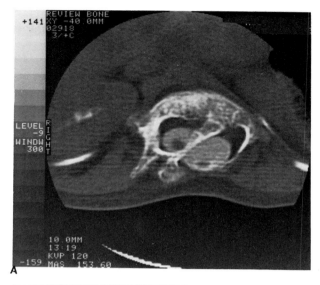

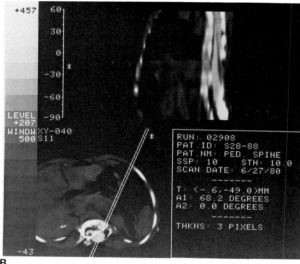

Figure 9.31. Diastometamyelia at T11-T12. *A*, Transverse section following metrizamide myelography shows bony spur, split spinal cord, and separate dural sacs in excellent detail using RE-VIEW (General Electric high resolution scan). Darker areas within the opacified sacs represent the separate portions of the spinal cord. *B*, A reformatted image in an oblique plane. (Reproduced by permission from A. Rusztyn et al. General Electric CT/T Clinical Symposium, Volume 3, Number 13, 1980.)

corresponding to the appearance of the heart in that short time interval. The solution is to gather data for each selected discrete interval within the cardiac cycle over many cycles. This is achieved by subdividing the cardiac cycle into discrete intervals (typically 100 ms) on the basis of the electrocardiogram and associating the data obtained during scanning with its appropriate interval within the cardiac cycle. The image obtained is a gated reconstruction based on information or data collected during a selected interval within the cardiac cycle over a specified number of cycles. The data may be collected either prospectively, by electrocardiographic control of the x-ray tube, or retrospectively, by taking the appropriate data for each interval within the cardiac cycle from a series of scans performed with simultaneous continuous recording of the electrocardiogram. The images corresponding to each interval within the cardiac cycle may also be grouped in their correct time sequence and shown in rapid sequence, permitting a real display of the cardiac cycle for a particular section through the heart.

Dual Energy Scanning

The attenuation of an x-ray beam in tissue depends upon the energy (kV) of the x-rays, the density and atomic number Z or chemical composition of the tissue, and the thickness of the tissue. The dependence of x-ray attenuation on the atomic number Z, or more correctly the average or effective atomic number $\bar{Z}$, reflects the relative contributions from the two different common causes of x-ray attenuation in tissue: the photoelectric effect and the Compton effect. As described in Chapter 2, there is a strong dependence of photoelectric absorption on the atomic number Z, whereas the Compton effect is nearly independent of Z.

If x-ray attenuation measurements of a tissue are performed for two different x-ray energies, it is possible to deduce the average or effective atomic number $\bar{Z}$ of the tissue. The x-ray attenuation can be expressed in terms of CT numbers when measurements are made by CT. This can be understood qualitatively by realizing that, by decreasing the energy of the x-ray beam, the attenuation from Compton scattering will not be significantly affected, but a measurable increase in the total x-ray attenuation will occur because of the increased x-ray absorption from photoelectric effects at the lower energy. Using formulas for the known Z dependence for Compton and photoelectric effects, the average or effective atomic number $\bar{Z}$ of the tissue can be estimated. This necessitates two scans, one done at a lower kVp, typically 80–90, and another at a second, higher kVp, typically 120–140. This results in a higher radiation dose to the patient, especially from the lower kVp scan.

A second technique for obtaining dual energy measurements from a single scan has been developed. This involves the use of thin metal foils covering alternate slits of the detector collimators. The detec-

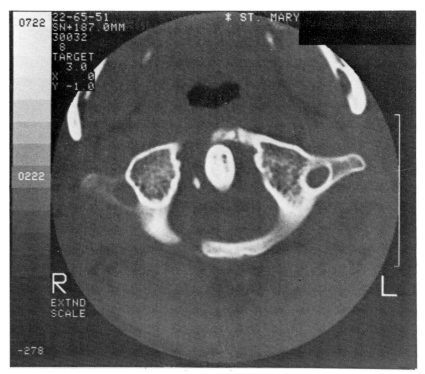

Figure 9.32. High resolution target scan with extended CT scale illustrating a Jefferson's fracture of C1.

tor readings associated with the covered slits are separated from those of the uncovered slits by computer software programs prior to processing. Two different pictures can then be formed, one identified with the covered slits and one with the uncovered slits. The image associated with the covered slits results from filtering or hardening the x-ray beam, leaving primarily the higher energy or kV components. The image derived from the uncovered slits represents the lower energy or kV contributions as well. From the differences between these two images (i.e., the differences in the CT numbers), it is possible to deduce the effective atomic number Z of the tissue.

OTHER TOMOGRAPHIC TECHNIQUES

Ultrafast Transmission Scanning

Even the most rapid CT units described in this text are limited to performing scans of single cross-sections in about 1 s. A significantly faster scanning time necessitates a dramatic change in technology and an entirely new and quite different generation of high speed body imagers. One such dramatic approach has been the development of a system called the Dynamic Spatial Reconstructor (DSR) by the Biodynamics Research Unit at the Mayo Clinic.

Dynamic Spatial Reconstruction The DSR is a multiple x-ray source, high speed transaxial imaging system for cylindrical scanning. Twenty-eight x-ray tubes are used to obtain up to 240 simultaneous contiguous body sections 1 mm in thickness in a cylindrical volume up to 37 cm in diameter and 25 cm high (axial) in as little as 10 ms. It is a fast volume scanner. The 28 x-ray tubes are mounted in a semicircular arrangement at 6° intervals over 168° (28 × 6°) in a circular gantry. There is an opposing semicircular arc of 28 x-ray imaging chains (one corresponding to each x-ray tube) mounted in the same gantry. In the usual positioning, the x-ray sources will be under the patient table and the imaging chains above it. The gantry has the capability of rotating about the patient at a rate of 1.5° in 1/60 s. This corresponds to a full rotation of 360° in 4 s, or 15 rpm.

A schematic diagram of a single imaging chain for the system is shown in Figure 9.33. The cone-shaped x-ray beam passes through the patient and strikes a 30 × 30 cm (12 × 12 inch) fluorescent screen. The crystals in the fluorescent screen convert

Further Applications 237

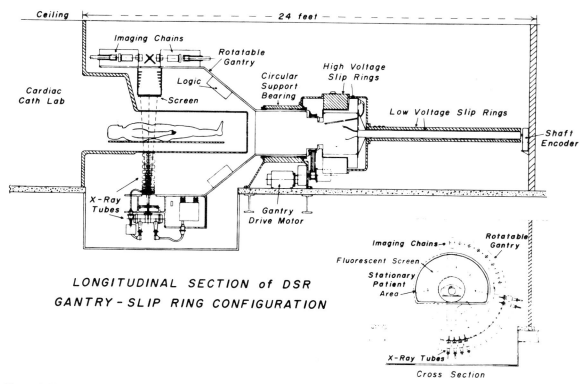

Figure 9.33. Diagram of proposed DSR system. The patient lies on a horizontal radiolucent table, which can be moved in three directions for optimal positioning. Twenty-eight x-ray sources are mounted along a semicircle below the patient so that corresponding projection images are formed on a 12-inch-wide semicircular fluorescent screen suspended above the patient. Image intensifier video camera chains are positioned behind the fluorescent screen as indicated in axial perspective in inset (right lower corner). Mechanical rotation of the entire circular structure permits scanning at many angles of view over a range up to 360°. Slip rings mounted along the horizontal shaft permit continuous rotation at 15 rpm. The gantry would be located in a room separated from the patient area by a soundproof wall. Patients and clinicians would see only a stationary tunnel opening in one wall of laboratory. (Reproduced by permission from E. L. Ritman et al. Quantitative imaging of the structure and function of the heart, lungs, and circulation. Mayo Clinic Proceedings 53:3–11, 1978.)

the x-ray photons into light photons (3,000–5,000 usable light photons for every x-ray photon at 70kV). The light signal from the fluorescent screen is then reflected off a mirror and focused onto an image intensifier. The input screen of the image intensifier is on a photocathode or photoemissive metal (usually a combination of cesium and antimony compounds). The photocathode emits photoelectrons in a number proportional to that of the light photons from the fluorescent screen. The photoelectrons are then focused by a series of positively charged electrodes. The photoelectrons are also accelerated by a potential difference between the photocathode and the output screen. The output fluorescent screen of an image intensifier is typically silver-activated zinc sulfide. The accelerated electrons produce more light than was present at the input screen, and this light is concentrated over a smaller area, further increasing the intensity of the output image. An optical lens system then couples this output light to a television camera. The imaging chain is similar to that employed in fluoroscopy. One exception is that the fluorescent screen and the photocathode of the image intensifier are not directly coupled. The x-ray information received by a single imaging chain represents a single view.

The use of a large, semicircular imaging surface, 30 cm high by about 200 cm long, precludes the use of the more typical solid-state detectors used in commercial CT units. The requirement for cross-sections 1 mm thick would necessitate the use of about 1 million discrete detectors. The preamplification and switching electronics required for this large number of detectors would present a major technical problem.

During scanning, the 28 x-ray tubes are activated individually and sequentially by pulses .34 ms long. This total sequence takes approximately 10 ms (28 × .34 ms). The sequence may be repeated 60 times per s, that is, every $16\frac{2}{3}$ ms. This leaves a dead time (no x-ray tubes activated) of 6⅔ ms between sequences. This is an entirely electronic sequence, with no mechanical motion involved in the scanning.

In the high temporal resolution configuration, 60 cyclindrical volumes can be scanned in a second. A single scan can be performed in 10 ms. This is an exclusively electronic scan over 168°. However, with only 28 views in this configuration, the high temporal resolution is offset by lower spatial and density resolution.

The interdependence of these parameters permits improvement in the spatial and density resolution at the expense of temporal resolution. A medium temporal, spatial, and density scan can be performed. This involves some mechanical as well as electronic scanning. If the gantry is rotated, additional views may be obtained every 1/60 s (corresponding to the time between activation sequences of the x-ray tubes), during which time interval each x-ray tube (and its corresponding imaging chain) will have rotated 1.5°. Each time an x-ray tube is activated, a view is obtained. Allowing for four activation sequences of 10 ms each with three intervening dead times of 6⅔ ms, a total of 112 (4 × 28) views may be obtained in 60 ms as the gantry rotates through 4.5° (views obtained at 0°, 1.5°, 3.0°, and 4.5°). In another 1/16 s the gantry would rotate through a full 6°, so that all but the lead x-ray tube would be in the same positions previously occupied by x-ray tubes at 0° rotation. Thus, all the x-ray tubes except the leading one would merely repeat views identical to those obtained at 0°.

It is also possible to perform a low temporal, high spatial, and high density scan. The gantry rotates through 360° in approximately 2.14 s. In the first 60 ms, 112 views are obtained as described above. As the gantry rotation continues, the leading tube obtains a new view every 1/60 s or 1.5°, so that a total of 240 views are obtained over 360°. The views in the first 168° are obtained by electronic scanning, and those in the remaining 192° by mechanical scanning. Only the leading tube is activated after the first 112 views, since the other tubes would merely duplicate a view already obtained, adding no new views or information. Thus, a combination of electronic and mechanical scanning allows for a tradeoff between temporal resolution and spatial/density resolution.

Figure 9.34 illustrates the mechanical rotation for programmable angles of view per scan.

In cardiac imaging the high temporal resolution scans allow accurate imaging to within 1 mm. The endocardium moves at about 100 mm per s during systole. Higher spatial/density resolution permits visualization of major coronary artery branches, detection of 5% changes in wall thickness, and time-dependent or static density changes such as 1% difference between normal and infarcted tissue.

The actual thickness of the individual cross-sections within the cylindrical volume can be arbitrarily varied after scanning (Figure 9.35). The television camera in each imaging chain scans the output of the corresponding image intensifier to detect the variation in the intensity of the x-ray beam along each of the 250 parallel scanning lines (slices) of raster of each 60-per-s video field. Each line is a horizontal line perpendicular to the x-ray beam and to the axis of the cylinder. The line separation is 1 mm, so that the entire 25-cm length (height) of the cylinder is covered. The voltage variations along each line are converted to appropriate digital values by an analog-to-digital converter for 200 to 1,000 equispaced points along each line. There is a corresponding line for each view recorded by each imaging chain. If the 1-mm lines are maintained, 1-mm thin slices result. Adjacent lines may be combined by averaging the digital values for corresponding points within the different lines, resulting in thicker slices. The larger total digital values as a result of the summation result in a better signal-to-noise ratio and concomitant improved density resolution. The thicker slices, however, may result in poorer spatial resolution.

Scanning Electron Beam Systems The use of multiple x-ray tubes permits the DSR to perform a purely electronic (nonmechanical) scan in a high temporal resolution mode. However, higher spatial and density mode scans require some mechanical motion as well.

One alternative approach to ultrafast scanning is based on the replacement of the conventional Coolidge x-ray tubes by scanning electron beam systems. These are based on the use of an electron beam, which is magnetically deflected along a circular anode ring or target surrounding the patient. X-rays are produced when the electron beam strikes a point on the target and are shaped into an appropriate fan beam by a suitable collimation.

A design based on such an approach was proposed by Iinuma et al. (1977). Their design features a large, bell-shaped generator housing containing an electron gun, a doughnut-like target, and a complicated beam deflection system. The x-ray beam that is generated as the electron beam strikes the target surface is directed perpendicularly to the electron beam. This permits an intense x-ray microbeam to

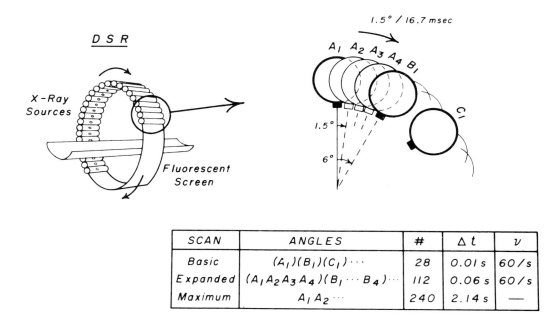

Figure 9.34. Mechanical rotation for programmable angles of view per scan. Each of 28 electronically scanned x-ray sources of the DSR is separated from its neighboring source by 6°. At a gantry rotation speed of 15 rpm, a .01-s, 28-view electronic scan is performed at 1.5° angular increments every 1/60 s. Consequently, after four 28-view scans, 112 angles of view will be recorded, with each view separated by 1.5°. In the 60-ms duration of this combined electronic and mechanical circumferential scanning procedure, movement of the heart of less than 1 mm is expected to occur during diastole. This mode of scanning is expected to be suitable for obtaining higher spatial and density resolution static images of the diastolic phase of a single heartbeat, and of the lungs during a transient breath-holding period than can be obtained by electronic scanning alone. However, the 60 ms required for mechanical scanning is too long to permit stop-action imaging of the heart during systole, when at least 5 mm of movement would be expected. If exact reproducibility of successive heartbeats can be achieved during 15 s of combined electronic and 360° mechanical scanning, with breath-holding, maximum spatial and density resolution reconstructions throughout an "average" heart cycle could be obtained. The column headings #, Δt, and ν indicate number of angles of view, duration of each scan, and number of such scans per second, respectively. Each letter indicates a location of one x-ray source. A, B, C, etc., indicate the 28 locations during the first .01-s scan; A_2, B_2, C_2, etc., indicate the 28 locations during the second .01-s scan, and so forth. (Reproduced by with the permission from E. L. Ritman et al. Quantitative imaging of the structure and function of the heart, lungs, and circulation. Mayo Clinic Proceedings 53:3–11, 1978.)

be projected continuously at high speed to an arbitrary tomographic imaging position. The system is designed to permit axial cross-sections to be obtained in as rapidly as 10 ms.

Scanning electron beam systems have also been proposed and developed by Haimson (described by Hsu, 1981) and by Boyd (1981). The latter system has been termed a cardiovascular CT (CVCT) scanner.

Emission Computed Tomography

General Description Emission computed tomography (ECT) is a tomographic imaging technique for obtaining transaxial sectional images based on the distribution of gamma ray or positron-emitting radionuclides within organs and structures. In transmission CT the tomographic image is a map of the spatial distribution of the x-ray attenuation coefficients; in ECT the sectional image portrays the spatial distribution of a previously administered radionuclide.

Tomographic imaging techniques for displaying the distribution of a radionuclide in the body were actually developed prior to transmission CT. Initially, however, ECT was used in only a relatively small number of institutions. Several factors have contributed to the more recent rapid growth in the development and application of ECT: 1) the increasing availability of small, high capability computers that are relatively inexpensive compared to earlier computers; 2) the application of many of the techniques, such as the mathematics of cross-sectional image reconstruction, developed in transmission CT to ECT; and 3) clinical evidence of the usefulness of ECT.

Two different approaches have been employed to obtain sectional images by ECT. Gamma ray emission computed tomography, also referred to as single-photon counting (SPC) or single-photon emission computed tomography (SPECT), is based on the distribution of radionuclides which decay by the direct emission of a gamma ray. Positron emission computed tomography, also referred to as positron emission tomography (PET) and annihilation coincidence detection (ACD), is a map of radionuclides which decay by the emission of a positron. Subsequently the positron interacts with an electron, resulting in the mutual annihilation of positron and electron, with the formation of two coincident photons which travel in opposite directions (180° apart). These different approaches are each discussed in greater detail later in this section.

In conventional or nontomographic techniques used in nuclear medicine, the images, referred to as scans when obtained with a rectilinear scanner and as scintigrams when obtained with a gamma camera, are severely distorted due to several factors: 1) a contribution to the recorded counts which form the image from radionuclide activity in sections both overlying and underlying the region of interest (this is the result of the projection nature of the image, in which three dimensions are compressed into two); 2) a variation in the field of view of the collimator as a function of the depth, or distance between the detector and source of radiation (i.e., the solid angle subtended at the detector by different points in the object to be imaged varies with the distance between

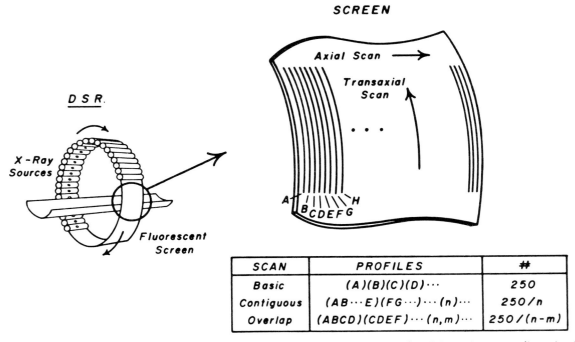

Figure 9.35. Programmable image slice thickness and slice spacing. Each x-ray source of the DSR projects a two-dimensional image of the chest onto a fluorescent screen. The fluorescent image generated on the back of the screen is scanned by a television camera to capture variation in x-ray intensity along each of 250 parallel scanning lines (slices) of the raster of each 60-per-s video field. Voltage variations of the video signal generated as each "horizontal" line is scanned are converted to digital values at 200–1,000 equispaced points along each line. Averaging of digital values obtained at corresponding sample positions along adjacent "horizontal" lines increases the slice thickness and signal-to-noise ratio of resultant values, with a corresponding increase in contrast resolution but a concomitant decrease of axial spatial resolution. Capital letters indicate individual "horizontal" video-scan lines, and parentheses indicate video lines in each profile (where n is the number of video lines per slice thickness and m is the number of video lines overlapped between adjacent slice profiles of each transaxial scan). The symbol # indicates number of slices (transaxial scans) per axial scan. (Reproduced by permission from E. L. Ritman et al. Quantitative imaging of the structure and function of the heart, lungs, and circulation. Mayo Clinic Proceedings 53:3–11, 1978.)

the point and the detector); 3) the attenuation of the gamma radiation by tissues lying between the section of interest and the detector cannot practically be accounted for (Ter-Pogossian, 1977, 1981).

ECT offers three significant advantages over the imaging techniques of conventional nuclear medicine: 1) ECT allows a third dimension to be added to the image; 2) contrast within the section of interest is not reduced by the superimposition of activity originating from outside this section; 3) ECT can provide an accurate quantitative description of the distribution of the radionuclide in the section imaged (Ter-Pogossian, 1980).

The basic apparatus of an ECT unit can be divided into two components: 1) a data acquisition system, which includes radiation detectors and a gantry that allows the appropriate mechanical motions for data sampling for image reconstruction, and 2) an electronics and computer system, which records and processes the data and performs image reconstruction.

In both transmission CT and ECT, the contrast resolution, and to a lesser extent the spatial resolution, of the final reconstructed image are limited by the total number of photons collected by the detector system. Practically, the number of such image-forming photons is limited by the acceptable radiation dose to the patient. In transmission CT the radiation dose during a single scan is essentially limited to the section being imaged. However, in ECT there is a radiation dose to all the tissues in which the radionuclides have accumulated, not merely the section being scanned. Furthermore, since the decay of radionuclides is isotropic (the decay products are emitted in all directions), only a fraction of the radionuclides that undergo decay in a section during a scan are detected. Finally, only a very small fraction of the radionuclides undergo decay during the time of the scan, while data are being collected. Therefore, in ECT (as in conventional nuclear medicine imaging techniques) only a small fraction of the radiation dose the patient receives contributes to image formation. In contrast, the dose utilization in transmission CT is significantly better, patient irradiation only occurring in the section being imaged and only during the scanning time.

Because of these inherent limitations of imaging with radionuclides, the total number of image-forming photons in a typical ECT examination is approximately 4 orders of magnitude less than in transmission CT (about 10^6 photons per section in ECT compared to about 10^{10} photons per section in transmission CT). Therefore, the contrast and spatial resolution of ECT are approximately an order of magnitude less than that for transmission CT.

The basic principles of ECT have been described by several authors (Phelps, 1977; Goodwin, 1980; Ter-Pogossian, 1981). The excellent review by Phelps (1977) also provides descriptions and pictures of the principal ECT devices to 1977.

Gamma Ray Emission Computed Tomography A number of different approaches have been developed to achieve tomographic images in nuclear medicine. Some of these approaches are actually blurring (or defocusing) techniques in which images of structures outside a section of interest are defocused while structures in the section of interest remain in focus. These blurring tomographs have not been as clinically useful in nuclear medicine as in conventional radiography.

Gamma ray ECT can be divided into two types: 1) horizontal or longitudinal tomography, in which the section imaged is parallel to the long axis of the patient; and 2) transaxial or transverse axial tomography, in which the section imaged is perpendicular to the patient's long axis.

Several approaches have been devised to achieve longitudinal tomography (Goodwin, 1980). The first rectilinear scanners using focused collimators possessed a limited longitudinal tomographic capability, since sources above and below the tomographic section were imaged less sharply. Other techniques for performing longitudinal tomography have been developed based on modifications of the collimator design (e.g., coded apertures, seven pinholes, and rotating slant-hole collimators).

Transaxial tomographic systems or ECT devices basically consist of a mechanical gantry that supports the radiation detection system and contains a mechanical system that directs the motion or motions of the detector system about the patient to collect data profiles at different angles. Both multicrystal detectors and rotating gamma cameras have been employed. There is associated electronic circuitry and a computer system. These devices generally can be used with common commercially available radioisotopes such as technetium-99m.

Multicrystal Detector Systems The simplest form of gamma ray ECT consists of a single collimated detector or two opposing collimated detectors, which undergo translational and rotational motions similar to those of the original EMI Mark I transmission CT unit. Such a system was first developed by Kuhl and Edwards in 1963, several years prior to the development of a transmission CT unit. This first ECT scanner, the Mark I, has been described in Chapter 1 and is illustrated in Figure 1.17.

Kuhl and Edwards not only pioneered the technique of multicrystal ECT but have continued the development through the Mark II, Mark III, and Mark IV units. The Mark IV, designed exclusively for head scanning, has a detector system that uses a four-sided arrangement of 32 independent collimated sodium iodide scintillation detectors, eight detectors on each side about the patient. The detectors rotate together as a unit, detecting, processing, and displaying the data as the study is performed. The outputs of the scintillation crystals are detected and amplified by photomultiplier tubes. A 360° rotation requires 50 s.

The first commercially marketed multicrystal transaxial ECT unit was the Cleon-710 Brain Imager developed by Union Carbide Imaging Systems (formerly Cleon Corporation). The head unit employed 12 detectors arranged approximately in a circle (more accurately, a 12-sided array). A scan time of 2–5 min was required to obtain enough data to reconstruct a single slice. Union Carbide, which acquired Cleon in 1976, has closed the Imaging Systems Division, so Cleon instruments are no longer being manufactured.

Other multicrystal ECT units have been developed commercially (Phelps 1977; Goodwin, 1980).

Rotating Gamma Camera Systems To obtain the capability of obtaining multiple slices during a scan, several systems have been developed which use one or two gamma cameras of relatively conventional design. Linear data sampling is done by the positioning logic of the gamma camera. A gamma camera (Anger camera) consists of a relatively large scintillation crystal with several photomultiplier tubes in different positions behind the front of the crystal. The relative strength of the scintillation or light signal that reaches each photomultiplier tube is related to its distance from the point in the crystal at which a scintillation occurred. By comparing the relative size of the signal in each photomultiplier tube, the camera logic can identify the spatial location of the scintillation in the crystal. Therefore, only camera rotation about the patient is required.

Rotating gamma camera ECT systems have been developed by Budinger et al., Keyes et al., Searle Radiographics and Baylor College of Medicine, and General Electric Medical Systems. These are described by Phelps (1977) and Goodwin (1980).

Limitations Cormack (1973) has discussed the physical limitations of gamma ray ECT, which include: 1) attenuation of the gamma radiation by tissues between the source of radiation and the detector, and 2) the variation in the field of view of the detector with the distance between the detector and the radiation source. However, these limitations may not preclude obtaining satisfactory images. With respect to the first limitation, the solid angle subtended at the detector by different points in the object usually does not vary that greatly. Thus, by using a suitable attenuation correction in an appropriate reconstruction algorithm, it may be possible to obtain an adequate map of the distribution of radionuclides in the section (Budinger and Gullberg, 1974).

In addition, the uniformity of the field of view of the detector can be improved by the use of long focus collimators. Alternatively, the response of the collimator may be averaged throughout the object being imaged. An example of the latter approach is the Union Carbide-Cleon unit. The motion of the 12 detectors (equally spaced in an array or circle about the patient) is rather complex. The detectors not only scan the patient in a rectilinear fashion (translation), but the individual detectors move in and out (toward and away from the patient). The latter motion provides the averaging effect for each individual collimator/detector.

At present, gamma ray ECT units require a relatively long time, of the order of several minutes, to obtain images of satisfactory quality.

Positron Emission Computed Tomography
Basic Principles The basic principles and features of positron ECT have been discussed by Ter-Pogossian (1977, 1981; Ter-Pogossian et al., 1980). The design of specific positron ECT devices has been described by Ter-Pogossian (1981), Ter-Pogossian et al. (1975, 1978), Phelps (1977), and Goodwin (1980).

There are three general types of radionuclide decay characterized by the decay particles: gamma ray, electron, and positron emission. In gamma ray emission the daughter nucleus following decay has the same atomic number Z as the parent radioactive nucleus. An example is the most commonly used radioisotope in nuclear media, technetium-99m (m stands for the metastable state), which undergoes decay with the emission of a photon of 140-keV energy. The gamma ray is neutral in charge, and the atomic number of the decay daughter nucleus is the same as the parent radionuclide.

Radionuclides that decay with the emission of either an electron or a positron are collectively referred to as beta emitters, a beta particle being either a negatively charged electron (β⁻) or its antiparticle, a positively charged positron (β⁺).

Electron or β⁻ decay is characterized by the emission of an electron. The daughter nucleus following decay has an atomic number greater than the parent radionuclide by one. Electrical charge is thus preserved, since the sum of the charges of the daughter nucleus and the electron is equal to the charge of the parent radionuclide. This form of radioactivity is usually seen in those nuclei which have a relative excess of neutrons compared to protons; that is, the ratio of neutrons to protons is unstable, there being a relative excess of neutrons, or alternatively a relative deficiency of protons. In electron decay a neutron is converted into a proton and an electron (and a neutral particle called a neutrino, or, more correctly, an antineutrino, $\bar{\nu}$). The electron is expelled from the nucleus, whereas the proton remains in the nucleus. The ratio of neutrons to protons is thus decreased in the daughter nucleus, since there is one less neutron and one more proton in the nucleus. An example is iodine-131, which undergoes beta decay to xenon-131m with emission of an electron.

In positron decay a positron is emitted. The daughter nucleus following decay has its atomic number decreased by one compared to the parent radionuclide. Electrical charge is preserved, since the sum of the charges of the daughter nucleus and the positron is equal to the charge of the parent radionuclide. This type of radioactivity is found in those nuclei which have a relative shortage of neutrons compared to protons; that is, the ratio of neutrons to protons is unstable, there being a relative shortage of neutrons, or alternatively a relative excess of protons. In positron decay a proton is converted into a positron and a neutron (and a neutrino). The positron is expelled from the nucleus, and the neutron remains in the nucleus. The ratio of neutrons to protons is thus increased in the daughter nucleus, since there is one more neutron and one less proton in the nucleus.

Both electrons and positrons possess a certain amount of kinetic energy (energy of motion) after being expelled from the nucleus. This kinetic energy is rapidly dissipated by excitation and ionization interactions. For electrons and positrons the linear energy transfer (LET), the rate at which energy is lost by the electron or positron and deposited into tissues, is in the range of 1–10 keV per micron of electron path. Thus the electron or positron is rapidly brought to rest at a very short distance from the site of radionuclide decay.

Nothing of further significance occurs when an electron is brought to rest. However, a very important phenomenon occurs when the positron has lost its kinetic energy. A positron is a form of antimatter, which does not normally coexist side by side with ordinary matter. When the positron is brought to rest, it interacts with its own opposite or antiparticle, an electron. The positron and electron then undergo the phenomenon of annihilation, whereby the two particles are converted into electromagnetic energy in the form of two photons, called annihilation radiation or annihilation photons. The two annihilation photons travel in approximately colinear paths (180° apart from each other), and each carries an energy of about 511 keV. The total energy of the two photons is about 1.02 MeV, which is the energy corresponding to the combined masses of the electron and positron. The photons are formed simultaneously at the same point and travel at the speed of electromagnetic radiation (the speed of light). This is illustrated in Figure 9.36.

A number of biochemical elements have isotopes that undergo positron decay. These isotopes can be used in the examination of biological systems. Typically they have short half-lives, permitting their safe administration in relatively large quantities. Furthermore, their decay by positron emission enhances their value for imaging by ECT.

The technique of positron ECT, or positron emission tomography (PET), is proving to be more important than gamma ray ECT in cerebral examinations. PET techniques can yield a great deal of valuable physiological and biochemical information as well as anatomical detail. The term PET is often used to describe not only positron ECT specifically but also the use of certain radionuclides with biochemical properties that are well suited for the study of biological systems in general, and in particular the examination of cerebral function integrity (Ter-Pogossian et al., 1980).

The nearly colinear directions of the annihilation photons permit detection of the annihilation radiation by the use of two opposing scintillation crystal detectors connected by a coincidence circuit. The coincidence circuit records an event only if both crystals detect the annihilation photons simultaneously or coincidentally.

Advantages and Limitations The method of coincidence detection used in positron ECT may be thought of as an electronic collimation, since the two detectors will record an event only from a limited volume element lying along the straight line joining

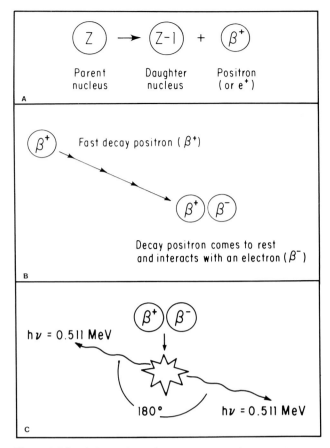

Figure 9.36. *A*, In positron decay a parent nucleus containing Z protons is transformed into a daughter nucleus that contains only $Z - 1$ protons but one more neutron. The excess positive charge is carried off in the form of a positron (β^+ or e^+), which is a positively charged electron, or antielectron. *B*, The positron is decelerated by collisions with atoms in its path until it comes to rest and interacts with an electron (β^- or e^-). *C*, The interaction between the position (β^+) and electron (β^-) results in annihilation of both with the formation of two colinear photons, each having energy $h\nu$ of about .511 MeV.

the two detectors. The two detectors in coincidence thus define a field of view comprising all the straight line paths between them. This field of view or detector sensitivity is nearly uniform in the region between the two detectors.

The total attenuation of the two annihilation photons can be readily estimated in positron ECT. The total amount of tissue attenuating the two photons is simply equal to the total thickness or diameter of the object along the line joining the two detectors. This facilitates correction or compensation for the photon attenuation.

The electronic collimation in positron ECT permits collimation without eliminating photons. This is in distinction to the physical collimation used in gamma ray ECT, where photons that do not travel in the direction selected by the collimator are eliminated.

Another advantage of positron ECT is that the high energy (511 keV) of the annihilation photons make them relatively penetrating in tissue. The half-value thickness for 511-keV photons is about 7 cm in water compared to 4 cm for 140-keV photons (Ter-Pogossian, 1977).

Electronic collimation through coincidence detection carries some disadvantages. The combined efficiency (E_c) of the two coincidence detectors is equal to the product of the efficiencies of each detector (E_1 and E_2):

$$E_c = E_1 \times E_2 \qquad (9.5)$$

Thus, if each detector has an efficiency of .7, the combined efficiency is .49. In gamma ray ECT, in contrast, the total efficiency is simply the efficiency of the individual detector. Thus, in positron ECT the detector efficiency should be relatively high. Since the annihilation photons are high in energy and relatively penetrating, the crystal must be thick along one direction to increase the probability of photon capture. Crystals constructed from material with a high atomic number are therefore preferred. As an example, when activated sodium iodide crystals are employed, the crystals are 5–8 cm thick in the direction of detection (Ter-Pogossian, 1981).

A major source of noise in positron ECT is random coincidences. These arise by chance when two uncorrelated photons are detected nearly simultaneously and recorded as coincidence events. The frequency of these random coincidence events increases with the random single counting rates in each detector and with the coincidence resolving time (the time that may separate two events observed by the two detectors and recorded as a coincidence event). The noise may be reduced by decreasing the coincidence resolving time. However, there are practical limitations on how much this time may be reduced, since it is determined by several factors. These include the time to form a light pulse in the crystal, the response time of the photomultiplier tube, and the resolving time of the electronic circuitry after the photomultiplier tube. In scintillation detectors the resolving time may vary from about ½–30 ns (1 ns = 10^{-9} s), according to Ter-Pogossian (1981).

Unfortunately, whereas the frequency of random coincidences increases as the product of the sin-

Further Applications

gle rate in each detector, the true coincidence rate only increases linearly with count rate. In a typical PET system, the number of coincidence events identified by a pair of detectors is typically less than 1% of the number of single events recorded by each detector (Ter-Pogossian, 1981).

The effect of random coincidences may be decreased in the following ways: 1) operating the coincidence system at low counting rates, 2) reducing the coincidence resolving time, and 3) subtracting the random coincidences by measuring the single rates in each detector or measuring the random counts directly.

The spatial accuracy of positron ECT is limited by two factors: 1) the two annihilation photons are not precisely colinear, and 2) the positrons travel a variable distance from the radionuclide before undergoing annihilation. This distance is a function of the positron's kinetic energy and the electron density of the tissue. The combined effects of these factors result in a fundamental uncertainty of about 2–3 mm in the relative position of the straight line joining the detectors and the source of the positrons (Ter-Pogossian, 1981).

Positron ECT also has two disadvantages compared to gamma ray ECT: 1) positron ECT is limited to use with positron-emitting radionuclides, and 2) the radiation dose to the patient includes a contribution not only from the annihilation radiation but also from the kinetic energy of the positrons.

Detectors Multiwire proportional counters possess the advantages of high spatial resolution and relatively low cost. However, they have the significant disadvantages of relatively low sensitivity in detecting the high energy annihilation photons and a very long coincidence resolving time (of the order of 200 ns). Therefore, they have not been used in any practical way in positron ECT.

The best detection system for positron ECT at this time is the scintillation crystal and photomultiplier tube. The properties and relative advantages and disadvantages of the different types of scintillation detectors for positron ECT have been discussed by Ter-Pogossian (1981).

The most commonly used crystal in positron ECT to date has been activated sodium iodide (NaI(Tl)). Its advantages include high light output, relatively high atomic number and density, and relatively short decay time. A disadvantage is that it is hygroscopic (absorbs water readily), so that it must be enclosed in a watertight envelope.

Bismuth germanate (BGO) crystals have also been employed. Its advantages compared to NaI(Tl) include a significantly higher mean atomic number and density, so that smaller detectors can be used, and its lack of hygroscopicity, so that it does not have to be protected against environmental humidity. BGO, however, has two significant disadvantages compared to NaI(Tl): its light output is a great deal less, and it has a much longer decay time. Coincidence resolving times with BGO are limited to the order of about 10–20 ns.

Cesium fluoride (CsF) has also been proposed as a detector. Its advantages include an effective atomic number and density greater than those of NaI(Tl) (but less than bismuth germanate), and an extremely fast decay time, which allows coincidence resolving times much less than 1 ns. The latter feature is very useful for dynamic studies, where the effect of random coincidences significantly affects the signal-to-noise ratio. Another advantage of such a fast coincidence time is that it permits construction of devices based on time-of-flight techniques. In this approach the difference in the arrival times of the two photons at the detectors is used to localize the particular point along the path at which the annihilation occurred. The disadvantages of cesium fluoride include its hygroscopicity and its relatively poorer light emission compared to sodium iodide.

Designs The simplest design for a positron ECT scanner consists merely of two opposing detectors undergoing a synchronous mechanical motion, which allows adequate linear and angular sampling. Such a system has a slow data acquisition rate and permits only one slice to be obtained per scan.

In the evolution of positron ECT units, several different geometries have been used. These have been described by Phelps (1977), Goodwin (1980), and Ter-Pogossian (1981). Both translational and rotational motions have been used.

Although positron cameras have been developed over a 25-year period in several institutions, their commercial development has been more recent. Three basic geometries have characterized the commercial development: 1) parallel-opposed multicrystal arrays, 2) a hexagonal arrangement of multicrystal arrays, and 3) single or multiple rings of crystals. The use of multiple detectors allows more rapid data acquisition, so scanning can be performed more rapidly. In addition, simultaneous data acquisition for multiple slices is possible through the use of multiple rings of crystal detectors. More slices per scan could also be obtained by using more photomultiplier tubes with each crystal, and by increasing the length of the crystals along the long axis of the patient. Simultaneous multislice capability is particularly helpful for imaging with radioisotopes with very short half-lives compared to the examination time, so that all the slices are compatible, that is, obtained for comparable densities of radionuclide distribution throughout the slices.

An example of a scanner employing parallel-opposed multicrystal arrays is the Massachusetts General Positron Camera, the initial PC-1 and later the PC-11 developed by Brownell and others. The PC-11 has two banks of 140 NaI crystals, each crystal 2 cm in diameter by 3.8 cm thick, arranged in two 12 × 12 arrays (less the corner crystals). Each crystal in this array is in coincidence with each of the crystals in a 5 × 5 array in the opposite bank. The detectors rotate about the patient, obtaining data at 29 different angles. Up to 23 slices can then be reconstructed, with a spacing between slices of 1.4 cm.

Hexagonal array geometry has been pioneered over the years by Ter-Pogossian and others at Washington University. These have been called positron emission transaxial tomographs (PETT), beginning with the PETT-I. The PETT-III was adapted commercially with modifications as the ECAT by ORTEC, Inc. The ECAT is a single slice scanner containing 66 NaI crystals arranged in six banks with 11 crystals per bank. Each detector is in coincidence with a crystal in the opposing (180° apart) bank. There is a total translation of 4 cm of the crystal arrays in steps of 5.7 or 11.4 mm. The crystal arrays then rotate through an angular increment of 4°, 7.5°, or 10° and translation is repeated, Successive rotations are performed through a total angle of 60°. The resolution of this system is determined by the number of samples. In addition, resolution can be improved by the use of "shadow shields," or collimation in front of the detectors. This collimation reduces the sensitivity but improves the spatial resolution. The ECAT allows for cardiac gating by the use of a buffer memory, which divides or partitions the data collected during different phases of the cardiac cycle.

The disadvantages associated with the PETT-III and the ECAT include: 1) imaging of only one slice at a time, 2) a complex mechanical motion which limits rapid (less than 10 s) data acquisition, and 3) a hexagonal distribution of detectors, which is not the most efficient utilization of annihilation radiation (radiation between the arrays is not detected).

The PETT-IV retains a hexagonal array geometry with NaI(Tl) crystals, but each crystal is elongated along the patient axis. Each crystal is also optically coupled to two photomultiplier tubes, which are in turn connected to an Anger or gamma camera-type logic. This gometry permits localization of the scintillation within the crystal and permits multislice capability.

The PETT-V consists of a circular array of 48 NaI(Tl) crystals, each fitted with two photomultiplier tubes. Adequate sampling is achieved by a rotation of the circular array of detectors and a wobbling motion of the detector circle. The PETT-V also incorporates the Anger-type logic of PETT-IV, which permits data acquisition for seven transverse slices simultaneously.

Multiple ring devices have been developed by several groups (Phelps, 1977; Goodwin, 1980). An example is the Therascan-3128 by Atomic Energy of Canada, Ltd. (AECL). The Therascan consists of two rings, each having 64 BGO detectors. The two rings permit simultaneous imaging of three slices; the central slice is a result of cross-coincidences between rings. Data samples can be increased by rotating the rings 2.8°. Static scan resolution is about .8 cm; the dynamic 1-s scan resolution is about 1.5 cm.

The Scanditronix Instrument Corporation of Sweden has manufactured a device with four rings, with 96 BGO crystals per ring, that can obtain up to seven simultaneous slices. A wobbling movement of the detectors allows for more data samples.

Positron-Emitting Radioisotopes A major problem in positron ECT has been the necessity of producing the positron-emitting radionuclides close to the site of patient administration. This is a result of the short half-lives of positron emitters. As examples, the clinically useful positron emitters carbon-11, nitrogen-13, and oxgyen-15 have respective half-lives of 20.34, 9.96, and 2.05 min.

Since positron emitters, as previously described, are characterized by having an excess number of protons, they are generally manufactured by bombarding a stable nucleus with accelerated protons, deuterons (hydrogen-2 nuclei), or helium nuclei. This generally necessitates the use of a cyclotron, a device that accelerates positively charged particles or nuclear species and uses them to bombard atoms. This is an expensive and complicated proposition. The cyclotron must be located in or near the hospital, and a team of chemists is needed to synthesize the desired radiopharmaceuticals. Prospects have been improved by the more recent development by several companies of relatively compact cyclotrons for hospital use. Some of these have been described by Goodwin (1980).

Performance Performance is a measure of how well a positron ECT device provides a nearly linear relationship between the actual concentration of positron emitters and the reconstructed image of the positron activity from the acquired data. Ter-Pogossian (1981) has listed the main factors interfering with this linearity: 1) the reconstruction algorithm, 2) counting data, 3) random coincidences, 4) scattered radiation, and 5) nonlinearity of positron ECT electronic circuitry.

The contribution to nonlinearity from the first factor can be minimized by selection of a well designed reconstruction algorithm. The effect of the second factor can be reduced obtaining an adequate number of counts. As discussed earlier, the effect of random coincidences can be decreased by use of a relatively low count rate, reducing the coincidence resolving time, and subtracting out the measured contribution of random coincidences. Proper collimation can reduce the effect of scattered radiation. Nonlinearity of electronic circuitry can be decreased by improvement in design.

Ter-Pogossian (1981) has stated that positron ECT devices at present may provide quantitative values with better than 10% accuracy for objects larger than the spatial resolution of the device. Data acquisition times of the order of a few seconds are possible, facilitating dynamic studies.

Ultrasound

Historical Background

The initial quantitative description dealing with the propagation of sound was by Sir Isaac Newton (1642–1727). Lord John William Strutt Rayleigh, (1842–1919) published the two volumes of his book *The Theory of Sound*, describing the physics of sound waves, in 1877–1878.

The Austrian physicist Christian Doppler (1803-1853) published in 1842 his *Über das farbige Licht der Doppelsterne* (*Concerning the Colored Light of Double Stars*), which contained his first statement of the Doppler effect. In this work he theorized that, since the pitch (apparent frequency) of sound from a moving source varies for a stationary observer, the color of light from a star should change, depending on the velocity of the star relative to the earth. The Doppler effect is a description of the effect that velocity has on the observed frequency of light and sound waves.

The brothers Pierre (1859–1906) and Jacques Curie discovered the piezoelectric effect in 1880. The piezoelectric effect is the physical basis for the use of ultrasound transducers to generate and detect ultrasound.

The sinking of the Titanic in 1912 was one of several incidents that provoked discussion and work in the development of methods for identifying obstacles at sea. The Englishman E. G. Richardson thought of transmitting a beam of underwater sound and then detecting the echoes reflected by submerged objects. This idea was explored during World War I.

It was the French physicist Paul Langevin (1872–1946) who in 1917 finally achieved success in using the pulse-echo technique for detecting submarines. This was the foundation of sonar (*so*und *n*avigation *a*nd *r*anging). With the development of the means for generating and detecting higher frequency ultrasound, pulse-echo techniques were used in the nondestructive testing of metallic structures. These methods were advanced by Firestone in the United States and Desch in Britain.

In the 1920s the initial connection between ultrasonics and radiology was made as publications began to explore the effects of ultrasound on biological systems. In the 1930s interest was aroused in potential therapeutic applications of ultrasound, but the efforts were not well directed.

The Russian S. Y. Sokolov during this time proposed techniques for medical diagnosis. Another Russians, I. E. Elpiner, began his work on the biophysics of ultrasound at this time.

During World War II a great many technical advances were made in sonar, and an increased interest developed in the biological effects of ultrasound. The first description of an ultrasonic scanner was by the Austrian K. T. Dussik in 1947 and was based on detecting and recording transmitted ultrasound. A receiver was placed in line with a beam of ultrasound directed through a patient's head. The first recordings were made in 1937 and were in the form of a plane, with higher intensities of transmitted ultrasound being portrayed in darker tones. Apparent initial success in imaging the ventricles was misleading; the skull fortuitously had an ultrasound transmission pattern that simulated the shape and appearance of normal ventricles. Although limited progress has been made in transmission scanners, the basic approach to ultrasound imaging has been based on reflection techniques.

In 1947, Douglas H. Howry, then an intern at Denver General Hospital, began construction of the first pulse-echo system designed for medical application. He completed a scanner with W. R. Bliss in 1949, and the first cross-sectional images were made in 1950 and 1951. Howry constructed a compound scanner (one using a combination of scanning motions) in 1954 in which the patient was submerged in a water tank made from a gun turret. The use of a water tank was necessitated by the inability of ultrasound to travel through air.

Ludwig and Struthers in 1949 first used pulse-echo technique to detect gallstones. A group in Minneapolis led by J. J. Wild, an Englishman with a background in radar, with J. M. Reid demonstrated echoes in an excised brain tumor (1952). Later a tumor was detected in vivo by scanning across the intact scalp through a craniotomy. Their initial work was based on information obtained along a single line-of-sight ultrasound path (amplitude mode). Wild and Reid went on to use two-dimensional scan techniques.

Echocardiography was originated by I. Edler in the mid-1950s. In this technique the relative motions of cardiac structures are observed along a single line-of-sight path of the ultrasound.

The Scottish obstetrician Ian Donald developed the first direct contact two-dimensional ultrasonic scanner in the early 1960s. Direct fluid coupling between patient and transducer was used, obviating the need for water tanks. Holmes built a similar device in 1965, and in 1964 Wells constructed the first scanner with two articulated arms (ajointed arm).

Sophisticated water bath scanners were developed by the ultrasonic Research Section established by George Kossoff in the National (formerly Commonwealth) Acoustic Laboratories in Sydney, Australia, in 1959. Kossoff's group developed the gray scale display for two-dimensional imaging. Different shades of gray are assigned in the two-dimensional image to echoes of different strength or amplitude. This permits a great deal more quantitative information to be displayed. The commercial introduction of gray scale ultrasound in the mid-1970s was greatly responsible for the rapid increase in the utilization of ultrasound imaging in clinical diagnosis.

General Principles Diagnostic ultrasound is a tomographic imaging modality that does not utilize ionizing radiation. High frequency mechanical or pressure waves generated by a vibrating crystal transducer travel through physical material, including body tissue, causing alternating high (compressive) and low (rarefactive) variations in the molecular distribution, and hence the density, of the material.

Sound waves audible to humans are in the range of 10 Hz to 20 kHz. By definition, ultrasound has a frequency above 20 kHz. Diagnostic ultrasound employs frequencies in the general range of 1–10 MHz. The velocity of sound is not constant but depends on the nature of the substance propagating the acoustic energy. In tissue this ranges from about 1,540 m per s for an average ultrasound velocity in soft tissues to about 3,500 m per s for bone. The velocity of sound in a substance is generally inversely related to its compressibility; in other words, more compressible substances propagate sound waves more slowly than substances that are less compressible. In easily compressible materials the different molecules interact weakly; they are poorly bound and may be thought of as coupled by loose springs. Thus, any change affecting one group of molecules is transmitted relatively slowly to the other molecules. In substances that are incompressible, the different molecules are strongly interacting (tightly coupled). Any change or force affecting one group of molecules is transmitted rapidly to the other molecules in the substance.

Since ultrasound obeys Equation 2.1, for a velocity of 1500 m per s, frequencies of 1 and 10 MHz will have corresponding wavelengths of 1.5 mm and .15 mm. The wavelength represents the distance between two regions of compression, or alternatively between two rarefactive regions. The frequency range of 1–10 MHz is used because ultrasound has poor penetration (rapid attenuation) at higher frequencies and poor spatial resolution because of the increasing wavelength at lower frequencies.

Ultrasound is generated by electrically exciting a crystal transducer, which resonates (vibrates) at a specific frequency. The principle of piezoelectricity (pressure electricity) underlying this technique for generating ultrasound was discovered by the Curie brothers in France in the 1880s. In the piezoelectric effect, when a voltage is applied to the faces of certain crystalline materials, the material is shortened or lengthened, depending upon the polarity of the voltage. The pressure causes a slight separation between the center of the negative charges and that of the positive charges. Conversely, when a mechanical pressure is applied that deforms the crystal, an electrical voltage is produced between the faces of the crystal. The polarity of the electrical voltage depends upon whether the distance between the crystal faces has increased or decreased. The piezoelectric effect is a property of certain naturally occurring crystalline materials, such as quartz and Rochelle salt, and certain polycrystalline ceramics such as barium titanate, lead titanate zirconate (PZT), and lead metaniobate.

Transducer is a general term applied to any device that is capable of transforming energy from one form into another. In ultrasound the transducer is the vibrating or resonating crystal, which can function as a transmitter or receiver for ultrasound. As a transmitter it converts electrical energy into ultrasound energy; as a receiver the ultrasound or acoustic energy is converted into an electrical signal.

The actual resonant frequency of the transducer is determined by the crystal thickness, the distance between the two faces of the wafer-shaped crystal. To achieve maximum energy coupling between an electrical circuit and the crystal, the crystal thickness should be one-half of the wavelength of the ultrasound wave in the crystal, so that the vibrations or reflections of acoustic energy from the two crystal faces reinforce one another. The corresponding frequency that produces internal wavelengths twice the thickness of the crystal is the natural or resonant frequency. If a frequency other than its resonant frequency is applied to a crystal, it will oscillate at the applied frequency, but usually rather weakly. For a constant level of electrical energy, the mechanical vibrations of the crystal will become stronger (increase in amplitude) as the applied frequency approaches the resonant frequency. The maximum energy transfer from the electrical oscillator circuit to the crystal occurs when the applied electrical frequency equals the crystal resonant frequency.

In practice, a single voltage spike is applied to the crystal transducer, which then vibrates at its resonant frequency, with rapidly decreasing amplitude as the crystal vibrations are mechanically dampened. In effect, from the large number of frequency components which together comprise the applied electrical spike or pulse, the crystal "recognizes" and is excited by those frequencies at or near its resonant frequency.

Of great practical consequence is the fact that an ultrasound transducer is not a frequency-variable device. It cannot be turned to different frequencies the way that the kV of an x-ray unit may be varied. Selection of a different frequency involves changing the transducer.

The techniques of medical ultrasound are based on those of sonar, the localization of objects in water with sound. The concepts of sonar are also similar to those of radar. A pulse of energy (acoustic energy in medical ultrasound or sonar, electromagnetic energy in the microwave range in radar) is transmitted along a straight line path. The transmitter only emits energy for the duration of a pulse and is then silent. Reflections of this pulse from distant structures or targets retrace this straight line path and are detected by an antenna or receiver. Following transmission of the pulse of energy, the transmitter may serve as the receiver. In ultrasound the crystal transducer typically vibrates for about 1 μs following electrical excitations. The crystal then functions as receiver to convert the reflected ultrasound energy into electrical energy for approximately 1 ms before transmitting another ultrasound pulse. The duty cycle represents the ratio of the time the crystal functions as a transmitter to the time it is a receiver (typically 1:1000).

The actual ultrasound pulse is a wave packet, typically two or three wavelengths long; that is, two or three complete oscillations are present. This is primarily determined by the dampening of the crystal, or how long it resonates. Since the axial resolution (the resolution parallel to the beam or along the line of sight) is determined by the length of this packet, the time of vibration should not be excessive. The wave packet is the probe that localizes the target, and the target cannot be localized better than the size of the probe. The off-axis or perpendicular resolution is related to the width of the beam. The sound beam can be focused. That is, its energy can be concentrated in a smaller area at a given depth or, more practically, over a range of depths. This can improve the off-axis resolution. Focusing is generally incorporated into a particular transducer, as is the frequency. The actual thickness of the tissue slice being imaged at any location within the cross-section is the diameter of the ultrasound beam at that location. This beam diameter can be reduced by focusing. Since focusing is not uniform throughout the slice, the thickness of the cross-section is also nonuniform.

The energy of the ultrasound is attenuated exponentially in its passage through tissue, analogous to the attenuation of x-rays. The attenuation occurs because of scattering, absorption, and dissipation by heating. Medical information, including images, is derived from the reflections of the acoustic pulse which are detected and recorded. Information about the total attenuation, including absorption, of ultrasound can be derived by examining the relative intensities of the reflected echoes as a function of distance for different acoustic paths.

The ultrasound beam is characterized by a near zone, called the Fresnel zone, and a far zone, the Fraunhofer zone. These zones are named after two early 19th century pioneers in optics, Augustin-Jean Fresnel (1788–1827), a French physicist, and Joseph von Fraunhofer (1787–1826), a German optician and physicist. Since the physical wave theory that describes the properties of ultrasound or mechanical waves was initially derived from optics, the study of light, not only the mathematics but much of the terminology used in optics is applied to acoustic waves as well. The wavelengths of ultrasound waves, of the order of 1 mm, are much larger than the wavelengths of typical x-rays, which are typically 10^{-8} mm at about 120 kV. Thus, ultrasound is best described as a wave, whereas diagnostic x-rays are best conceptualized and treated as discrete quanta of energy following ray paths.

In the near zone, the acoustic energy travels as a parallel wave of constant cross-sectional area equal to the area of the transducer. In the far zone, the acoustic energy is characterized as a diverging wave, similar to a spherical wave diverging outward from a point source. The length T of the Fresnel zone is given by

$$T = \frac{D^2}{4\lambda}, \qquad (9.6)$$

where D is the diameter of the transducer and λ is the wavelength. This equation tells us that the larger the ratio of the transducer diameter to the wavelength, the larger the near zone.

The angle θ of divergence or the dispersion angle in the far or Fraunhofer zone is given by

$$\sin \theta = \frac{1.22\lambda}{D}. \qquad (9.7)$$

This equation tells us that the larger the ratio of the transducer diameter to the wavelength, the smaller the divergence of the acoustic beam. Thus, a larger ratio of the transducer diameter to the wavelength gives a relatively long parallel beam which diverges slowly in the far zone. A smaller ratio results in a shorter parallel or near beam and relatively rapidly divergent far beam. The ultrasound wave can be focused, or narrowed, within the near zone.

Following electrical excitation, the transducer emits a single acoustic pulse which follows a straight line or line-of-sight path. It is actually a pencil beam of variable cross-sectional area initially identical to the area of the transducer, then narrowing in the portion of the near zone where it is focused, and then widening or diverging in the far zone. The slice thickness varies in a corresponding way. When the incident sound beam encounters interfaces between different types of tissues or local inhomogeneities within the tissue, collectively called targets, part of the sound beam is reflected. If the interfaces or inhomogeneities are larger than the cross-sectional area of the beam, the reflection is termed specular. This type of reflection is similar to a ball bouncing off a wall and is the type of echo that defines large boundaries or surfaces. The angle of reflection of the sound will be equal to the angle of incidence, where both are measured with respect to a perpendicular to the plane of the reflecting surface. If the incident beam is perpendicular to the interface, the reflected sound will also be perpendicular and will retrace the path of the incident beam. In doing so it will intercept the transducer, which now functions as a receiver that converts the acoustic or pressure signal from the transducer into an electrical signal that can be processed (amplified, made into video, or digitized). The time from initiation of the ultrasound pulse to reception of the reflected wave is equal to the time for the wave to reach the target and be reflected back to the transducer. The time t involved is an indication of the distance d of the target from the transducer as follows

$$d = \frac{t}{2v}, \qquad (9.8)$$

where v is the velocity of sound in tissue, and the factor of 2 accounts for the roundtrip path of the sound wave.

In addition to information about target localization, the size of the reflected echo is measured to give quantitative information about the nature of the target. The acoustic properties of a tissue are described in terms of its acoustic impedance, defined by

$$Z = \rho v, \qquad (9.9)$$

where ρ is the density in grams per cubic centimeter, and v is the velocity expressed in centimeters per second.

Echoes or reflections arise when there are abrupt changes in the acoustic impedance of a tissue. The greater the relative difference in the acoustic impedances between two tissues (i.e., the greater the acoustic mismatch), the larger is the reflected portion of the ultrasound beam at the interface between the two tissues. This is expressed mathematically as follows:

$$R = \left(\frac{Z_1 - Z_2}{Z_1 + Z_2}\right)^2, \qquad (9.10)$$

where R is the fraction of the incident energy that is reflected at the interface between two tissues with acoustic impedances Z_1 and Z_2. The differences in acoustic impedance between different soft tissues is small, and so only a small part of the incident energy is reflected from boundaries between soft tissues.

Since both the density of air and sound velocity in air are much less than the corresponding values for soft tissues, the fraction of energy reflected is very large. In fact it is almost identical to 1, implying that there is nearly total reflection of the acoustic energy at an interface with air. This necessitates coupling the transducer to the body through a fluid rather than air, and it precludes the penetration of ultrasound beyond air. Similarly, the much greater density of bone and velocity of sound in bone compared to soft tissue result in nearly total reflection of sound at an interface of bone and soft tissue. Bone is also nearly opaque to ultrasound.

Nonspecular echoes arise from interfaces smaller than the acoustic beam and are independent of the size of the target. These are generally weaker echoes but can give important information about the tissue texture.

Imaging Techniques The different techniques employed in diagnostic ultrasound are listed in Table 9.1.

Amplitude, Brightness, and Motion Modes The amplitude mode (A-mode) displays information about the echoes received from targets along a single line of sight. The horizontal axis of an oscilloscope is used to represent time or distance along the line of sight, and the vertical axis is used to represent the magnitude of the reflected echo. This is illustrated in Figure 9.37.

In the brightness mode (B-mode), the magnitude of the reflected echo is represented as a dot of variable brightness on the oscilloscope face at the corresponding distance along the horizontal axis or line of sight. Only a single line is shown on the oscilloscope face. B-mode is not used as such in clinical practice except in the common M-mode or B-scan.

The motion mode (M-mode) employs a B-mode trace to look at moving targets such as the structures of the heart. The amplitude and rate of change of the motion associated with particular targets can be identified and analyzed by a continuous trace of the reflections from these targets displayed on the oscil-

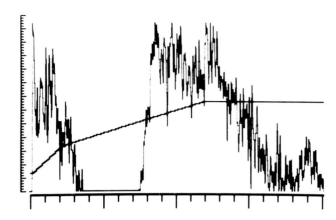

Figure 9.37. An ultrasound A-mode trace. The abscissa represents transmission time or distance (1-cm markers are indicated); the ordinate or represents the magnitude of the reflections or echoes. The flat portion of the graph is due to a fluid path (urine-filled bladder). The superimposed trace is a time compensation gain curve, which indicates the compensation in the receiver to offset ultrasound attenuation in tissue.

loscope face or on a strip chart recorder. An example of an M-mode trace is illustrated in Figure 9.38.

The A-, B-, and M-modes give only one-dimensional information about target reflections, corresponding to the line of sight of the ultrasound pulse. A two-dimensional, cross-sectional image requires information along multiple lines of sight. This is accomplished with B-scanning by building up an image from a series of individual B-mode lines. There are several approaches to B-scanning.

Static B-Scanning In the traditional B-scan technique, the patient is manually scanned with a single transducer or an articulated scanning arm. This

Table 9.1. Ultrasound techniques

A-Mode (amplitude)
B-Mode (brightness)
M-Mode (motion)
B-Scan
    Manual scanning with an articulated arm
    Real time or dynamic imaging
    Automated scanning
Doppler
    Continuous
    Pulsed

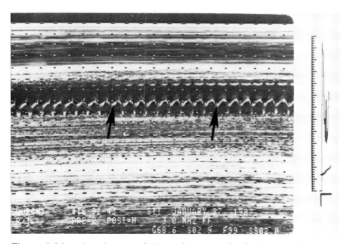

Figure 9.38. An ultrasound M-mode trace of a fetal heart. The fluctuating line (arrows) represents motion of the heart.

generally takes several seconds, and a static B-scan image is obtained. The arm has three segments and three corresponding joints that allow orientation of the transducer along any arbitrary axis in space. The angle between the different arm segments can be accurately measured by different means. This permits accurate determination of the orientation of the line of sight of each acoustic data line and of the entire scan section. The echoes along each line of sight can be displayed with proper orientation on the electrical display, the oscilloscope in early B-scan units now having been replaced by a television monitor. Rotation and angulation of the scanning arm permit the selection of a scan section at any arbitrary orientation.

The television monitor is part of the technique of gray scale imaging, introduced in commercial units in 1974. Previously, echoes of different magnitude were all displayed equally; there was no difference in their appearance. The only alternative was to reject entirely echoes of a certain magnitude or less. With gray scale imaging, the magnitude of echoes can be displayed by different shades of gray. Prior to display on the television monitor, echoes are converted into electrical signals, which are stored on a scan converter. This is a square matrix of about a million elements, each of which represents a small area in the cross-section being imaged. The size of the signal corresponding to an echo can be stored in analog or digital form, more recent scan converters being of the digital type. The electrical image on the scan converter is read and transformed into a visual image on the television monitor. The video signal can also be displayed on another television monitor for photography, as in CT. Gray scale static B-scans are shown in Figures 9.39 and 9.40.

Real Time (Dynamic B-Scanning) An alternative method of B-scanning is real time or dynamic imaging. In this technique, sequential images are each generated in a fraction of a second (typically 1/30 to 1/10 s) using single or multiple transducers located at the end of a cable containing electrical wiring. Handling of the transducer(s) is thus considerably easier than in a static B-scanner, facilitating rapid changes in the scanning plane. However, the location and angulation of the scanning plane are not identifiable on the display monitor.

There are several approaches to real time imaging. A rocking transducer can form a sector format

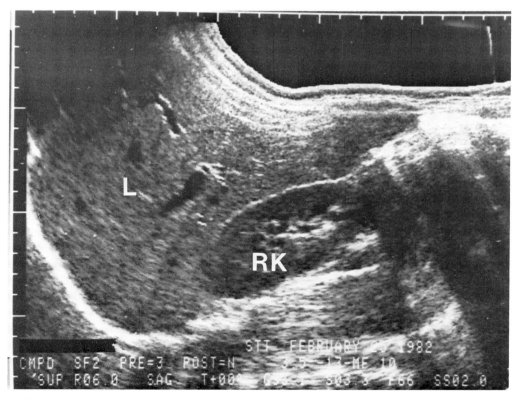

Figure 9.39. Longitudinal gray scale ultrasound scan through the liver (*L*) and right kidney (*RK*).

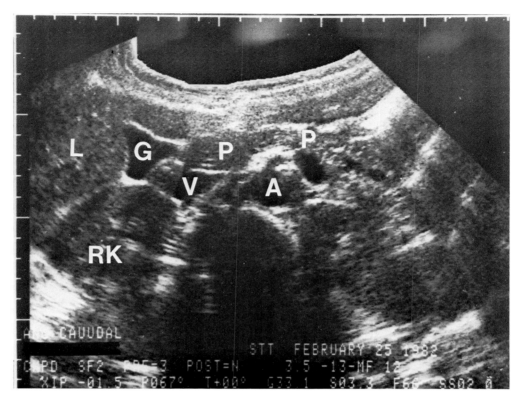

Figure 9.40. Transverse gray scale ultrasound scan through the upper abdomen showing the liver (*L*), right kidney (*RK*), gallbladder (*G*), vena cava (*V*), pancreas (*P*), and aorta (*A*).

image from the acoustic lines it generates as it moves through an arc (Figure 9.41). One or more transducers moving through a circle can each generate a sector format acoustic image during part of the circular path (Figure 9.42). A parabolic acoustic mirror can convert the rotary motion of transducers at its focus to a linear sweep motion across the patient, forming a rectangular image (Figure 9.43). An oscillating acoustic mirror can be used to reflect the ultrasound beam at different angles, so that the ultrasound beam is swept through the patient (Figure 9.44).

In a linear array of small transducer elements (typically 64–256), groups of small adjacent elements can be sequentially energized, each group producing a line of information in a rectangular image format (Figure 9.45). A phased array is a short array of transducer elements (typically 16–32) that are energized in phase as a collective transducer. Each element contributes to each line of information, and the acoustic beam is electronically steered through a sector (Figure 9.46).

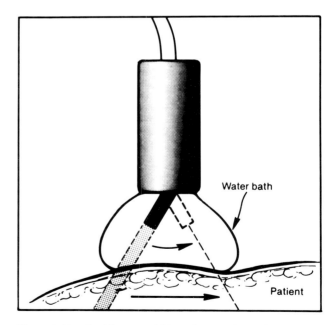

Figure 9.41. Rocking or wobbling ultrasound transducer with a water bath. A sector format image is generated.

Basic Principles of Computed Tomography

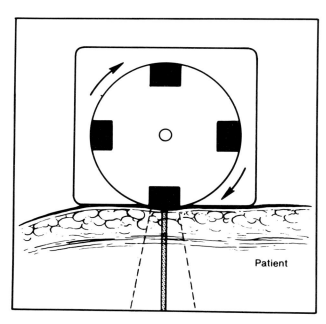

Figure 9.42. Rotating transducers on a wheel in direct contact with the patient generate a rectangular format image.

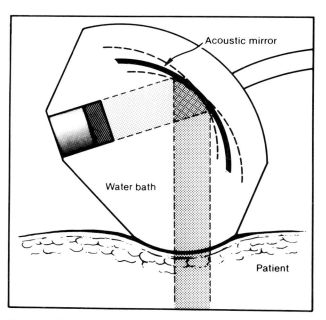

Figure 9.44. Stationary ultrasound transducer and a rocking acoustic mirror. This generates a rectangular format image.

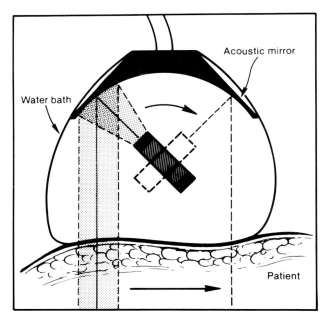

Figure 9.43. Two rotating ultrasound transducers at the focus of a parabolic acoustic mirror will sweep out a rectangular format image by reflecting the sound beam off the mirror.

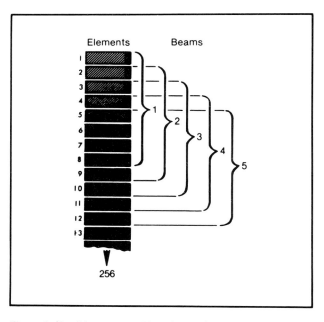

Figure 9.45. Linear array. Transducer elements in a group are simultaneously excited, generating a single line of acoustic information. The group thus acts as a single transducer. In this example eight elements are in the group. After all the information is received from this single acoustic beam, another group of light elements is simultaneously excited. This is repeated for an array with 256 elements so that a rectangular format image is obtained.

Further Applications 255

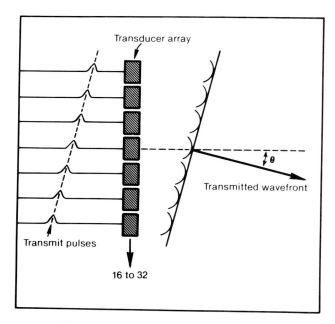

Figure 9.46. Phased array. A relatively smaller number of transducer elements (e.g., 16–32) comprise the array. All of the elements are used to generate each line of acoustic information (in distinction to a linear array where different groups of elements generate different lines). The individual elements are excited at slightly different times (phased). The individual acoustic waves associated with each element are superimposed to form a wavefront that generates a single line of acoustic information. By changing the phasing sequence of the individual elements, the angle θ of the wavefront is altered and a new line of acoustic information is obtained. The image, therefore, has a sector format.

Advantages and disadvantages of static B-scanning and real time ultrasound are listed in Tables 9.2–9.4.

Automated Scanning The last approach to B-scanning is automated scanning. In this technique, images similar to static B-scans are produced in a fraction of the usual time by means of multiple transducers, each of which travels through a water path to the patient.

Doppler Techniques A final application of ultrasound to medicine involves Doppler techniques.

Table 9.2. Advantages of static B-scanning

Wide imaging field of view
Compound imaging or registration of target echoes from multiple different angles
Identification of the location and orientation of the scanning plane
Automatic indexing of changes in position of the scanning plane
Good spatial and contrast resolutions
Relatively high density of acoustic lines of information

Table 9.3. Disadvantages of static B-scanning

Long scanning time per image
Absence of dynamic information
Delay and difficulty in obtaining optimal orientation of the scanning plane
Inconvenience of using an articulated, multijointed scanning arm

These are based on the Doppler effect. When sound is reflected from a moving target, the frequency f of the sound wave is shifted by an amount Δf as follows:

$$\Delta f = f \times \frac{v}{c} \cos \theta, \qquad (9.11)$$

where v is the velocity of the moving target, c the wave velocity, and θ the angle between the path of the wave and the direction of motion of the target. The frequency shift is positive or negative, depending on whether the target is moving toward or away from the wave.

Continuous Doppler ultrasound employs two side-by-side transducers. One is continuously emitting ultrasound, the second receiving it. This permits constant surveillance of moving structures. Both the velocity of a moving structure and the rate at which the velocity of a moving structure changes can be detected. In fetal monitoring the rate at which fetal cardiac structures such as heart valves and muscle change velocity is detected. The continuous nature of the ultrasound does not permit spatial localization.

A pulsed Doppler transducer can be used which permits analysis of the shift of the frequencies within the pulse from a specific location.

Nuclear Magnetic Resonance Imaging

Historical Background Magnetic resonance occurs when atomic electrons or nuclei respond to the application of magnetic fields by absorbing or emitting electromagnetic radiation. When the electrons of an atom are involved, the process is referred to as electron spin resonance (ESR) or electron paramagnetic resonance (EPR); when the atomic nuclei are involved, the process is called nuclear magnetic resonance (NMR).

Table 9.4. Advantages of real time ultrasound

Visualization of motion in abdomen
Ultrasonic accessibility through small or difficult-to-reach acoustic portals without having to move the patient
Direct in utero orientation to the fetus
Intra-abdominal orientation to organs and structures
Rapid survey capability

Table 9.5. Disadvantages of real time ultrasound

Restricted size of the field of view in a single frame
Limitations in compound scanning
Difficulty in localization of the scanning plane on hard copy images
No capability for automatic indexing of changes in position of the scanning plane
Density of acoustic lines inversely related to frame rate and generally lower than static B-scans

ESR is generally observed only in a restricted class of substances: the transition elements with unfilled electronic shells, free radicals (atomic or molecular fragments), and various paramagnetic defects and impurity centers. The first experimental observation of ESR was made in 1944 by the Soviet physicist Yevgeny K. Zavoysky (1907–1976) in several concentrated salts in the iron group.

The initial experimental observations and measurements of NMR were performed in 1946. A group at Stanford University headed by Felix Bloch and including William W. Hansen and Martin E. Packard observed NMR with protons of water. They employed the method of nuclear induction to measure the electrical signal induced in a coil by a precessing nuclear magnetization.

Independently, a group at Harvard including Edward Purcell, Robert V. Pound and Henry C. Torrey identified NMR in protons of paraffin. They measured the energy transferred between a resonant electrical circuit and a nuclear magnetic sample.

Bloch and Purcell received the Nobel Prize in Physics in 1952 for their work in NMR.

Magnetic resonance phenomena have been studied extensively in physics and chemistry, and a wide variety of engineering and practical applications have evolved based on magnetic resonance principles.

The potential for medical applications of NMR was first described by Raymond Damadian, who in 1971 reported differences in the relaxation times (a magnetic resonance parameter described below) of tumor and normal tissue in rats. The possibility for achieving images with nuclear magnetic resonance was proposed by Damadian in a patient application in 1972. The first two-dimensional images with NMR were achieved by Paul Lauterbur in 1973. This was done by using magnetic field gradients in multiple different directions relative to the object to study magnetic resonance signals and combining these one-dimensional projections to form a two-dimensional image. This is similar to projection reconstruction techniques in transmission CT.

In 1974 Lauterbur demonstrated cross-sectional images of animals. A human wrist was imaged in vivo with NMR by Hinshaw and others in 1977. EMI showed a head scan in 1978. The first commercially available whole body NMR scanner, the FONAR (focused NMR) QED 80, was introduced by the Fonar Corporation in 1980. Other units have been sponsored or developed commercially by companies including Diasonics, General Electric, Picker International, and Technicare.

Basic Principles of NMR The attenuation of electromagnetic radiation by tissue via absorption and scattering is highly dependent upon frequency. The body appears relatively transparent to the higher frequencies or energies associated with the gamma rays of radioisotope imaging, making emission CT feasible. At diagnostic x-ray frequencies (corresponding to those energies used in conventional radiography and transmission CT), both Compton scattering and photoelectric absorption increase, the latter becoming dominant as the x-ray energy is further decreased. Body tissue is essentially opaque to electromagnetic frequencies in the range from soft (low energy) x-rays down to microwave frequencies, precluding effective imaging of the tissues at these frequencies. Optical and infrared frequencies lie within this range, and imaging techniques, such as thermography, that employ these frequencies are limited to studying the surface or superficial structures. The body again becomes transparent at microwave frequencies. Another form of electromagnetic attenuation may then occur in the presence of a large, constant magnetic field. This involves the absorption of energy from the radiofrequency fields associated with the electromagnetic radiation by the naturally occurring magnetic nuclei within atoms of the body. This phenomenon of NMR can be used to obtain cross-sectional body images.

Atomic nuclei are composed of positively charged protons and neutrons. The neutrons are nearly identical in mass to protons but are electrically neutral. The term nucleon is used to describe either a proton or a neutron. The atomic number Z responsible for the chemical properties of the atom is equal to the number of protons. The atomic mass A is effectively due to the total mass of the protons and neutrons, the negatively charged electron having only about 1/1,837 the mass of the proton or neutron, Atoms with the same atomic number but different numbers of neutrons are called isotopes.

Both protons and neutrons are in orbit within the nucleus, just as the earth revolves about the sun,

Further Applications 257

and the electrons can be considered to be in orbit about the nucleus. This imparts a physical quantity called angular momentum to the particle or object. This is analogous to the property of momentum (the product of mass and velocity) in linear motion. Angular momentum is a vector quantity; it is associated with a direction as well as a magnitude. Angular momentum is a function of the mass of the rotating object, the radius of rotation, and the angular frequency and direction of the rotation. The angular frequency w is expressed in terms of the number of radians per second. In a 360° rotation, the number of radians is equal to 2π (the number of radii that it takes to equal the circumference).

The nucleons also rotate about their own axes, as the earth (or an electron) rotates about its axis, and this imparts to each nucleon a certain intrinsic angular momentum, referred to as its spin. This revolution or rotation of electrical charge results in the formation of a magnetic moment or magnet. Although the neutron has no net electrical charge, it may be envisioned as having components of rotating charge that give it a net magnetic moment.

Pairs of protons or neutrons are aligned in the nucleus so that their spins and magnetic moments cancel out. However, a nucleus with an odd number of neutrons and/or protons will have a net angular momentum called the spin of the nucleus, as well as an associated magnetic moment. There are over 100 such nuclear species with a net spin and magnetic moment. These include a number of naturally occurring atomic nuclei in tissues, including hydrogen-1, hydrogen-2, carbon-13, nitrogen-14, nitrogen-15, oxygen-17, fluorine-19, sodium 23, phosphorus-31, sulfur-33, chlorine-35, potassium-39, and calcium-43. It is the presence of these nuclei in body tissues that permits imaging by NMR. Hydrogen-1 nuclei, or protons, are by far the most abundant of the naturally magnetic nuclei, and NMR imaging has been primarily concentrated on mobile proton imaging. Mobile protons are those in free water, fat, or oil in the soft tissues.

Usually, the spins and magnetic moments of individual nuclei are randomly oriented with respect to one another, so that they cancel each other out. The vector sum of all the magnetic moments, or the net magnetization, averages out to zero.

Magnetic moments, however, tend to orient along external magnetic fields, like the needle of a compass. Individual nuclear magnetic moments precess or resonate (similar to a spinning top) about an external magnetic field (Figure 9.47). The component

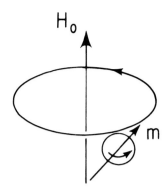

Figure 9.47. An individual nuclear magnetic moment m precesses about the external magnetic field H_0.

of this magnetic moment that projects onto the magnetic field is associated with an energy state because of the interaction between the magnetic moment and the external magnetic field. When this component is parallel (pointing in the same direction) with the magnetic field, it is in a low energy state; when it is antiparallel (pointing in the opposite direction), it is a high energy state. The larger the external magnetic field, the greater the magnitude of the energy involved. There are more magnetic moments in the low energy state than in the high energy state. The ratio of the number in the high energy to that in low energy state is governed by a fundamental law of statistical theory, the Boltzmann distribution. This ratio decreases as the energy difference between the low and high energy states increases. Since there are naturally more individual magnetic moment components parallel to the external magnetic field than antiparallel, there is a net total magnetic moment or magnetization M which is parallel to the external static magnetic field H_0 (Figure 9.48). This net magnetic moment is proportional to the strength of the external magnetic field and to the spin density (or density of magnetic nuclei).

The energy difference ΔE between the parallel and antiparallel states of the magnetic moment relative to the static external magnetic field H_0 is given by

$$\Delta E = hf = \frac{h\gamma}{2\pi}H_0, \tag{9.12}$$

where

$$f = \frac{\gamma}{2\pi}H_0. \tag{9.13}$$

In Equations 9.12 and 9.13, h is Planck's constant, the resonant frequency f is the frequency of the elec-

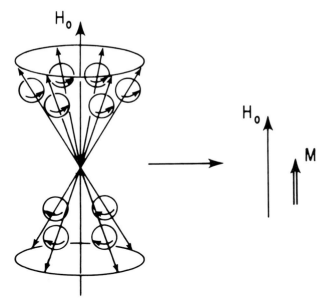

Figure 9.48. Individual magnetic moments may have a vector component parallel or antiparallel to the external magnetic field H_0. Parallel components represent low energy interaction states between the magnetic moment and the external magnetic field; antiparallel components represent high energy states. For a large number of individual nuclear magnetic moments, the individual vector components perpendicular to the magnetic field H_0 cancel, leaving only the components parallel and antiparallel to the magnetic field. In the natural state there will be more components in the low energy parallel state than in the higher energy antiparallel state. This results in a net magnetization M parallel to the external magnetic field H_0.

tromagnetic wave associated with the energy ΔE (as described in Equation 2.2), and γ is the gyromagnetic (or magnetogyric) ratio. The gyromagnetic ratio is a constant for a particular nucleus or isotope, so that the magnetic moments for various nuclear species will have different resonant frequencies in the same magnetic field H_0. The resonant frequency is so called because the nucleus can resonate or change back and forth between the two energy states separated by ΔE (Figure 9.49).

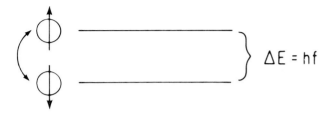

Figure 9.49. The two different resonant states separated by the energy difference $\Delta E = hf$ are illustrated.

The strength or magnitude of a magnetic field can be expressed in gauss units, named after the German mathematician Johann Friedrich Carl Gauss (1777–1855). As an example, the magnetic field of the earth at its surface is typically about .6 gauss. An alternative system uses tesla units (T), where 1 T is equal to 10,000 gauss. Tesla are named after the Croatian-born physicist Nikola Tesla (1856–1943). Tesla are used in nearly all works involving strong magnetic fields (including NMR), whereas the gauss is more useful with small magnets.

The subject to be imaged is placed in a static external magnetic field, typical magnitudes in NMR imaging ranging from .1–.35 T. These correspond to proton resonance radiofrequencies of 4.26–30 MHz. Consider a tissue containing magnetic moments (e.g., protons) being irradiated with a pulse of radiofrequency f corresponding to the energy at the resonant frequency defined by the magnetic field H_0 and the gyromagnetic ratio γ, according to Equation 9.12. Those magnetic moments in the lower energy state will be able to absorb the radiofrequency energy and flip to the higher energy state antiparallel to the magnetic field H_0. If the radiofrequency pulse is sufficiently strong, then enough nuclei will be flipped to reverse the direction of the total magnetic moment or magnetization from parallel to antiparallel to the field. After the radiofrequency pulse is completed, the magnetic moments or spins will begin to flip back or relax to their initial equilibrium value in the magnetic field in an experimental fashion with a characteristic relaxation time T_1. This will result in an emission of energy at the resonant frequency that can be detected, for example, by a radiofrequency coil in which it induces a signal. The emitted energy is usually irradiated away or dissipated thermally by coupling to other nearby atoms.

The application of a radiofrequency pulse at the resonant frequency also causes a transient alignment of the transverse (relative to the magnetic field H_0) components of the magnetic moments. This net transverse component of magnetization actually rotates or precesses about the field H_0 at a frequency called the Larmor precession frequency. This Larmor precession frequency f is related to the external magnetic field H_0 by the Larmor equation

$$f = \frac{\gamma}{2\pi} H_0, \tag{9.14}$$

or alternatively

$$\omega = \gamma H_0, \tag{9.15}$$

Further Applications

where $\omega = 2\pi f$ is the angular frequency. This is illustrated in Figure 9.50. The Larmor precession frequency defined by Equations 9.14 and 9.15 is identical to the resonant frequency defined by Equation 9.13.

Following cessation of the radiofrequency pulse, this transverse component of the magnetization is lost as the individual transverse components again become randomly oriented in an exponential fashion. This occurs with a characteristic relaxation time T_2.

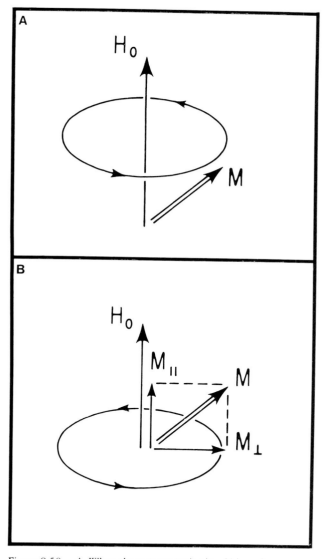

Figure 9.50. *A*, When the net magnetization M is no longer parallel to the external field H_0, it will precess about the field. *B*, M can be expressed in terms of its two vector components: $M_\parallel$, which is parallel (or antiparallel) to the external magnetic field H_0; and $M_\perp$, which is the transverse component that is perpendicular to the external magnetic field.

The radiofrequency pulse is in the form of a pulsed radiofrequency magnetic field H_1 applied at right angles to the static magnetic field H_0 (which lies along the Z axis). H_1 has a frequency equal to the Larmor frequency and is usually considerably smaller than H_0 in magnitude. The net magnetization M which lay along the direction parallel to H_0 then precesses or rotates about H_1 and away from the Z direction. This is illustrated in Figure 9.51. This rotating magnetization represents a rotating magnetic field which will induce an electrical signal in a receiving coil. This is the principle of nuclear induction, first used by Bloch. The induced electrical signal is called the free induction decay.

Fundamental Parameters of NMR   The basic parameters or physical quantities measured in NMR are the magnetic moment or spin density ρ, the spin-lattice relaxation time T_1, the spin-spin relaxation time T_2, and the chemical shift δ.

Magnetic Moment or Spin Density   The magnitude of the NMR signal is proportional to the spin or magnetic moment density ρ, which is related to the density of free protons that may respond to the radiofrequency signal. Thus, areas containing few free protons, such as bone or air, will yield very small NMR signals.

Spin-Lattice Relaxation Time (T_1) T_1, termed the spin-lattice or longitudinal relaxation time, characterizes the interaction between the magnetic moment and its environment (lattice). It is the exponential time constant at which the component of magnetization along the direction of the external magnetic field grows or decays to an equilibrium value. This occurs because of the interaction between the nuclear moment or spin with its physical environment. T_1 was originally introduced to describe the return to equilibrium of the spins with a lattice of neighboring molecules in a crystal. The radiofrequency pulse causes a depolarization (loss of magnetization) or reversal of the magnetization (antiparallel to the magnetic field). After cessation of the pulse, the nuclei in the radiofrequency-irradiated sample repolarize or recover their initial magnetization in an exponential fashion with the time constant T_1. The spin-lattice relaxation time is a function of the local magnetic field, temperature, viscosity, and strength of the interaction between the proton nucleus and the surrounding atoms and molecules. It is the characteristic time for the nuclear magnetic moments to regain thermal equilibrium (the equilibrium or Boltzmann distribution at a given temperature among different energy states) with their environment for a particular energy interaction, in this

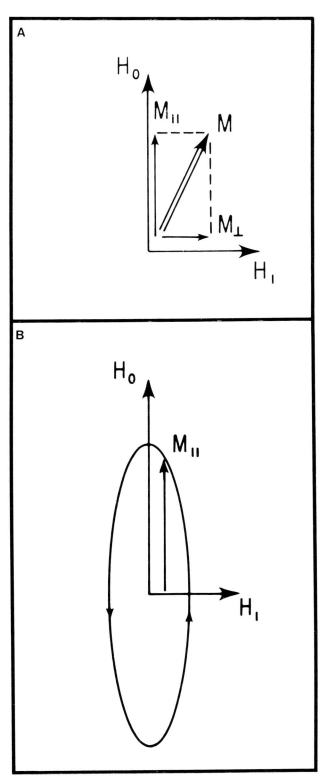

Figure 9.51. Application of a magnetic field H_1 (arising from a radiofrequency pulse) perpendicular to H_0 will result in precession of the $M_\parallel$ component of M illustrated in A to precess about H_1, as shown in B.

case between magnetic moments and an external magnetic field. It is a measure of molecular motion.

The magnitude of the NMR signal is inversely proportional to T_1. If a tissue has a large value for T_1, it will repolarize and emit energy slowly. Since energy emission stops with the next radiofrequency pulse, if T_1 becomes comparable to the time between pulses there will be less total energy emission.

Spin-Spin Relaxation Time T_2, called the spin-spin relaxation time, characterizes the interaction of a magnetic moment with other neighboring magnetic moments. It is the time constant describing the exponential decay of the transverse (perpendicular to the external magnetic field) component of the magnetization after cessation of the radiofrequency pulse. It occurs as a result of the interaction between nuclei with opposing spins. T_2 indicates the time for the individual transverse components of magnetization to again become randomly oriented with respect to each other. The width (full-width-at-half maximum) of the NMR signal is inversely proportional to T_2.

Relationship between T_1 and T_2 For simple liquids such as water, T_1 and T_2 are equal. Rapidly changing internal magnetic fields are equally effective in flipping or inverting the magnetic moments or spins for longitudinal relaxation and in dephasing them to eliminate the transverse magnetization, thus achieving transverse or off-axis relaxation. T_1 and T_2 are both approximately 3–5 s for pure water.

In solids, the atoms and molecules are relatively fixed in position. Internal magnetic fields therefore change or fluctuate slowly and are relatively ineffective in inverting or flipping the magnetic moments or spins, so that longitudinal relaxation is rather prolonged. T_1 may be of the order of minutes, or perhaps even hours, for solids at low temperatures. Ice has a value of T_1 of the order of minutes. The relatively static internal magnetic fields of solids are very efficient, however, in causing transverse relaxation, so that T_2 is shortened considerably compared to liquids. Ice, for example, has a T_2 of the order of tens of microseconds.

In summary, T_1 and T_2 are approximately equal in simple liquids. In solids, T_1 is prolonged and T_2 is shortened. Therefore,

$$T_1 \text{ (solid)} > T_1 \text{ (liquid)} = T_2 \text{ (liquid)}$$
$$> T_2 \text{ (solid)}. \quad (9.16)$$

There have been reports that T_1 and T_2 are elevated in neoplastic or other abnormal tissue compared to normal tissues.

Chemical Shift The chemical shift (δ) is a shift in the Larmor frequency that results when various nuclei and their magnetic moments interact with slightly different magnetic fields. The shift arises as a result of electrons screening the magnetic moments slightly from the magnetic field, thereby altering the resonant frequency. The degree of shielding depends on the specific nature of the local environment of the nucleus involved. This differs with various chemical compounds. In NMR spectroscopy, the chemical shift yields structural information. Chemical shifts are generally reported in fractional shifts expressed in parts per million (ppm).

Techniques of Imaging with NMR An image of any object may be defined as a graphical representation of the spatial distribution of a physical property or properties of the object. In conventional radiography and transmission CT, the property represented is the linear attenuation coefficient, related to the interactions between diagnostic x-rays and matter. In radioisotope imaging or scintigraphy, including emission CT, it is the distribution of radiopharmaceuticals. In ultrasonography it is the nature and distribution of echo-producing targets. The physical property that is to be measured and recorded for NMR imaging may be either the density of the nuclear magnetic moments, a relaxation time (either T_1 or T_2), or a combination of these parameters. In general, it is the interaction between magnetic moments and externally applied magnetic fields that is to be studied.

The NMR imaging technique permits cross-sectional imaging of the spatial distribution of magnetic nuclei, particularly hydrogen or protons. The images are thus basically distribution density maps of the mobile protons contained in body water and liquids. NMR imaging is noninvasive and uses no ionizing radiation. It also penetrates bone and air without difficulties or artifacts. No definite biological hazards have been identified to date. Finally, the technique allows the electronic selection of an imaging plane of any desired thickness at any arbitrary location and orientation, whether transverse, sagittal, coronal, or oblique.

The formation of an image usually involves an interaction between the object to be imaged and a radiation field, the latter having a wavelength comparable to or less than the smallest feature that must be distinguished. The spatial detail, and hence the resolution, of an image generally cannot be better than the wavelength of the radiation that is used to generate the image. The wavelengths of the radiofrequency radiation described are of the order 10–100 m, precluding any collimation of the radiation into a narrow beam. The radiation thus has intrinsically limited spatial resolution, which is completely inadequate for medical imaging. NMR circumvents this apparently overwhelming limitation by taking advantage of locally induced interactions; that is, the interactions are restricted to spatially discrete regions. Lauterbur has pointed out that in the presence of a second field that restricts the interaction of the object with the first field, the resolution becomes independent of wavelength.

To construct a tomographic image based on an NMR parameter, it is necessary to measure the value of that parameter for individual small regions (volume elements or voxels) within the tissue cross-section. This requires the capability to identify and distinguish each such small individual subvolume or voxel within the larger volume. The usual method for achieving this is based on the use of magnetic field gradients superimposed on the main external field H_0. A magnetic field gradient represents a linear variation ΔH in the strength or size of the magnetic field along a particular direction or axis. In addition, this magnetic field gradient may be varied in time as well, either by changing the direction of the gradient or by modulating the gradient along a particular direction. By selectively applying fields that vary in magnitude in a defined way with distance and time, a known map of the magnetic field is established in the sample (the term sample is often used in NMR, as in physics and chemistry, to denote the volume being studied). As the magnetic field H_0 varies, there is a corresponding variation in the resonant frequency ω_0. The intensity of the magnetic field as a function of time is thus determined for each voxel within the sample. Therefore, the gradient fields permit signal information, for example, ρ, T_1, T_2, to be localized to individual voxels in the sample; that is, the magnetic field gradients provide the spatial localization or discrimination required for construction of an NMR image.

If there were no magnetic field gradients, the entire sample or region undergoing exposure would experience the same magnetic field H_0. The resonant or Larmor frequency ω_0 would be the same throughout the entire sample. Therefore, the signal detected would represent a combination or summation of signals from all the individual voxels in the entire volume; spatial discrimination would not be present.

Several different approaches to the use of magnetic field gradients have been developed. The different approaches represent variations in the method of gradient production (the number of magnetic coils used), the sequence in which the different gradients are applied, and whether or not the changing gradient is pulsed or steady.

In the first practical NMR images achieved by Lauterbur (1973), a magnetic field gradient was applied along different directions. A projection was obtained for each different field direction, analogous to the projection obtained in transmission CT. An image was synthesized by using a computer to combine the different projections. This is a projection-reconstruction method for NMR imaging. There is, however, a significant difference between this technique and transmission CT. The narrowly collimated pencil beam of CT irradiates a thin section for imaging, whereas in this NMR imaging technique the entire object within the NMR probe coil is irradiated. Thus, the method described does not provide a thin image section. It is a projection image (like a conventional or computed radiograph) onto a plane perpendicular to the axis about which the field gradients are applied.

One approach for obtaining thin image sections involves the application of a time-varying or alternating magnetic field gradient, rather than a static gradient (Hinshaw, 1976). This approach is somewhat more complicated to conceptualize. Basically, the NMR signal is modulated with the alternating field gradient, typically 100 Hz, except in one cross-section whose position and thickness may be varied. The modulated signals are then filtered out so that the remaining NMR signals are only from the defined section. Again a computer is used for processing the data.

Just as the application of a single alternating field gradient permits selection of a defined plane (actually a thin section), the use of two mutually perpendicular alternating field gradients allows selection of a defined or sensitive line (actually a strip). By extension of this principle, the application of three mutually perpendicular alternating field gradients defines a sensitive point (actually a small volume element). After filtration of the modulated signals, the remaining NMR signal represents information from the sensitive point. By changing the intersection of the three alternating field gradients, the sensitive point may be moved throughout an imaging plane, thereby scanning the plane. This is the single-sensitive-point method (Hinshaw, 1976), also referred to as spin mapping. Its advantages are that it is simple, direct, and does not require a computer for reconstruction.

Its disadvantage is that as a point-by-point sequential method it is slow.

By replacing one of the three alternating gradients in the single-sensitive-point method with a static gradient, the NMR signal obtained after filtering is a one-dimensional projection along a sensitive line. After measuring the free induction decay, described earlier, following a radiofrequency pulse, Fourier transformation is performed on this signal to transform it from a time-varying signal to a frequency-dependent signal. This sensitive line is scanned throughout the entire imaging plane to obtain an NMR image of the plane. The advantage of this multiple-sensitive-point method is a significant decrease in scanning time compared to the single-sensitive-point method.

In addition to the methods described, other approaches to NMR imaging that utilize field gradients have been devised. In general, these may be classified in terms of the region defined by individual data collections. These methods may then be classified as: 1) point-by-point methods, 2) line methods, 3) plane methods, and 4) volume methods. These classes involve successively faster data acquisition rates, but with a concomitant increase in the complexity of data processing.

Other methods for tomographic imaging with NMR have been devised which do not require the use of field gradients. In the technique of focused nuclear resonance (FONAR) developed by Damadian et al. (1976), the object is placed in a static inhomogeneous magnetic field. This field is designed so that only a small region or volume element of the object, located in a saddle-shaped region of the field, is at the resonance frequency. This volume element is moved throughout an image plane, and the NMR signal is recorded sequentially. Like the single-sensitive-point method, this technique is simple and direct, but slow.

An essential feature of any NMR imaging technique is to have a homogeneous, high intensity magnetic field. Two types of magnets have been used for NMR imaging. Resistive magnets, which have to be cooled by air or water, are capable of producing magnetic field intensities sufficient for proton NMR imaging. These are relatively lower strength, of the order of .1 T (1,000 gauss). Superconducting magnets employ unusual materials that have nearly zero electrical resistance (compared to the more conventional metallic conductors like copper) and can conduct very large currents. However, these materials operate only at extremely low temperatures (just above absolute zero), and this necessitates cryogenic cooling. Superconducting magnets are capable of generating significantly larger magnetic field intensities, of the order of 1–3 T (10,000–30,000 gauss), than resistive magnets. Superconducting magnets not only permit proton NMR imaging but can be used for detecting chemical shifts in the study of individual molecular species.

Biological Effects NMR imaging employs three different electromagnetic fields: 1) a static magnetic field H_0 of moderate strength, which is used to align the magnetic moments of the protons or other nuclei; 2) smaller and rapidly varying magnetic fields or pulsed field gradients ΔH, which are used for spatial localization; 3) radiofrequency pulses, whose magnetic component H_1 is responsible for the precession of the magnetization, or equivalently the change in energy states of the magnetic moments.

There are several potential side effects or biological hazards associated with NMR imaging. The rapidly changing magnetic fields (ΔH and H_1) are capable of inducing electrical currents in tissue. The organ systems most likely to be affected are probably the heart and the nervous system, both of which might be susceptible to small electrical currents. A potential hazard, therefore, might be a cardiac arrhythmia in a patient with heart disease. To date it would seem that the electrical currents involved are too small to produce such a noticeable side effect in these organs.

A second potential hazard is that the currents induced in tissues by the changing magnetic fields may result in the significant production of heat in the tissues. This might become a significant problem in tissues where there is relatively low blood flow to remove excess heat. Metallic implants, such as surgical clips and prostheses, might constitute a closed conducting loop through which electrical currents could flow, with resulting resistive losses causing heating of the implant. This problem has been studied by Davis et al. (1981), who were not able to detect significant heating in implanted surgical clips during NMR exposure.

Another hazard is the potential effect of a large, static magnetic effect on tissues.

Finally, the potential might exist for DNA or chromosomal damage from either the static magnetic field H_0, the pulsed field gradient ΔH, or the radiofrequency field H_1. This potential effect has been investigated in the laboratory by Wolff et al. (1980), who were unable to detect genetic damage in the conditions used for NMR imaging.

Further investigation of potential biological hazards from NMR imaging is necessary.

Microwave Computed Tomography

Microwaves lie between radiowaves and infrared radiation in the electromagnetic spectrum, with wavelengths of the order of centimeters. Correspondingly, the frequency range lies between the lower frequency radiowaves and the higher frequency infrared.

Bragg et al. (1977) investigated the use of microwaves in monitoring and diagnosing pulmonary edema. Using microwave frequencies from 300–950 MHz, they were able to demonstrate excellent correlation between changes in microwave reflection and pulmonary physiological indicators of developing pulmonary edema. Reflected energy was measured (as in ultrasound) rather than transmitted energy. Microwaves are capable of penetrating both soft tissue and air, in contrast to ultrasound, which does not penetrate air. The experiment did not result in the production of images.

A CT imaging technique based on measurements of microwave transmissions through biological tissues has been proposed by Rao, Santosh, and Gregg (1980). Tissue phantoms were suspended in a tank of fluid, which was coupled to a microwave source and an opposing microwave detector. The phantoms underwent translational and rotational motions within the tank while being exposed to microwave energy at a frequency of 10.5 GHz (1 GHz = 10^9 Hz).

An appropriate computational algorithm was used based on the assumptions that microwaves travel in straight lines, like x-rays, and that their attenuation follows a simple exponential law, also like x-rays. The complicated reflection and diffraction patterns seen in microwave propagation in a heterogeneous medium (unlike x-rays) were neglected. Images were obtained with an estimated spatial resolution of 2 cm.

Work is continuing in this technique, and its long-term future remains to be determined.

REFERENCES AND SUGGESTED READINGS

Computed Radiography

Amtey, S. R., Morgan, C., Cohen, G., et al. Applications of digital processing in computed radiography. *In* Recent and Future Developments in Medical Imaging II. Proc. SPIE 206:190–192, 1979.

Brody, W. R., Macovski, A., Lehmann, L., et al. Intravenous angiography using scanned projection radiography: Preliminary investigation of a new method. Investigative Radiology 15:220–223, 1980.

Brody, W. R., Cassell, D. M., Sommer, F. G., Lehmann, L. A., Macovski, A., Alvarez, R. E., Pelc, N. J., Riederer, S. J., and Hall, A. L. Dual-energy projection radiography: Initial clinical experience. American Journal of Roentgenology 137:201–205, 1981.

Brody, W. R., and Macovski, A. Dual-energy digital radiography. Diagnostic Imaging, pp. 19–25, October, 1981.

Cohen, G., Wagner, L. K., Amtey, S. R., et al. Contrast-detail-dose evaluation of computed radiography: Comparison with computed tomography (CT) and conventional radiography. In Applications of Optical Instrumentation in Medicine VII. Proc. SPIE 173:41–47, 1979.

Foley, W. D., and DiBianca, F. A. Computed radiography. In T. H. Newton and D. G. Potts (eds.), Radiology of the Skull and Brain: Technical Aspects of Computed Tomography, Vol. 5, Chap. 128, Part XVIII, pp. 4312–4325. C. V. Mosby, St. Louis, 1981.

Foley, W. D., Lawson, T. L., Scanlon, G. T., Heeschen, R. C., and DiBianca, F. Digital radiography of the chest using a computed tomography instrument. Radiology 133:231–234, 1979.

Katragadda, C. S., Fogel, S. R., Cohen, G., Wagner, L. K., Morgan, C., Handel, S. F., Amtey, S. R., and Lester, R. G. Digital radiography using a computed tomographic instrument. Radiology 133:83–87, 1979.

Kruger, R. A., Anderson, R. E., Koehler, P. R., Nelson, J. A., Sorenson, J. A., and Morgan, T. A method for noninvasive evaluation of cardiovascular dynamics using a digital radiographic device. Radiology 139:301–305, 1981.

Lawson, T. L., Foley, W. D., Imray, T. J., Stewart, E. T., Wilson, C. R., and Youker, J. E. Abdominal computed radiography: Evaluation of low-contrast lesions. Investigative Radiology 15:215–219, 1980.

Sommer, F. G., and Brody, W. R. Contrast resolution of line-scanned digital radiography. Journal of Computer Assisted Tomography 6:373–377, 1982.

Sommer, F. G., Brody, W. R., Gross, D., and Macovski, A. Renal imaging with dual energy projection radiography. American Journal of Roentgenology 138:317–322, 1982.

Zonneveld, F. W. The scanogram: Technique and applications. Medicamundi 25:25–28, 1980.

Reformatted Images in Nontransverse Planes

Baker, H. L. The clinical usefulness of routine coronal and sagittal reconstructions in cranial computed tomography. The President's Address. Radiology 140:1–9, 1981.

Bergstrom, M. and Sundman, R. Picture processing in computed tomography. American Journal of Roentgenology 127:17–21, 1976.

Berland, L. Dissecting aortic aneurysm. General Electric CT/T Clinical Symposium, Vol. 4, No. 3, 1981.

Boroff, R. D., and Pribram, H. F. W. Coronal reconstruction in computerised tomography. Surgical Neurology 9:85–93, 1978.

Brant-Zawadzki, M. N., Minagi, H., Federle, M. P., and Rowe, L. D. High resolution CT with image reformation in maxillofacial pathology. American Journal of Roentgenology 138:477–483, 1982.

Brant-Zawadzki, M., Jeffrey, R. B., Minagi, H., and Pitts, L. H. High resolution CT of thoracolumbar fractures. American Journal of Roentgenology 138:699–704, 1982.

Federle, M. P., Moss, A. A., Boyd, D. P., and Royal, S. A. Coronal and sagittal reconstructions using a 4.8 second CT body scanner: Developments and applications. American Journal of Roentgenology 133:625–632, 1979.

Foley, W. D., Lawson, T. L., and Quiroz, F. Sagittal and coronal image reconstruction: Application in pancreatic computed tomography. Journal of Computer Assisted Tomography 3:717–721, 1979.

Gale, M. E., and Pugatch, R. D. Sagittal and coronal CT reconstruction for demonstration of subcarinal adenopathy. Journal of Computer Assisted Tomography 6:249–253, 1982.

Glenn, W. V., Johnston, R. J., Morton, P. E., and Dwyer, S. J. Image-generation and display techniques for CT scan data. Thin transverse and reconstructed coronal and sagittal planes. Investigative Radiology 10:403–416, 1975.

Glenn, W. V., Johnston, R. J., Morton, P. E., and Dwyer, S. J. Further investigation and initial clinical use of advanced CT display capability. Investigative Radiology 10:479–489, 1975.

Glenn, W. V., Rhodes, M. L., Altschuler, E. M., Wiltse, L. L., Kostanek, C., and Kuo, Y. M. Multiplanar display computerized body tomography applications in the lumbar spine. Spine 4:282–352, 1979.

Glenn, W. V., Harlow, C. A., Dwyer, S. J., Rhodes, M. L., and Parker, D. L. Image manipulation and pattern recognition. In T. H. Newton and D. G. Potts (eds.), Radiology of the Skull and Brain: Technical Aspects of Computed Tomography, Vol. 5, Chap. 129, Part XVII, pp. 4326–4354. C. V. Mosby, St. Louis, 1981.

Goldberg, H. I., Moss, A., Tilles, R., Federle, M. P., and Jeffrey, R. B. Caudate lobe liver mass—Value of sagittal and coronal reconstruction. General Electric CT/T Clinical Symposium, Vol. 3, No. 5, 1980.

Harris, L. D., Robb, R. A., Yuen, T. S., and Ritman, E. L. Display and visualization of three-dimensional reconstructed anatomic morphology: Experience with the thorax, heart, and coronary vasculature of dogs. Journal of Computer Assisted Tomography 3:439–446, 1979.

Hirschy, J. C., Leue, W. M., Berninger, W. H., Hamilton, R. H., and Abbott, G. F. CT of the lumbosacral spine: Importance of tomographic planes parallel to vertebral end plate. American Journal of Roentgenology 126:47–52, 1981.

Jelden, G., Sufka, B., Arnold, J., Rodriguez-Antunez, A., Doering, E., Lavik, P., and Turnbull, R. New dimensions in computed tomography. Radiology 123:213–215, 1977.

Lancourt, J. E., Glenn, W. V., and Wiltse, L. L. Multiplanar computerized tomography in the normal spine and in the diagnosis of spinal stenosis. A gross anatomic-computerized tomographic correlation. Spine 4:379–390, 1979.

Leonardi, M., Barbina, V., Fabris, G., and Penco, T. Sagittal computed tomography of the orbit. Journal of Computer Assisted Tomography 1:511–512, 1977.

Maravilla, K. R. Computer reconstructed sagittal and coronal computed tomography head scans: Clinical applications. Journal of Computer Assisted Tomography 2:189–198, 1978.

Naidich, T. P., Yu, R. H., King, D. G., and Wholahan, J. D. Superimposition reformatted CT for preoperative lesion localization and surgical planning. Journal of Computer Assisted Tomography 4: 693–696, 1980.

Peters, T. M. Enhanced display of three-dimensional data from computerized x-ray tomograms. Computers in Biology and Medicine 5:49–52, 1975.

Pevsner, P. H., Kreel, L., King, D. C., and Wilson, P. Multiple axis image reconstruction from axial transverse data. Journal of Computer Assisted Tomography 3:279–281, 1979.

Rhodes, M. L., Glenn, W. V., and Azzawi, Y. M. Extracting oblique planes from serial CT sections. Journal of Computer Assisted Tomography 4:649–657, 1980.

Schulz, R. A., Joseph, P. M., and Hilal, S. K. Frontal and lateral views of the brain reconstructed from EMI axial slices. Radiology 125:701–710, 1977.

Smith, W. P., and Levine, E. Sagittal and coronal CT image reconstruction: Application in assessing the inferior vena cava in renal cancer. Journal of Computer Assisted Tomography 4:531–535, 1980.

Dynamic Computed Tomography

Axel, L. Imaging technology. Diagnostic Imaging, 4–7, August 1980.

Axel, L. Cerebral blood flow determination by rapid-sequence computed tomography. A theoretical analysis. Radiology 137:679–686, 1980.

Berland, L. Dissecting aortic aneurysm. General Electric CT/T Clinical Symposium, Vol. 4, No. 3, 1981.

Berninger, W. H., and Redington, R. W. Dynamic computed tomography. In T. H. Newton and D. G. Potts (eds.), Radiography of the Skull and Brain: Technical Aspects of Computed Tomography, Vol. 5, Chap. 125, Part XVIII, pp. 4261–4285. C. V. Mosby, St. Louis, 1981.

Berninger, W. H., Axel, L., Norman, D., Napel, S., and Redington, R. W. Functional imaging of the brain using computed tomography. Radiology 138:711–716, 1981.

Cipriano, P. R., Nassi, M., Ricci, M. T., Reitz, B. A. and Brody, W. R. Acute myocardial ischemia detected in vivo by computed tomography. Radiology 140:727–731, 1981.

Cohen, W. A., Pinto, R. S., and Kricheff, I. I. Dynamic CT scanning for visualization of the parasellar carotid arteries. American Journal of Roentgenology 138: 905–909, 1982.

Coin, C. G., and Chan, Y. S. Computed tomography arteriography. Journal of Computer Assisted Tomography 1:165–168, 1977.

Dobben, G. D., Valvassori, G. E., Mafee, M. F., and Berninger, W. H. Evaluation of brain circulation by rapid rotational computed tomography. Radiology 133: 105–111, 1979.

Drayer, B. P., Heinz, E. R., Dujovny, M., Wolfson, S. K., and Gur, D. Patterns of brain perfusion: Dynamic computed tomography using intravenous contrast enhancement. Journal of Computer Assisted Tomography 3:633–640, 1979.

Dunn, V., Wing, S. D., Miller, F. J., et al. Hemodynamic studies using a CT scanner. Journal of Computer Assisted Tomography 3:173–177, 1979.

Fike, J. R., Cann, C. E., and Berninger, W. H. Quantitative evaluation of the canine brain using computed tomography. Journal of Computer Assisted Tomography 6:325–333, 1982.

Glazer, G. M., Axel, L., Goldberg, H. I., and Moss, A. A. Dynamic CT of the normal spleen. American Journal of Roentgenology 137:343–346, 1981.

Godwin, J. D., Herfkins, R. L., Skiöldebrand, C. G., Federle, M. P., and Lipton, M. J. Evaluation of dissections and aneurysms of the thoracic aorta by conventional and dynamic CT scanning. Radiology 135:125–133, 1980.

Godwin, J. D., and Webb, R. W. Dynamic computed tomography in the evaluation of vascular lung lesions. Radiology 138:629–635, 1981.

Godwin, J. D., Turley, K., Herfkins, R. J., and Lipton, M. J. Computed tomography for follow-up of chronic aortic dissections. Radiology 139:655–660, 1981.

Gur, D., Drayer, B. P., Borovetz, H. S., Griffith, B. P., Hardesty, R. L., and Wolfson, S. K. Dynamic Computed tomography of the lung: Regional ventilation measurements. Journal of Computer Assisted Tomography 3:749–753, 1979.

Hacker, H., and Becker, H. Time controlled computed tomographic angiography. Journal of Computer Assisted Tomography (Computed Tomography) 1:405–409, 1977.

Hayman, L. A., Evans, R. A., and Hinck, V. C. Rapid high dose (RHD) contrast cranial computed tomography: A concise review of normal anatomy. Journal of Computer Assisted Tomography 3:147–154, 1979.

Heinz, E. R., Dubois, P., Osborne, D., Drayer, B., and Barrett, W. Dynamic computed tomography study of the brain. Journal of Computer Assisted Tomography 3:641–649, 1979.

Heinz, E. R., Dubois, P. J., Drayer, B. P., et al. A preliminary investigation of the role of dynamic computed tomography in renovascular hypertension. Journal of Computer Assisted Tomography 4:63–66, 1980.

Hirschy, J. C. Thoracic CT angiography: Dynamic sequential scanning of the chest. General Electric CT/T Clinical Symposium, Vol. 4, No. 6, 1981.

Ishikawa, I., Onouchi, Z., Saito, Y., Kitada, H., Shinoda, A., Ushitani, K., Tabuchi, M., and Suzuki, M. Renal cortex visualization and analysis of dynamic CT curves of the kidney. Journal of Computer Assisted Tomography 5:695–701, 1981.

Koehler, P. R., and Anderson, R. E. Computed angiotomography. Radiology 137:843–845, 1980.

Ladurner, G., Zilkha, E., Sager, W. D., Iliff, L., Du Boulay, G., Lechner, H., and Marshall, J. Dynamic investigations using computer tomography. In P. Gerhardt and E. van Kaick (eds.), Total Body Computerized Tomography. International Symposium, Heidelberg, 1977, pp. 370–374. Georg Thieme, Stuttgart, 1979.

Marchal, G., Baert, A. L., and Wilms, G. Intravenous pancreaticography in computed tomography. Journal of Computer Assisted Tomography 3:727–732, 1979.

Mori, K. W. Dynamic scanning in the evaluation of superior vena cava syndrome. General Electric CT/T Clinical Symposium, Vol. 4, No. 2, 1981.

Moss, A. A., Dean, P. B., Axel, L., Goldberg, H. I., Glazer, G. M., and Friedman, M. A. Dynamic CT of hepatic masses with intravenous and intraarterial contrast material. American Journal of Roentgenology 138:847–852, 1982.

Norman, D., Axel, L., Berninger, W. H., Edwards, M. S., Cann, C. E., Redington, R. W., and Cox, L. Dynamic computed tomography of the brain: Techniques, data analysis, and applications. American Journal of Neuroradiology 2:1–12, 1981.

Reese, D. F., McCullough, E. C., and Baker, H. L., Jr. Dynamic sequential scanning with table incrementation. Radiology 140:719–722, 1981.

Traupe, H., Heiss, W. D., Hoeffken, W., and Zulch, K. J. Hyperperfusion and enhancement in dynamic computed tomography of ischemic stroke patients. Journal of Computer Assisted Tomography 3:627–632, 1979.

Turner, R. J., Young, S. W., and Castellino, R. A. Dynamic continuous computed tomography: Study of retroaortic left renal vein. Journal of Computer Assisted Tomography 4:109–111, 1980.

Wing, S. D., Anderson, R. E., and Osborn, A. G. Dynamic cranial computed tomography: Preliminary results. American Journal of Roentgenology 134:941–945, 1980.

Young, S. W., Noon, M. A., Nassi, M., and Castellino, R. A. Dynamic computed tomography body scanning. Journal of Computer Assisted Tomography 4:168–173, 1980.

Applications of Computed Tomography in Radiation Therapy

Battista, J. J., Rider, W. D., and Van Dyk, J. Computed tomography for radiation therapy. International Journal of Radiation Oncology, Biology, and Physics 6:99–107, 1980.

Birkhead, B. M., Banks, T. E., and Short, D. B. Use of CT scans in manual radiotherapy treatment planning. Radiology 130;539–540, 1979.

Brizel, H. E., Livingston, P. A., and Grayson, E. V. Radiotherapeutic applications of pelvic computed tomography. Journal of Computer Assisted Tomography 3:453–466, 1979.

Chernak, E. S., Rodriguez-Antunez, A., Jelden, G. L., Dhaliwal, R. S., and Lavik, P. S. The use of computed tomography for radiation therapy treatment planning. Radiology 117:613–614, 1975.

Coffey, C. W. CT-assisted treatment planning systems in radiotherapy, Part 1. Comparison of conventional and CT-assisted systems. Applied Radiology 101:55–64, 1981.

Geise, R. A., and McCullough, E. C. The use of CT scanners in megavoltage photon-beam therapy planning. Radiology 124:133–141, 1977.

Goitein, M., Wittenberg, J., Mendiondo, M., Doucette, J., Friedberg, C., Ferrucci, J., Gunderson, L., Linggood, R., Shipley, W. U., and Fineberg, H. V. The value of CT scanning in radiation therapy treatment planning: A prospective study. International Journal of Radiology Oncology, Biology, and Physics 5:1787–1798, 1979.

Herskovic, A., Lee, S., and Padikal, T. Utilization of the computed tomography scanner in interstitial dosimetry. Radiology 135:781–782, 1980.

Hobday, P., Hodson, N. J., Husband, J., Parker, R. P., and Macdonald, J. S. Computed tomography applied to radiotherapy treatment planning: Techniques and results. Radiology 133:477–482, 1979.

Ibbott, G. S. Radiation therapy treatment planning and the distortion of CT images. Medical Physics 7:261, 1980.

Jelden, G. L., Chernak, E. S., Rodriguez-Antunez, A., Haaga, J. R., Lavik, P. S., and Dhaliwal, R. S. Further progress in CT scanning and computerized radiation therapy treatment planning. American Journal of Roentgenology 127:179–185, 1976.

Kijewski, P. K., and Bjarngard, B. E. The use of computed tomography data for radiotherapy dose calculations. International Journal of Radiation Oncology, Biology, and Physics 4:429–435, 1978.

Kubota, K., Itoh, M., Yamada, K., Endo, S., and Matsuzawa, T. Some devices for computed tomography radiotherapy treatment planning. Journal of Computer Assisted Tomography 4:697–699, 1980.

Lammerts, J. H. Therapy planning from CT data, Medicamundi 26:93–97, 1981.

Lee, K. R., Mansfield, C. M., Dwyer, S. J., Cox, H. L., Levine, E., and Templeton, A. W. CT for intracavity radiotherapy planning. American Journal of Roentgenology 135:809–813, 1980.

McCullough, E. C. Potentials of computed tomography in radiation therapy treatment planning. Radiology 129:765–768, 1978.

McCullough, E. C. Computed tomography in radiation therapy treatment planning. In T. H. Newton and D. G. Potts (eds.), Radiology of the Skull and Brain: Technical Aspects of Computed Tomography, Vol. 5, Chap. 127, Part XVIII, pp. 4301–4311. C. V. Mosby, St. Louis, 1981.

Morgan, C. L., Calkins, R. F., and Cavalcanti, E. J. Computed tomography in the evaluation, staging, and therapy of carcinoma of the bladder and prostate. Radiology 140:751–761, 1981.

Pilepich, M. V., Perez, C. A., and Prasad, S. Computed tomography in definitive radiotherapy of prostatic carcinoma. International Journal of Radiation Oncology, Biology, and Physics 6:923–926, 1980.

Prasad, S. C., Glasgow, G. P., and Purdy, J. A. Dosimetric evaluation of a computed tomography treatment system. Radiology 130:777–781, 1979.

Prasad, S. C., Pilepich, M. V., and Perez, C. A. Contribution of CT to quantitative radiation therapy planning. American Journal of Roentgenology 136:123–128, 1981.

Ragan, D. P., and Perez, C. A. Efficacy of CT-assisted two-dimensional treatment planning: Analysis of 45 patients. American Journal of Roentgenology 131:75–79, 1978.

Smith, V., Parker, D. L., Stanley, J. H., Phillips, T. L., Boyd, D. P., and Kan, P. T. Development of a computed tomographic scanner for radiation therapy treatment planning. Radiology 136:489–493, 1980.

Sontag, M. R., Battista, J. J., Bronskill, M. J., and Cunningham, J. R. Implications of computed tomography for inhomogeneity corrections in photon beam dose calculations. Radiology 124:143–149, 1977.

Sternick, E. S., Lane, F. W., and Curran, B. Comparison of computed tomography and conventional transverse axial tomography in radiotherapy treatment planning. Radiology 124:835–836, 1977.

Tatcher, M., and Palti, S. Evaluation of density correction algorithms for photobeam dose calculations. Radiology 141:201–205, 1981.

Van Dyk, J., Battista, J. J., Cunningham, J. R., Rider, W. D., and Sontag, M. R. On the impact of CT scanning on radiotherapy planning. Computerized Tomography 4:55–64, 1979.

Van Dyk, J., Battista, J. J., and Rider, W. D. Half body radiotherapy: The use of computed tomography to determine the dose to lung. International Journal of Radiation Oncology, Biology, and Physics 6:463–470, 1980.

Van Houtte, P., Piron, A., Lustman-Marechal, J., Osteaux, M., and Henry, J. Computed axial tomography (CAT) contribution for dosimetry and treatment evaluation in lung cancer. International Journal of Radiation Oncology, Biology, and Physics 6:995–1000, 1980.

High Resolution Computed Tomography

Blumenfeld, S. M., and Glover, G. Spatial resolution in computed tomography. In T. H. Newton and D. G. Potts (eds.), Radiology of the Skull and Brain: Technical Aspects of Computed Tomography, Vol. 5, Chap. 112, Part XVI, pp. 3918–3940. C. V. Mosby, St. Louis, 1981.

Brant-Zawadzki, M. N., Minagi, H., Federle, M. P., and Rowe, L. D. High resolution CT with image reformation in maxillofacial pathology. American Journal of Roentgenology 138:477–483, 1982.

Brant-Zawadzki, M., Jeffrey, R. B., Minagi, H., and Pitts, L. H. High resolution CT of thoracolumbar fractures. American Journal of Roentgenology 138:699–704, 1982.

Dihlmann, W., Graeper, J. P., Buchmann, F., and Zimmer, H. Practical application of the CT target scan. Medicamundi 25:89–94, 1981.

Littleton, J. T., Shaffer, K. A., Callahan, W. P., and Durizch, M. L. Temporal bone: Comparison of pluridirectional tomography and high resolution computed tomography. American Journal of Roentgenology 137:835–845, 1981.

Nathanson, A. M. Destructive lesions of the base of the skull. General Electric CT/T Clinical Symposium, Vol. 4, No. 13, 1981.

Rusztyn, A., Chuang, S., Fitz, C. R., and Harwood-Nash, D. General Electric CT/T Clinical Symposium, Vol. 3, No. 13, 1980.

Shaffer, K. Cholesteatoma. General Electric CT/T Clinical Symposium, Vol. 3, No. 6, 1980.

Shaffer, K. A., Haughton, V. M., and Wilson, C. R. High resolution computed tomography of the temporal bone. Radiology 134:409–414, 1980.

Shaffer, K. A., Volz, D. J., and Haughton, V. M. Manipulation of CT data for temporal-bone imaging. Radiology 137:825–829, 1980.

Vaisman, V. Herniated disk in the lumbar spine. General Electric CT/T Clinical Symposium, Vol. 4, No. 7, 1981.

Weinstein, M. A., Modic, M. T., Risius, B., Duchesneau, P. M., and Berlin, A. J. Visualization of the arteries, veins, and nerves of the orbit by sector computed tomography. Radiology 138:83–87, 1981.

Gated Scanning

Alfidi, R. J., Haaga, J. R., MacIntyre, W. J., Bacon, K. T., and Ferrario, C. M. Gated computed tomography of the heart. Computed Axial Tomography 1:51–57, 1977.

Berninger, W. H., Redington, R. W., Doherty, P., Lipton, M. J., and Carlsson, E. Gated cardiac scanning: Canine studies. Journal of Computer Assisted Tomography 3:155–163, 1979.

General Electric Company. CT/T continuum. Research in clinical application. General Electric Publication No. 5058, 1979.

Harell, G. S., Guthaner, D. F., Breiman, R. S., Morehouse, C. C., Seppi, E. J., Marshall, W. H., and Wexler, L. Stop-action cardiac computed tomography. Radiology 123:515–517, 1977.

Higgins, C. B. Computed tomography of the heart. Radiology 140:525–526, 1981.

Lackner, K., and Thurn, P. Computed tomography of the heart: ECG-gated and continuous scans. Radiology 140:413–420, 1981.

Morehouse, C. C., Brody, W. R., Guthaner, D. F., Breiman, R. S., and Harell, G. S. Gated cardiac computed tomography with a motion phantom. Radiology 134:213–217, 1980.

Sagel, S. S., Weiss, E. S., Gillard, R. G., Hounsfield, G. N., Jost, G. T., Stanley, R. J., and Ter-Pogossian, M. M. Gated computed tomography of the human heart. Investigative Radiology 12:563–566, 1977.

Dual Energy Scanning

Akutagawa, W. M., Huth, G. G., Levis, R. E., Drianis, G. C., and Davis, R. L. Increased tissue differentiation using color display of multiple-energy CT scans. Radiology 134:739–756, 1980.

Alvarez, R. E., and Macovski, A. Energy-selective reconstructions in x-ray computerized tomography. Physics in Medicine and Biology 21:733–744, 1976.

Brooks, R. A. A quantitative theory of the Hounsfield unit and its application to dual energy scanning. Journal of Computer Assisted Tomography 1:487–493, 1977.

Brooks, R. A., and Di Chiro, G. Split-detector computed tomography: A preliminary report. Radiology 126:255–257, 1978.

Cho, Z. H., Tsai, C. M., and Wilson, G. Study of contrast and modulation mechanisms in x-ray/photon transverse axial transmission tomography. Physics in Medicine and Biology 20:879–889, 1975.

Di Chiro, G., Brooks, R. A., Kessler, R. M., Johnston, G. S., Jones, A. E., Herdt, J. R., and Sheridan, W. T. Tissue signatures with dual-energy computed tomography. Radiology 131:521–523, 1979.

Dubal, L., and Wiggli, U. Tomochemistry of the brain. Journal of Computer Assisted Tomography 1:300–307, 1977.

Fenster, A. Split xenon detector for tomochemistry in computed tomography. Journal of Computer Assisted Tomography 2:243–252, 1978.

Genant, H. K., and Boyd, D. Quantitative bone mineral analysis using dual energy computed tomography. Investigative Radiology 12:545–551, 1977.

Hounsfield, G. N. Computerized transverse axial scanning (tomography): Part I, Description of system. British Journal of Radiology 46:1016–1022, 1973.

Isherwood, I., Pullan, B. R., Rutherford, R. A., and Strang, F. A. Electron density and atomic number determination by computed tomography. British Journal of Radiology 50:613–619, 1977.

Kan, W. C., Wiley, A. L., Wirtanen, G. W., Lange, T. A., Moran, P. R., Paliwal, B. R., and Cashwell, R. J. High Z elements in human sarcomata: Assessment by multienergy CT and neutron activation analysis. American Journal of Roentgenology 135:123–129, 1980.

Larsson, S., Bergström, M., Dahlqvist, I., Israelsson, A., and Lagergren, C. A method for determining bone mineral content using Fourier image reconstruction and dual source technique. Journal of Computer Assisted Tomography 2:347–351, 1978.

Latchaw, R. E., Payne, T. J., and Gold, L. H. A. Effective atomic number and electron density as measured with a computed tomography scanner: Computation and correlation with brain tumor histology. Journal of Computer Assisted Tomography 2:199–208, 1978.

Latchaw, R. E., Payne, J. T., and Loewenson, R. B. Predicting brain tumor histology: Change of effective atomic number with contrast enhancement. American Journal of Roentgenology 135:757–762, 1980.

Marshall, W. H., Easter, W., and Zatz, L. M. Analysis of the dense lesion at computed tomography with dual kVp scans. Radiology 124:87–89, 1977.

Marshall, W. H., Alvarez, R. E., and Macovski, A. Initial results with prereconstruction dual-energy computed tomography (PREDECT). Radiology 140:421–430, 1981.

McDavid W. D., Waggener, R. G., Dennis, M. J., Sank, V. J., and Payne, W. H. Estimation of chemical composition and density from computed tomography carried out at a number of energies. Investigative Radiology 12:189–194, 1977.

Riederer, S. J., and Mistretta, C. A. Selective iodine imaging using K-edge energies in computerized x-ray tomography. Medical Physics 4:474–481, 1977.

Ritchings, R. T., and Pullan, B. R. A technique for simultaneous dual energy scanning. Journal of Computer Assisted Tomography 3:842–846, 1979.

Rutherford R. A., Pullan, B. R., Isherwood, I., and Young, I. M. Measurement of effective atomic number and electron density using an EMI scanner. Neuroradiology 11:15–21, 1976.

Rutt, B., and Fenster, A. Split-filter computed tomography: A simple technique for dual energy scanning. Journal of Computer Assisted Tomography 4:501–509, 1980.

Zatz, L. M. The effect of the kVp level of EMI values. Radiology 119:683–688, 1976.

Ultrafast Transmission Scanning

Boyd, D. P. Transmission computed tomography. In T. H. Newton and D. G. Potts (eds.), Radiology of the Skull and Brain: Technical Aspects of Computed Tomography, Vol. 5. Chap. 130, Part XIX, pp. 4357–4371. C. V. Mosby, St. Louis, 1981.

Boyd, D., Cann, C. E., Genant, H. K., Gould, R., Kaufman, L., Parker, D., and Stanley, J. A proposed multi-source CT densitometer, for ultra-accurate mineral determination throughout the human body (abstract). Journal of Computer Assisted Tomography 3:856, 1979.

Drew, P. G. The DSR: Is it worth it? Diagnostic Imaging, pp. 12, 43–44, February 1981.

Hsu, T. Scanning electron beam CT systems. Applied Radiology 10(2):86–88, 1981.

Iinuma, T. A., Tateno, Y., Umegaki, Y., and Watanabe, E. Proposed system for ultrafast computed tomography. Journal of Computer Assisted Tomography 1:494–499, 1977.

Ritman, E. L., Robb, R. A., Johnson, S. A., Chevalier, P. A., Gilbert, B. K., Greenleaf, J. F., Sturm, R. E., and Wood, E. H. Quantitative imaging of the structure and function of the heart, lungs, and circulation. Mayo Clinic Proceedings 53:3–11, 1978.

Ritman, E. L., Kinsey, J. H., Robb, R. A., Harris, L. D., and Gilbert, B. K. Physics and technical considerations in the design of the DSR: A high temporal resolution volume scanner. American Journal of Roentgenology 134:369–374, 1980.

Ritman, E. L., Harris, L. D., Kinsey, J. H., and Robb, R. A. Computed tomographic imaging of the heart: The dynamic spatial reconstructor. Radiologic clinics of North America 18:547–556, 1980.

Robb, R. A., and Ritman, E. L. High speed synchronous volume computed tomography of the heart. Radiology 133:655–661, 1979.

Emission Computed Tomography

Brooks, R. A., and Di Chiro, G. Principles of computer assisted tomography in radiographic and radioisotopic imaging. Physics in Medicine and Biology 21:689–732, 1976.

Brooks, R. A., Sank, V. J., and Di Chiro, G. Design of a high resolution positron emission tomograph. The Neuro-PET. Journal of Computer Assisted Tomography 4:5–13, 1980.

Budinger, T. F. Physical attributes of single photon tomography. Journal of Nuclear Medicine 21:579–592, 1980.

Budinger, T. F., and Gullberg, G. T. Three dimensional reconstruction of isotope distributions. Physics in Medicine and Biology 19:387–389, 1974.

Budinger, T. F., Derenzo, S. E., Gullberg, G. T., Greenberg, W. L., and Huesman, R. H. Emission computer assisted tomography with single-photon and positron annihilation photon emitters. Journal of Computer Assisted Tomography (Computed Tomography) 1:131–145, 1977.

Budinger, T. F., Derenzo, S. E., Greenberg, W. L., et al. Quantitative potentials of dynamic emission computed tomography. Journal of Nuclear Medicine 19:309–315, 1978.

Buonocore, E., and Hubner, K. F. Positron-emission computed tomography of the pancreas: A preliminary study. Radiology 133:195–201, 1979.

Capp, M. P. Radiological Imaging—2000 A.D. New Horizons Lecture. Radiology 138:541–550, 1981.

Chung, V., Chak, K. C., Zacuto, P., and Hart, H. E. Multiple photon coincidence tomography. Seminars in Nuclear Medicine 4:345–354, 1980.

Cormack, A. M. Reconstruction of densities from their projections, with applications in radiological physics. Physics in Medicine and Biology 18:195–207, 1973.

Cowan, R. J., and Watson, N. E. Special characteristics and potential of single photon emission computed tomography in the brain. Seminars in Nuclear Medicine 4:335–344, 1980.

Ericson, K., Bergstrom, M., and Eriksson, L. Positron emission tomography in the evaluation of subdural hematomas. Journal of Computer Assisted Tomography 4:737–745, 1980.

Goodwin, P. N. Recent developments in instrumentation for emission computed tomography. Seminars in Nuclear Medicine 4:322–334, 1980.

Gustafson, D. E., Berggren, M. J., Singh, M., and Dewanjee, M. K. Computed transaxial imaging using single gamma emitters. Radiology 129:187–194, 1978.

Hoffman, E. J., Phelps, M. E., Mullani, N. A., Higgins, C. S., and Ter-Pogossian, M. M. Design and performance characteristics of a whole-body positron transaxial tomograph. Journal of Nuclear Medicine 17:493–502, 1976.

Hoffman, E. J., and Phelps, M. E. An analysis of some of the physical aspects of positron transaxial tomography. Computers in Biology and Medicine 6:345–360, 1978.

Hoffman, E. J., Huang, S. C., and Phelps, M. E. Quantitation in positron emission computed tomography: 1. Effect of object size. Journal of Computer Assisted Tomography 3:299–308, 1979.

Huang, S. C., Hoffman, E. J., and Phelps, M. E. Quantitative positron emission tomography: 2. Effects of inaccurate attenuation correction. Journal of Computer Assisted Tomography 3:804–814, 1979.

Huang, S. C., Hoffman, E. J., Phelps, M. E., and Kuhl, D. E. Quantitation in positron emission computed tomography: 3. Effect of sampling. Journal of Computer Assisted Tomography 4:819–826, 1980.

Isenberg, J. F., and Simon, W. Radionuclide axial tomography by half back-projection. Physics in Medicine and Biology 23:154–158, 1978.

Kay, D. B., Keyes, J. W., and Simon, W. Radionuclide tomographic image reconconstruction using Fourier transform techniques. Journal of Nuclear Medicine 15:981–986, 1974.

Kuhl, D. E., and Edwards, R. Q. Image separation radioisotope scanning. Radiology 80:653–661, 1963.

Kuhl, D. E., and Edwards, R. Q. Cylindrical and section radioisotope scanning of the liver and brain. Radiology 83:926–936, 1964.

Kuhl, D. E., Pitts, F. W., Sanders, T. P., and Mishkin, M. M. Transverse section and rectilinear brain scanning with Tc-99m pertechnetate. Radiology 86:822–829, 1966.

Kuhl, D. E., and Sanders, T. P. Characterizing brain lesions with use of transverse section scanning. Radiology 98:317–328, 1971.

Kuhl, D. E., Edwards, R. Q., Ricci, A. R., et al. The Mark IV system for radionuclide computed tomography of the brain. Radiology 121:405–413, 1976.

Kumar, B., Miller, T. R., Siegel, B. A., Mathias, C. J., Markham, J., Ehrhardt, G. J., and Welch, M. J., Positron tomographic imaging of the liver: 68 Ga iron hydroxide colloid. American Journal of Roentgenology 136:685–690, 1981.

Maeda, T., Matsuda, H., Hisada, K., Tonami, N., Mori, H., Fujii, H., Hayashi, M., and Yamamoto, S. Three-dimensional regional cerebral blood perfusion images with single-photon emission computed tomography. Radiology 140:817–822, 1981.

McIntyre, J. A. Plastic scintillation detectors for high resolution emission computed tomography. Journal of Computer Assisted Tomography 4:351–360, 1980.

Oldendorf, W. H. Future imaging methods. *In* The Quest for an Image of Brain. Computerized Tomography in the Perspective of Past and Future Imaging Methods, pp. 127–145. Raven Press, New York, 1981.

Osborne, D., Jaszczak, R., Coleman, R. E., and Drayer, B. Single photon emission computed tomography in the canine lung. Journal of Computer Assisted Tomography 5:684–689, 1981.

Phelps, M. E. Emission computed tomography. Seminars in Nuclear Medicine 7:337–365, 1977.

Stokely, E. M., Sveinsdottir, E., Lassen, N. A., and Rommer, P. A single photon dynamic computer assisted tomography (DCAT) for imaging brain function in multiple cross sections. Journal of Computer Assisted Tomography 4:230–240, 1980.

Syrota, A., Duquesnoy, N., Paraf, A., and Kellershohn, C. The role of positron emission tomography in the detection of pancreatic disease. Radiology 143:249–253, 1981.

Ter-Pogossian, M. M. Basic principles of computed axial tomography. Seminars in Nuclear Medicine 7:109–127, 1977.

Ter-Pogossian, M. M. Physical aspects of emission computed tomography. *In* T. H. Newton and D. G. Potts (eds.), Radiology of the Skull and Brain: Technical Aspects of Computed Tomography, Vol. 5, Chap. 131, Part XIX, pp. 4372–4388. C. V. Mosby, St. Louis, 1981.

Ter-Pogossian, M. M., Phelps, M. E., Hoffman, E. J., and Mullani, N. A. A positron-emission transaxial tomograph for nuclear imaging (PETT). Radiology 114:89–98, 1975.

Ter-Pogossian, M. M., Mullani, N. A., Hood, J. T., Higgins, C. S., and Ficke, D. C. Design considerations for a positron emission transverse tomography (PETT-V) for imaging of the brain. Journal of Computer Assisted Tomography 2:539–544, 1978.

Ter-Pogossian, M. M., Raichle, M. E., and Sobel, B. E. Positron-emission tomography. Scientific American 243:171–181, October 1980.

Ter-Pogossian, M. M., Ficke, D. C., Hood, J. T., Yamamoto, M., and Mullani, N. A. PETT VI: A positron emission tomograph utilizing cesium fluoride scintillation detectors. Journal of Computer Assisted Tomography 6:125–133, 1982.

Ultrasound

Baker, M., and Dalrymple, G. Biological effects of diagnostic ultrasound. A review. Radiology 126:479–484, 1978.

Birnholz, J. A critique of high speed imaging, with an introduction to the phased array. Applied Radiology 5:135–140, 1976.

Bom, N., Lancee, C. T., van Zwieten, G., Kloster, F. E., and Roelandt, J. Multiscan echocardiography. 1. Technical description. Circulation 48:1066–1074, 1973.

Carlson, E. Ultrasound physics for the physicians: A brief review. Journal of Clinical Ultrasound 3:71–80, 1975.

Christensen, E. E., Curry, T. S., and Dowdey, J. E. An Introduction to the Physics of Diagnostic Radiology, 2nd ed. Chap. 25, Ultrasound, pp. 361–394. Philadelphia, Lea & Febiger, 1978.

deVlieger, M., Holmes, J. H., Kazner, E., Kossoff, G., Kratochwil, A., Kraus, R., Poujol, J., and Strandness, D. E. (guest eds.), Handbook of Clinical Ultrasound. John Wiley & Sons, New York, 1978.

Feigenbaum, H. Echocardiography, 2nd ed. Lea & Febiger, Philadelphia, 1976.

Fleischer, A. C., and James, A. E. Introduction to Diagnostic Sonography. John Wiley & Sons, New York, 1980.

Goldberg, B. B. Abdominal Gray Scale Ultrasonography. John Wiley & Sons, New York, 1977.

Hobbins, J., and Winsberg, F. Ultrasonography in Obstetrics and Gynecoloy. Williams & Wilkins, Baltimore, 1977.

James, A. E. Ultrasound. Radiologic Clinics of North America 17, No. 3, 1979.

King, D. L. Real-time cross-sectional ultrasonic imaging of the heart using a linear array multi-element transducer. Journal of Clinical Ultrasound 1:196–200, 1973.

Krause, W., and Soldner, R. Ultrasonic imaging technique (B scan) with high image rate for medical diagnosis. Electromedica 4:1–5, 1967.

McDicken, W. N. Diagnostic Ultrasonics: Principles and Use of Instruments. John Wiley & Sons, New York, 1976.

Morgan, C. L., Trought, W. S., von Ramm, O. T., and Thurstone, F. L. Abdominal and obstetric applications of a dynamically focused phased array real time ultrasound system. Clinical Radiology 31:277–286, 1980.

Rose, J. L., and Goldberg, B. B. Basic Physics in Diagnostic Ultrasound. John Wiley & Sons, New York, 1979.

Sanders, R. C. (guest ed.) Ultrasound. Radiology Clinics of North America 13, No. 3, 1975.

Sanders, R. C., and James, A. E. The Principles and Practice of Ultrasonography in Obstetrics and Gynecology. Appleton-Century-Crofts, New York, 1980.

Sprawls, P. The Physical Principles of Diagnostic Radiology. Chap. 25, Ultrasound, pp. 309–332. University Park Press, Baltimore, 1977.

von Ramm, O. T., and Thurstone, F. L. Cardiac imaging using a phased array ultrasound system. 1. System design, Circulation 53:258–262, 1976.

Wells, P. N. T. In deVlieger, M., et al. (eds.), Handbook of Clinical Ultrasound, Section I, Chap. 1, pp. 3–13. John Wiley & Sons, New York, 1978.

Wells, P. N. T., and Ziskin, M. C. New Techniques and Instrumentation in Ultrasonography (Clinics in Diagnostic Ultrasound, Vol. 5). Churchill Livingstone, New York, 1980.

Nuclear Magnetic Resonance Imaging

Alfidi, R. J., Haaga, J. R., ElYousef, S. J., Bryan, P. J., Fletcher, B. D., Lipuma, J. P., Morrison, S. C., Kaufman, B., Richey, J. B., Hinshaw, W. S., Kramer, D. M., Yeung H. N., Cohen, A. M., Butler, H. E., Ament, A. E., and Lieberman, J. M. Preliminary experimental results in humans and animals with a superconducting, wholebody, nuclear magnetic resonance scanner. Work in progress. Radiology 143:175–181, 1982.

Andrew, E. R., Bottomley, P. A., Hinshaw, W. S., Holland, G. N., Moore, W. S., and Simaroj, C. NMR images by the multiple sensitive point method: Application to larger biological systems. Physics in Medicine and Biology 22:971–974, 1977.

Andrew, E. R., and Worthington, B. S. Nuclear magnetic resonance imaging. In T. H. Newton and D. G. Potts (eds.), Radiology of the Skull and Brain: Technical Aspects of Computed Tomography, Vol. 5, Chap. 132, Part XIX, pp. 4389–4405. C. V. Mosby, St. Louis, 1981.

Barriolhet, L. E. and Moran, P. R. Nuclear magnetic resonance (NMR) relaxation spectroscopy in tissues. Medical Physics 2:191–194, 1975.

Bloch, F. Nuclear induction. Physical Review 70:460–473, 1946.

Bloch, F., Hansen, W. W., and Packard, M. Nuclear induction. Physical Review 69:127, 1946a.

Bloch, F., Hansen, W. W., and Packard, M. The nuclear induction experiment. Physical Review 70:474–485, 1946b.

Bloembergen, N., Purcell, E. M., and Pound, R. V. Relaxation effects in nuclear magnetic resonance absorption. Physical Review 73:679–712, 1948.

Budinger, T. F. Nuclear magnetic resonance (NMR) *in vivo* studies: Known thresholds for health effects. Journal of Computer Assisted Tomography 5:800–811, 1981.

Buonanno, F. S., Pybett, I. L., Kistler, J. P., Vielma, J., Brady, T. J., Hinshaw, W. S., Goldman, M. R., Newhouse, J. H., and Pohost, G. M. Cranial anatomy and detection of ischemic stroke in the cat by nuclear magnetic resonance imaging. Radiology 143:187–193, 1982.

Capp, M. P. Radiological imaging–2000 A. D. New Horizons Lecture. Radiology 138:541–550, 1981.

Crooks, L. E., Grover, T. P., Kaufman, L., and Singer, J. R. Tomographic imaging with nuclear magnetic resonance. Investigative Radiology 13:63–66, 1978.

Crooks, L., Hoenninger, J., Arakawa, M., Kaufman, L., McRee, R., Watts, J., and Singer, J. H. Tomography of hydrogen with nuclear magnetic resonance. Radiology 136:701–706, 1980.

Crooks, L., Arakawa, M., Hoenninger, J., Watts, J., McRee, R., Kaufman, L., Davis. P. L., Margulis, A. R., and DeGroot, J. Nuclear magnetic resonance whole-body imager operating at 3.5 kGauss. Radiology 143:169–174, 1982.

Currie, C. M., Partain, C. L., Price, R. R., and James, A. E., Jr. The clinical potential of NMR—CT imaging. Diagnostic Imaging, pp. 46–50, November 1981.

Damadian, R. Tumor detection by nuclear magnetic resonance. Science 171:1151–1153, 1971.

Damadian, R. Apparatus and method for detecting cancer in tissue. U.S. Patent No. 3,789,832, March 1972.

Damadian, R., Zaner, K., Hor, D., and DiMaio, T. Human tumors detected by nuclear magnetic resonance. Procedings of the National Academy of Science of the U.S.A. 71:1471–1473, 1973.

Davis, P. L., Crooks, L., Arakawa, M., McRee, R., Kaufman, L., and Margulis, A. R. Potential hazards, in NMR imaging: Heating effects of changing magnetic fields on small magnetic implants. American Journal of Roentgenology 137:857–860, 1981.

Di Chiro, G. Editor's note. Journal of Computer Assisted Tomography 4:210, 1980.

Doyle, F. H., Pennock, J. M., Banks, L. M., McDonnell, M. J., Bydder, G. M., Steiner, R. E., Young, I. R., Clarke, G. J., Pasmore, T., and Gilderdale, D. J. Nuclear magnetic resonance imaging of the liver: initial experience. American Journal of Roentgenology 138:193–200, 1982.

Edelstein, W. A., Hutchinson, J. M., Johnson, G., and Redpath, T. Spin warp NMR imaging and applications to human whole-body imaging. Physics in Medicine and Biology 25:751–756, 1980.

Encyclopedia Britannica. Magnetic Resonance. In The Macropedia, Vol. 11, pp. 305–309, 15th ed., 1981.

Garroway, A. N., Grannell, P. K., and Mansfield, P. Image formation in NMR by a selective irradiative process. Journal of Physics C. Solid State Physics 7:1457–1462, 1974.

General Electric Company Medical Systems. NMR. An introduction. General Electric Publication No. 5251A, 1981.

Hansen, G., Crooks, L. E., Davis, P., DeGroot, J., Herfkens, R., Margulis, A. R., Gooding, C., Kaufman, L., Hoenninger, J., Arakawa, M., McRee, R., and Watts, J. In vivo imaging of the rat anatomy with nuclear magnetic resonance. Radiology 136:695–700, 1980.

Hawkes, R. C., Holland, G. N., Moore, W. S., and Worthington, B. S.: Nuclear magnetic resonance (NMR) tomography of the brain: A preliminary clinical assessment with demonstration of pathology. Journal of Computer Assisted Tomography 4:577–586, 1980.

Hawkes, R. C., Holland, G. N., Moore, W. S., Roebuck, E. J., and Worthington, B. S. Nuclear magnetic resonance (NMR) tomography of the normal heart. Journal of Computer Assisted Tomography 5:605–612, 1981.

Hawkes, R. C., Holland, G. N., Moore, W. S., Roebuck, E. J., and Worthington, B. S. Nuclear magnetic resonance (NMR) tomography of the normal abdomen. Journal of Computer Assisted Tomography 5:613–618, 1981.

Hazelwood, C. F., Cleveland, G., and Medina, D. Relationship between hydration and proton nuclear magnetic resonance relaxation times in tissues of tumor-bearing and non-tumor-bearing mice: Implications for cancer detection. Journal of the National Cancer Institute 52:1849–1853, 1974.

Heneghan, M. A., Biancaniello, T. M., Heidelberger, E., Peterson, S. B., Marsh, M. J., and Lauterbur, P. C. Nuclear magnetic resonance zeumatographic imaging of the heart: Application to the study of ventricular septal defect. Radiology 143:183–186, 1982.

Herfkens, R., Davis, P., Crooks, L., Kaufman, L., Price, D., Miller, T., Margulis, A. R., Watts, J., Hoenninger, J., Arakawa, M., and McRee, R. Nuclear magnetic resonance imaging of the abnormal live rat and correlations with tissue characteristics. Radiology 141:211–218, 1981.

Hinshaw, W. S. Image formation by nuclear magnetic resonance: The sensitive point method. Journal of Applied Physics 47:3709–3719, 1976.

Hinshaw, W. S., Bottomley, P. A., and Holland, G. N. Radiographic thin-section image of the human wrist by nuclear magnetic resonance. Nature 270:722–723, 1977.

Hinshaw, W. S., Andrew, E. R., Bottomley, P. A., Holland, G. N., and Moore, W. S. Display of cross sectional anatomy by nuclear magnetic resonance imaging. British Journal of Radiology 51:273–280, 1978.

Holland, G. N., Moore, W. S., and Hawkes, R. C. Nuclear magnetic resonance tomography of the brain. Journal of Computer Assisted Tomography 4:1–3, 1980.

Holland, G. N., Hawkes, R. C., and Moore, W. S. Nuclear magnetic resonance (NMR) tomography of the brain: coronal and sagittal sections. Journal of Computer Assisted Tomography 4:429–433, 1980.

Hollis, D. P., Economou, J. S., Parks, L. C., Eggleston, J. C., Saryan, L. A., and Czeisler, J. L. Nuclear magnetic resonance studies of several experimental and human malignant tumors. Cancer Research 33:2156–2160, 1973.

Hollis, D. P., Saryan, L. A., Eggleston, J. C., and Morris, H. P. Nuclear magnetic resonance studies of cancer. Relationship among spin-lattice relaxation times, growth rate, and water content of morris hepatomas, Journal of the National Cancer Institute 54:1469–1472, 1975.

Hounsfield, G. N. Computed medical imaging. Nobel lecture, December 1979. Journal of Computer Assisted Tomography 4:665–674, 1980.

Inch, W. R., McCredie, J. A., Knispel, R. R., Thompson, R. T., and Pintar, M. M. Water content and spin relaxation time for neoplastic and non-neoplastic tissues from mice and humans. Journal of the National Cancer Institute 52:353–356, 1974.

James, A. E., Partain, C. L., Coulam, C. M., and Rollo, F. D. Nuclear magnetic resonance imaging. Editorial. Applied Radiology 9(4):18, 1980.

James, A. E., Jr., Partain, C. L., Holland, G. N., Gore, J. C., Rollo, F. D., Harms, S. E., and Price, R. R. Nuclear magnetic resonance imaging: The current state. A review. American Journal of Roentgenology 138:201–210, 1982.

Johnson, C. C., and Guy, A. W. Nonionizing electromagnetic wave effects in biological materials and systems. Proceedings of the I.E.E.E. 60:692–716, 1972.

Kaufman, L., Crooks, L. E., and Margulis, A. R. (eds.). Nuclear Magnetic Resonance Imaging in Medicine, Igaku-Shoin, Tokyo, 1981.

Knispel, R. R., Thompson, R. T., and Pintar, M. M. Dispersion of proton spin-lattice relaxation in tissues. Journal of Magnetic Resonance 14:44–51, 1974.

Lauterbur, P. C. Image formation by induced local interactions: Examples employing nuclear magnetic resonance. Nature 242:190–191, 1973.

Lauterbur, P. C. Magnetic resonance zeumatography. Pure and Applied Chemistry 40:149–157, 1974.

Luiten, A. L. Nuclear magnetic resonance: An introduction. Medicamundi 26:98–101, 1981.

Mansfield, P. Carcinoma of the breast imaged by nuclear magnetic resonance (NMR). British Journal of Radiology 52:242–243, 1979.

Mansfield, P., and Maudsley, A. A. Medical imaging by NMR. British Journal of Radiology 50:188–194, 1977.

Mansfield, P., and Maudsley, A. A. Planar spin imaging by NMR. Journal of Magnetic Resonance 27:101–119, 1977.

Marx, J. L. NMR opens a new window into the body: The use of nuclear magnetic resonance for medical diagnosis hovers on the brink of practical application. Science 210:302–305, 1980.

Medina, D., Hazlewood, C. F., Cleveland, G. G., Chang, C. G., Spjut, H. J., and Moyers, R. Nuclear magnetic resonance studies on human breast dysplasias and neoplasms. Journal of the National Cancer Institute 54:813–818, 1975.

Moore, W. S., and Holland, G. N. The NMR CAT scanner—A new look at the brain. CT: The Journal of Computed Tomography 4:1–7, 1980.

Oldendorf, W. H. Future imaging methods. *In* The Quest for an Image of Brain. Computerized Tomography in the Perspective of Past and Future Imaging Methods, Chap. 9, pp. 127–145. Raven Press, New York, 1980.

Pake, G. E. Paramagnetic Resonance. An Introductory Monograph. W. A. Benjamin, New York, 1962.

Partain, C. L., Rollo, F. D., and James, A. E. Clinical NMR imaging. Diagnostic Imaging, 4–7, July 1980.

Partain, C. L., James, A. E., Watson, J. T., Price, R. R., Coulam, C. M., and Rollo, F. D. Nuclear magnetic resonance and computed tomography. Comparison of normal human body images. Radiology 136:767–770, 1980.

Pykett, I. L., Newhouse, J. H., Buonanno, F. S., Brady, T. J., Goldman, M. R., Kistler, J. P., and Pohost, G. M. Principles of nuclear magnetic resonance imaging. Radiology 143:157–168, 1982.

Ross, R. J., Thompson, J. S., Kim, K., and Bailey, R. A., Nuclear magnetic resonance imaging and evaluation of human breast tissue: Preliminary clinical trials. Radiology 143:195–205, 1982.

Slichter, C. P. Principles of Magnetic Resonance with Examples from Solid State Physics. Harper and Row, New York, 1963.

Smith, F. W., Reid, A., Hutchison, J. M. S., and Mallard, J. R. Nuclear magnetic resonance imaging of the pancreas. Radiology 142:677–680, 1982.

Weisman, I. D., Bennett, L. H., Maxwell, L. R., Woods, M. W., and Burk, D. Recognition of cancer in vivo by nuclear magnetic resonance. Science 178:1288–1290, 1972.

Wolff, S., Crooks, L. E., Brown, P., Howard, R., and Painter, R. B. Tests for DNA and chromosomal damage induced by nuclear magnetic resonance imaging. Radiology 136:707–710, 1980.

Young, I. R., Bailes, D. R., Burl, M., Collins, A. G., Smith, D. T., McDonnell, M. J., Orr, J. S., Banks, L. M., Bydder, G. M., Greenspan, R. H., and Steiner, R. E. Initial clinical evaluation of a whole body nuclear magnetic resonance (NMR) tomograph. Journal of Computer Assisted Tomography 6:1–18, 1982.

Zavoisky, Y. Journal of Physics USSR 9:211–245, 1945 (cited by Pake, 1962).

Microwave Computed Tomography

Bragg, D. G., Durney, C. H., Johnson, C. C. and Pedersen, P. Monitoring and diagnosis of pulmonary edema by microwaves: A preliminary report. Investigative Radiology 12:289–291, 1977.

Capp, M. P. Radiological imaging—2000 A.D. New Horizons Lecture. Radiology 138:541–550, 1981.

Larsen, L. E., and Jacobi, J. H. Microwave scattering parameter imagery of an isolated canine kidney. Medical Physics 6:394–403, 1979.

Rao, P. S., Santosh, K., and Gregg, E. C. Computed tomography with microwaves. Radiology 135:769–770, 1980.

Appendix I
ARTIFACTS

GEOMETRIC ARTIFACTS

Motion Artifacts
Aliasing Artifacts (Finite Sampling)
Inadequate Angular Sampling
Edge Gradient Streaks
Geometric Misalignment Artifacts
Hounsfield Partial Volume Effect

ALGORITHM ARTIFACTS

Point Spread Effect
Edge Enhancement Effects

ARTIFACTS ARISING FROM ATTENUATION MEASUREMENT ERRORS

Scanner Geometry
Scatter Radiation
Faulty Detectors
X-ray Source Variations
Nonlinearity in Measurements

BEAM HARDENING ARTIFACTS

PARTIAL VOLUME EFFECTS

VISUAL ILLUSIONS

REFERENCES AND SUGGESTED READINGS

An artifact is any distortion or error in an image that is unrelated to the subject being studied. Artifacts are relatively common in CT and may be considered as a source or type of noise. Their cause may not always be obvious. However, there are a number of different effects that may be responsible for artifacts in CT.

In contrast to CT imaging, artifacts are relatively uncommon in conventional radiography. Furthermore, their etiology is usually apparent. Artifacts in conventional radiography are frequently due to metallic or other foreign bodies external to the subject, to dirt or scratches involving the film-screen combinations, and to light leaks.

Because artifacts in CT often arise as a result of the interaction between the subject and the machine, it is useful to follow the example of Joseph (1981) and classify artifacts by the nature of the error made in the scanning process. In CT, artifacts may be produced by geometric effects or a machine peculiarity, by an inadequacy in the reconstruction algorithm, by an error in x-ray attenuation measurements, as a result of alterations in the energy spectrum of the x-ray beam (beam hardening) as it passes through the patient, because of partial volume effects, or by visual illusions.

Regardless of their etiology, however, most CT artifacts manifest as streaks (Figures A1.1–A1.3). Jo-

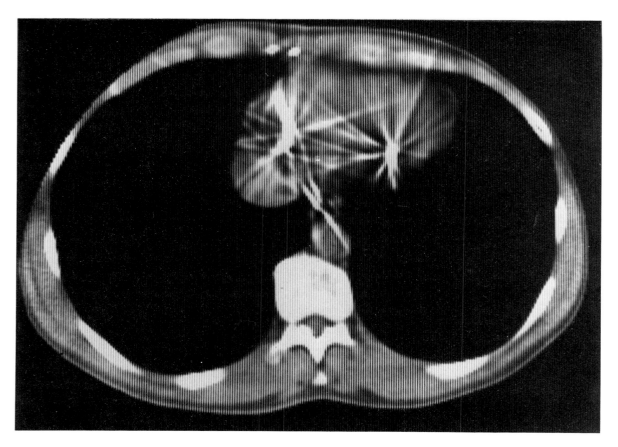

Figure A1.1. Streak artifacts arising from metallic surgical clips in the mediastinum.

seph (1981) has pointed out two reasons for this. First, each individual measurement involves the evaluation of a single ray or straight line path through the slice. This is a fundamental property of CT imaging and is independent of the algorithm used. Therefore, an error involving a single ray will affect primarily those pixels lying along that ray; thus, a streak is produced. Furthermore, in filtered backprojection an error in a ray is handled in the same way as a true value—it is filtered and back-projected along the direction of the ray. The second, more subtle cause for streak artifacts arises when there is an abrupt discrepancy or inconsistency between views, as might be seen with patient motion. With perfect data, the combination of filtering and back-projection results in a series of positive and negative contributions to the image along lines in such a manner that at every pixel the contributions from adjacent views are integrated to form the correct reconstruction. However, if rays from adjacent views are not consistent with each other, there will be an imbalance in the process of cancellations of positive and negative components, with a resultant streaking.

In general, the principle of smoothness applies in CT imaging. This principle states that the CT reconstruction algorithm is very sensitive to an error that causes an abrupt change from ray to ray or from view to view. In contrast, it is more insensitive or tolerant to errors that cause gradual changes from ray to ray or from view to view. An excellent presentation of the different types of artifacts has been written by Joseph (1981).

This appendix describes briefly some of the sources of artifacts found in CT.

GEOMETRIC ARTIFACTS

Geometric artifacts arise either when the different rays on which measurements are performed are not properly oriented in space with respect to one another or when the number of measurements made is inadequate. The most easily understood example

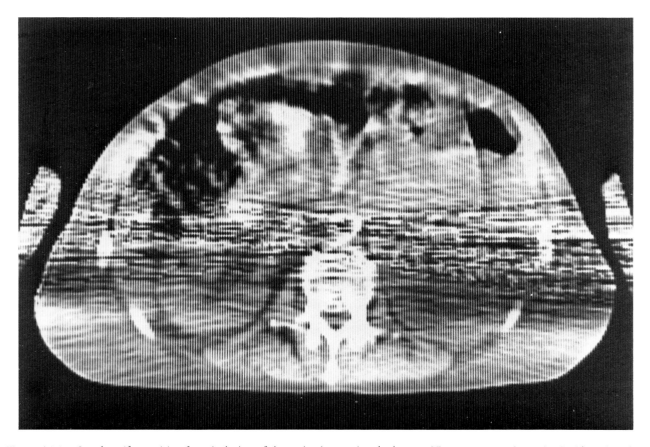

Figure A1.2. Streak artifacts arising from inclusion of the patient's arms in a body scan. The arms are at the patient's side rather than raised above the abdomen, and the bones are responsible for the artifact.

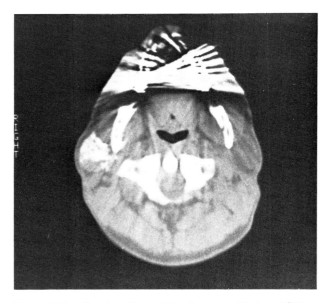

Figure A1.3. Streak artifacts arising from metallic dental fillings (contrast is in the parotid gland from sialography).

of a geometric artifact is that of patient motion. In this case rays measured at different times during the scan would not all have the appropriate location or orientation with respect to the patient. The rays may be regarded as being displaced. Other causes of geometric artifacts include errors associated with finite sampling or aliasing, inadequate angular sampling, edge gradient streaks, geometric misalignment artifacts, and the Hounsfield partial volume effect.

Motion Artifacts

There are a number of different types of patient motion that may result in image degradation. These include cardiac motion, respiration, peristalsis, and voluntary or involuntary muscular motion. The results of each type of motion can be additive. More rapid scan times may permit elimination of the artifacts associated with the slower motions.

With reference to the principle of smoothness discussed in the introduction, the pertinent question

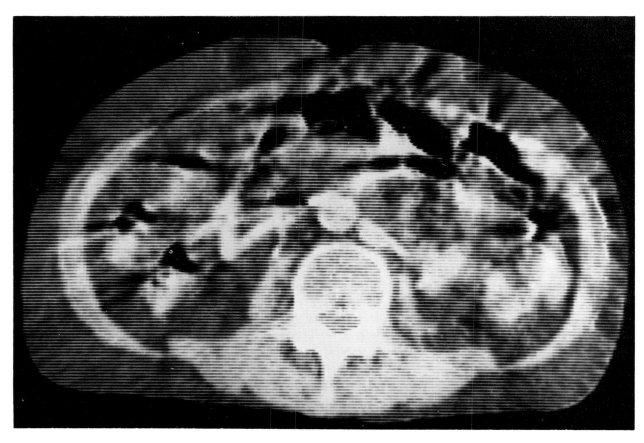

Figure A1.4. Artifacts arising from peristaltic motion in a 19-s scan.

in motion artifacts is whether or not there was significant patient motion between views. Abrupt motion is generally far more significant than gradual motion in causing artifacts. Figures A1.4 and A1.5 illustrate artifacts associated with two types of motion.

There is no generally satisfactory approach at present for handling or correcting artifacts associated with abrupt motion. On the other hand, many streaks arising as a result of gradual motion may be correctable, because the most significant problem arising from gradual motion is an inconsistency between the initial and last views. This problem may be treated by the technique of overscanning, or obtaining additional views (going beyond the usual 180° or 360° normal scan angle). Overscanning at least theoretically entails the collection of repeated views, that is, collecting the same views that were initially measured at the beginning of a scan. The collection of these additional final views gives information regarding the final position of the patient. An appropriate mixing of these initial and final overlapping views, perhaps

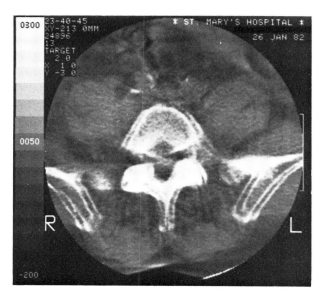

Figure A1.5. An apparent double contour artifact due to patient motion during a 10-s scan.

with some weighting factors attached to both sets of views, can reduce the inconsistency between the sets of data and reduce or eliminate the streak artifacts.

Aliasing Artifacts (Finite Sampling)

Aliasing has been described briefly in Chapter 8. Detailed descriptions and explanations for this phenomenon have been given by Brooks et al. (1978), Stockham (1979), Joseph et al. (1980), and Joseph (1981).

The Nyquist theorem requires that for adequate imaging of an object the spatial sampling frequency (rate) must be at least twice that of the highest spatial frequency present in the object. The latter frequency (or, equivalently, half of the sampling frequency) is referred to as the Nyquist frequency, ν_N.

Sampling consists of a set of discrete measurements. The successive samples are separated spatially by a finite spatial sampling interval T_s. When this interval is not less than half of the spatial wavelength associated with the highest spatial frequency present in the image (or, equivalently, when the sampling rate is not greater than at least twice the highest spatial frequency in the image), the artifact of aliasing may appear. The spatial wavelength is simply the inverse of the spatial frequency. Therefore,

$$T_s = \frac{1}{2} \frac{1}{\nu_N}. \tag{A1.1}$$

In aliasing, information at spatial frequencies higher than the Nyquist frequency appears superimposed on lower frequency information. This may be understood intuitively in the following way. When discrete samples are obtained of frequency components greater than the sampling rate, there is no way to identify the information as having a frequency greater than the sampling rate. The values or measurement data sampled from the higher frequencies are assumed to be associated with lower frequencies. The high frequency information will appear, incorrectly, at lower frequencies. The higher frequencies will masquerade themselves at lower frequencies; that is, they will adopt the appearance of the lower frequencies as an alias.

One method of eliminating aliasing is to increase the sampling rate. However, this entails an increase in data acquisition and scanning time as well as greater radiation dosage. Another approach is to eliminate or filter out those frequencies that exceed the Nyquist frequency. A practical method for achieving this is by choosing an appropriate width for the x-ray beam. As discussed in Chapter 8, the effective width of the x-ray beam is one factor determining the spatial resolution. The localization of an object is limited by the width of the sampling beam. The object may be detected as being in the path of the beam, as defined by the beam width (and height or section thickness), but it cannot be more precisely localized within the beam area. There is an upper limit to the spatial frequencies that can be detected by a particular finite beam width. As this beam width is increased, this limit is decreased. Higher frequencies are thus filtered by the beam width, and there is a zero response at frequencies exceeding a certain value ν_0, where

$$\nu_0 = \frac{1}{\text{beam width}}. \tag{A1.2}$$

Thus, the beamwidth filters out or suppresses frequencies above ν_0 prior to the sampling process. This permits elimination of aliasing artifacts by the suppression of the higher frequency components above the Nyquist frequency by setting ν_0 equal to the Nyquist frequency ν_N. By combining equations A1.1 and A1.2,

$$\text{sampling interval} = \tfrac{1}{2} \text{ beam width}. \tag{A1.3}$$

Therefore, the elimination of aliasing artifacts requires at least two data samples per beam width. Narrower beams can be used, permitting increased spatial resolution, but more data samples must be obtained to suppress aliasing. When aliasing artifacts appear, they are frequently seen as streaks associated with edges.

A problem that arises in third generation scanners is the fixed distance between rays (i.e., a fixed sampling interval). The number of rays in a view is a constant determined by the number of detectors in the array; the distance between rays or spatial sampling interval is fixed by the distance between detector elements. Data acquisition is increased by increasing the number of views (when a view is obtained by pulsing the tube) or the number of times the detector array obtains samples. Therefore, there can only be one sample per beam width, and aliasing artifacts would seem to present a problem. However, this problem can be reduced by a geometric modification. By offsetting the detector array by exactly one-quarter of the width of a detector element, opposing views (those 180° apart) will have rays that are slightly offset. These "interleave" rays will supply the additional data needed to suppress aliasing; that is, the data obtained in this manner are roughly equivalent to measuring two samples per beam width, thus satisfying Equation A1.3.

Inadequate Angular Sampling

The artifacts associated with an inadequate or limited number of views appear as very fine streaks that can be seen only at some distance from dense objects. This distance is related to the number of views and the spatial resolution.

An increase in the number of views or in the number of rays per view contributes more information to the process of image reconstruction. An increase in the number of rays per view (the sampling rate) may result in direct improvement of the spatial resolution, as described previously. However, an increase in the number of views (keeping the number of rays per view constant) does not lead directly to an increase in spatial resolution. What it does is to increase the diameter of the region over which a particular spatial resolution can be obtained. A limited number of views limits the area with a particular spatial resolution to a smaller diameter; increasing the number of views extends this diameter of higher spatial resolution.

Joseph (1981) has presented the formulas that have been derived for the minimum number of views in CT. For second generation translational-rotational units the minimum number of views N required is given by

$$N = \pi D \nu_0, \qquad (A1.4)$$

where D is the maximum patient diameter (or, equivalently, the maximum diameter over which the desired or required spatial resolution must be established) and ν_0 is the maximum resolvable spatial frequency (the spatial resolution expressed as a frequency).

For a 360° fan beam scanner this needs to be modified as follows

$$N = 2\pi D \nu_0 / (1 - \sin \psi/2), \qquad (A1.5)$$

where ψ is the opening angle of the fan.

Commercial scanners generally acquire too few views to satisfy Equations A1.4 and A1.5. For example, the General Electric CT/T 8800, with $D = 42$ cm, ν_0 approximating 10 cm^{-1} and $\psi = 30°$, would require 3500–4000 views by Equation A1.5, far more than the 288 views obtained in a 4.8-s scan or the 576 views obtained in a 9.6-s scan. However, Equations A1.4 and A1.5 represent a worst case situation, a high-density, sharp-edged object at the edge of the field of reconstruction. The artifact is actually rarely seen in clinical CT scanning.

If the number of views and the spatial resolution frequency ν_0 are fixed, the distance D from a sharp-edged dense object to the point where streaks will appear can be predicted from Equations A1.4 and A1.5.

The cause of the artifact associated with inadequate angular sampling can be understood intuitively. In the reconstruction of a dense pin or object, the contribution from each view would be a streak back-projected along the direction of the view. The superimposition of many different views results in a cancellation of the streaks by one another. However, the degree of completeness or the thoroughness of the cancellation is a function of the distance from the pin. At points close to the pin, the cancellation is complete. At points more distant from the pin this cancellation is incomplete or altogether absent. This occurs because the back projections from different views diverge geometrically and so cannot cancel each other out. The streaks thus become more evident. This has been illustrated in Figure 5.12.

Because the artifact can be reduced by increasing the number of views and reducing the maximum spatial frequency (reducing spatial resolution), it has also been referred to as view aliasing. However, there are significant differences. Ray aliasing (due to finite sampling) may be reduced by increasing the sampling rate (the density of ray samples); view aliasing is not decreased by increasing the sampling rate. However, view aliasing can always be suppressed by the use of a smoothing algorithm; this not true for ray aliasing. The effect of view aliasing is sometimes called view sampling.

View aliasing artifacts should not be mistaken for artifacts arising from metallic objects. The latter are due to aliasing and other edge effects, not to the angular spacing between views.

Edge Gradient Streaks

This has been described by Joseph (1981) as a purely "mathematical" artifact in which lucent streaks arise from the edges of dense objects with unusually straight shapes. Its origin is the interaction between the exponential law of radiation absorption and a smoothing effect introduced by the width of the x-ray beam. The artifact will not be present if the beam width is zero or the contrast between the object and its surroundings is small. It is a nonlinear effect because the contrast of the streaks depends approximately on the square of the object contrast. This artifact may contribute to the streaks between the petrous pyramids on head scans at lower levels.

Longer edges increase this artifact. It may be reduced by modification of the algorithm or by the utilization of a higher photon energy (harder) beam.

Geometric Misalignment Artifacts

These arise as a result of a mechanical misalignment of either the x-ray tube or the detectors and are dependent on the particular characteristics of each machine. In addition, the appearance of the artifact will depend on whether the scanning geometry involves a full circular (360°) rotation or a lesser rotation (e.g., 180°).

When the rotation is less than 360°, there is a tuning fork pattern with positive and negative streaks in the vertical (0°) direction. Most commonly this is due to a shift or mislocation of the mechanical center of rotation with respect to the center of coordinates that are used in reconstruction. Because of this difference between the true and assumed positions of the isocenter, the initial and final views will be inconsistent, and streak artifacts will arise.

A narrow pin phantom can be scanned to detect this error. The artifact can arise off-center when the position encoding device used is inaccurate. In this case the computer misinterprets the positions of off-center rays. Thus, several pins should be used. It may be difficult to distinguish the streaks associated with geometric misalignment from those associated with gradual patient motion.

In third and fourth generation systems there are so many detectors that mechanical alignment can be impractical, and software programs are designed to permit the computer to ascertain the precise position of the x-ray tube and detectors.

Hounsfield Partial Volume Effect

This is an effect described by Hounsfield which pertains only to translational-rotational systems with 180° of rotation. It is a subtle geometric effect manifested by streaks which result from the partial volume effect discussed in Chapter 2 and later in this appendix. The streaks result from an inconsistency between the initial and final views as a result of the partial volume effect, where dense objects (or air) only partly occupy the entire section thickness. It is complicated by the fact that the x-ray beam is divergent rather than parallel. The latter effect is particularly prominent in scanners that obtain two slices per scan, because it is necessary to angle each beam slightly with respect to its scan plane. As a result, a different fraction of the volume of an object will intercept the beam on the initial and final views. This difference is responsible for the inconsistency between initial and final views that causes the streaks. It may be suppressed by overscanning and by reducing slice width.

ALGORITHM ARTIFACTS

Algorithm artifacts are due to the details of the particular reconstruction algorithm used. These are a result of modifications and alterations employed in the basic back projection algorithm that permit image manipulation.

Point Spread Effect

This effect has been described by Koehler et al. (1979) in their discussion of the effect of CT viewer controls on anatomical measurements. The apparent size of an object changes as the CT window level is varied. This effect is increased when narrower window widths are used or for greater differences in density between the object and its background. An example is shown in Figure A1.6.

The effect may be complicated by a superimposed partial volume effect, which can be minimized by performing overlapping images and choosing the one that best depicts the full size of the object in cross-section.

Because of inherent limitations of resolution in CT, the edges of sharp objects are blurred. This causes the apparent size of an object to change as the window settings are varied. Consider the image of a point object in CT. A point object will be imaged as a blur of finite dimensions in conventional radiography or CT. The inherently poorer spatial resolution of CT compared to conventional radiography will result in a greater spreading of the image of a point object (i.e., a wider blur). The density of the blurred image will vary, decreasing more or less rapidly with distance from the center. The apparent size of the point object will be affected by the width of the point spread function at the window (or density) level and the window width selected. Decreasing the window level permits more peripheral, and less dense, portions of the blur to be displayed.

This artifact may be reduced by improved spatial resolution, so that the point spread function becomes narrower. It may also be reduced by appropriate selection and manipulation of the window settings.

Edge Enhancement Effects

Edge enhancement involves modification of the algorithm to permit display of abrupt edges. It involves

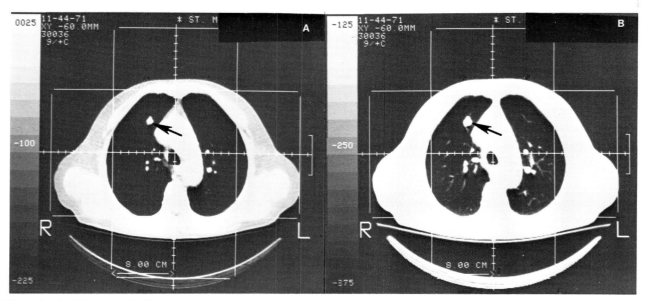

Figure A1.6. Point spread effect or dependence of the size of an object in the window settings. A, a pulmonary nodule (arrow) is identified with the window level set at −100 and a window width of 250 EMI units. B, the apparent size of the nodule (arrow) is increased when the window level is decreased to −250 and the width increased to 500.

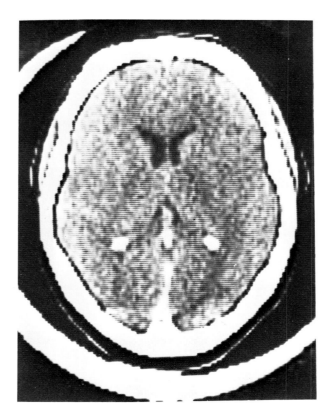

Figure A1.7. Edge enhancement effect. The lucency adjacent to the inner surface of the skull is an artifact, which suggests visualization of the cerebrospinal fluid in the subarachnoid space.

the enhancement of higher spatial frequency components of the images. As a consequence of this algorithm modification, however, very dense objects may appear to be surrounded by a lucent zone. This is a false lucency or artifact. In cranial CT this often results in the production of a lucency under the skull that suggests imaging of the subarachnoid space. This is illustrated in Figure A1.7. Lucent halos may appear around dense objects, and air pockets may be surrounded by dense rings.

The artifact produced by edge enhancement can be removed by eliminating the modifications in the algorithm, that is, by using a more "faithful" algorithm.

ARTIFACTS ARISING FROM ATTENUATION MEASUREMENT ERRORS

These artifacts are due to any derangement or malfunction involving the detector system so that an inaccurate measurement of the x-ray attenuation is made. The rays are correctly aligned, in contrast to geometric effects, but the actual numerical value is in error.

Scanner Geometry

There are three principal sources of error in attenuation measurements: scatter radiation, faulty detectors, and x-ray source errors. These have been described in detail by Joseph (1981).

Scatter Radiation Scatter radiation tends to be a greater problem in fourth generation scanners than in the other generations of scanning geometries. This occurs because in the fixed detectors and rotating x-ray tube geometry that characterize fourth generation scanners, each of the detectors must intercept and detect rays from multiple different angles of incidence. This has been described in Chapter 3 and is illustrated in Figure A1.8.

In contrast, in both translational-rotational systems (first and second generations) and in systems with rotating tube and detectors (third generation), a detector will intercept a ray at the same angle of incidence. This permits improved collimation and better scatter rejection.

Faulty Detectors A single faulty detector presents a greater problem in third generation scanners than in fourth generation units. The basis of this difference is the fact that in third generation systems a particular detector always samples the same ray in every view. In contrast, in a fourth generation system each detector samples different rays in each view. A faulty detector in a third generation system therefore results in the same bad ray in every view. In a fourth generation system a faulty detector results in a single bad view (because a view is defined by all the rays that a detector intercepts). A problem that produces a uniform error in a particular view is a great deal

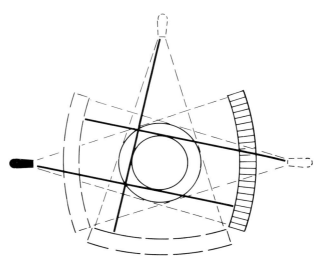

Figure A1.9. In third generation scanners a particular detector always intercepts the same ray in every view. This ray is always tangential to a circle. The more peripheral the detector, the greater the radius of the circle. A faulty detector thus leads to artifacts with a circular or ringlike configuration.

less significant than one that produces an error in the same ray in every view.

A faulty detector in a third generation system results in a circular or ring artifact, as described in Chapter 3. During a scan a specific ray will always be tangent to a particular circle. The ray effectively traces out a circle. This is illustrated in Figure A1.9. The errors associated with measurements of a particular ray in every view will thus result in a circular or ring artifact. A clinical example is shown in Figure A1.10. Even very small error measurements of the order of 0.1% may lead to ring artifacts.

In a fourth generation system a faulty detector results in a uniform inaccuracy for all ray measurements in a single view (defined by the faulty detector). This does not cause a significant distortion, rather just a small shift of CT numbers across the image.

In translational-rotational systems a detector measures a number of different rays during each translation, each such set of measurements constituting a view. This is more analogous to data collection in a fourth generation system than a third generation system. However, a first generation unit has, by definition, only a single detector, so that a detector error may present a significant problem. Second generation units that have a large number of detectors, however, may be a great deal more tolerant of an error in a single detector, spreading out the error or averaging it smoothly over the entire image.

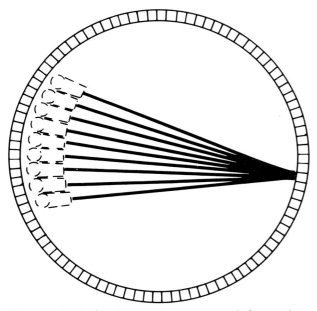

Figure A1.8. In fourth generation scanners each detector is capable of intercepting rays over a range of angles. A collection of such ray measurements constitutes a view. This limits scatter rejection.

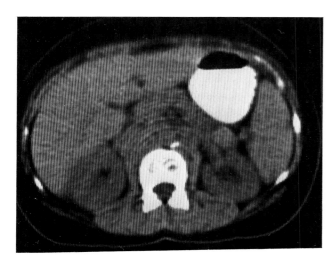

Figure A1.10. Clinical examples of circular or ring artifacts. *A*, gross artifacts in head scan. *B*, more subtle artifacts in body scan.

X-Ray Source Variations In third generation systems all the rays in a view are measured at the same time. Thus, a variation in the x-ray tube output affects all the rays in a view or measurement set in the same way, and third generation systems are relatively more tolerant of fluctuations in x-ray tube output than other generations.

In fourth generation systems the rays in a view are measured consecutively, so that any fluctuation in tube output will not affect all the rays uniformly. However, because the same fluctuation would not usually be expected to be repeated in a cyclic fashion from view to view, ring artifacts would not be expected. The effect of variations in the x-ray flux may also be reduced by monitoring the output with a reference detector which rotates with the tube. Variations can then be detected and appropriate corrections made by the computer.

Because translational-rotational units also measure rays sequentially in time, they are similar to fourth generation scanners in regard to variations in x-ray flux.

Nonlinearity in Measurements

Nonlinearity refers to a deviation in detector response from a linear relationship between the radiation intensity input and detector current output. The dynamic range of detectors (the ratio of the largest to the smallest signal intensity) may be as much as 10,000:1. Maintaining linearity over such a wide dynamic range puts a great demand on the technical requirements of the detectors.

Several factors may contribute to nonlinearity in CT detectors (Joseph, 1981). These include leakage current, saturation, hysteresis, and afterglow.

Leakage current is the nonzero detector output current that may be present without a radiation input. In third generation units using pulsed x-ray tubes, the leakage current may be measured between pulses and then subtracted from data measurements. Leakage becomes more significant for thicker or denser body parts when the input radiation (and output signal) are at low values.

Saturation refers to the inability of a detector to increase its output current above a certain level (the saturation level) as the input radiation intensity is increased. The output current is insufficient to depict higher radiation inputs accurately. Saturation is actually the opposite problem to leakage current. It becomes significant for thinner, less dense body parts when the input radiation intensity and output current are relatively high.

Hysteresis is a phenomenon in which the output of a detector depends on its history of previous radiation exposure as well as the present level of incident radiation intensity. It is common in detectors employing a scintillation crystal-photomultiplier tube combination.

Afterglow is a type of hysteresis that occurs in a scintillation crystal. This is an undesirable property of the crystal to continue emitting light after the termination of x-ray excitation. This is particularly significant in sodium iodide, where the computer must make corrections to compensate for it. Afterglow is comparatively less of a problem in calcium fluoride and bismuth germanate crystals.

Hysteresis may also be seen in gas ionization detectors (xenon cells) if there is not enough time between measurements to collect all the ions formed.

Hysteresis effects may be quite difficult to detect or correct in CT systems. Streak artifacts may result.

The effect of scattered radiation in CT can be significantly greater than in conventional radiography. The single effect of scatter on image quality in conventional radiography is to reduce image contrast by superimposing an additive component to the film exposure. In CT, however, scatter contributes a nonlinearity. This occurs because the measured signal in transmission CT is the logarithm of the detected x-ray intensity, and logarithms are not linear functions. Specifically, if I_T is the true signal and I_S the scatter,

$$\log(I_T + I_S) \neq \log I_T + \log I_S. \quad (A1.6)$$

The logarithm of a sum is not equal to the sum of logarithms. Therefore, even a uniform distribution of scatter would not contribute a constant additive background.

Three important ways to reduce the effects of nonlinearity are: 1) detector calibration, 2) reduction in the dynamic range of the detectors, and 3) incorporation of mathematical corrections to nonlinearity in the algorithm.

Calibration can be performed during scanning in translational-rotational units and fourth generation units. In these systems every detector intercepts rays that do not pass through the patient during scanning.

In third generation units all of the useful rays always pass through the patient during scanning. Therefore, long-term detector stability and accuracy are more important in third generation systems than in translational-rotational or fourth generation units.

Reduction of the dynamic range may be the most effective single way of reducing detector nonlinearities. The water bag, as used in the EMI Mark I scanner (illustrated earlier in Figure 2.32), accomplished this quite well by maintaining the total path length through the patient and water a constant. A water bag may reduce the dynamic range to a ratio of two or three to one. As discussed earlier in Chapter 2, the water bag also provides a built-in calibration for water and reduces beam hardening effects.

One substitute for a water bag has involved the packing of "bolus" material, simulating a water path, around the patient. The packing does provide a minimum path length through material (other than air) for all the x-rays. Another technique for simulating a water path involves the use of a "bow tie" filter between the x-ray tube and the patient. The filter is thinner in its midportion than at its periphery. Thus, there is more attenuation or contribution by the filter to a path length in the periphery, where the thickness of the patient is less, compared to the center where there is a greater patient thickness.

The most commonly employed method of correcting for nonlinearity is the use of a computer software correction. By measuring the transmitted x-ray intensity for different path lengths through a water phantom, the relationship between the intensity and the path length can be established. This might be expressed as a table. With this information the computer can then determine from an x-ray intensity measurement a water equivalent thickness that will take into account most of the causes of nonlinearity in the measurement. This permits a relatively good correction for a stable and reproducible cause of nonlinearity such as beam hardening. It is not as good for a less constant source of nonlinearity such as scatter, which shows more variation between patients.

This process for correcting nonlinearity is sometimes referred to alternatively as linearization, linearizing, or water correcting.

BEAM HARDENING ARTIFACTS

This phenomenon has been referred to earlier in Chapter 2 as well as in this appendix. The x-ray beam is not monochromatic or monoenergetic (containing a single wavelength or photon energy). Rather it is polychromatic, there being photons of different energy corresponding to different wavelengths or frequencies. The lower-energy photons are preferentially removed as the beam passes through the patient; that is, there is relatively more attenuation of the lower-energy components of the beam. Thus, the average photon energy of the beam progressively increases with path length. The beam is said to become harder, since it is more penetrating (relatively less attenuated) by tissue as its average photon energy increases. The energy spectrum, or the relative distribution of the energy components of the beam, is shifted so that relatively more photons have higher energy. The average or effective photon energy becomes greater.

Because of beam hardening, tissue closer to the detector side of the path length of a ray will be exposed to a beam with a higher effective energy than tissue closer to the tube side of the path length. Tissue on the exit side (detector side) of the beam will be exposed to fewer total photons than tissue on the entrance side (tube side), because a fraction of the photons will have been absorbed or scattered. However, the average or effective energy of the photons will be higher on the exit side of the beam.

At a particular point in the section being scanned, the average photon energy that the point "sees" will vary for different ray paths. When the point is closer to the exit side of a ray, it will "see" a beam with relatively high average photon energy. When the point is closer to the entrance side of a ray, it will "see" a beam with a larger number of photons but with a lower average photon energy.

The value of the linear attenuation coefficient μ depends upon the incident photon energy. There is a different value of μ for different photon energies as well as for different types of tissues. The "average" value of the linear attenuation coefficient ($\bar{\mu}$) for a voxel is a composite value which depends upon the energy distribution of the photons in the beam (i.e., the energy spectrum of the beam). When the energy spectrum is altered, $\bar{\mu}$ will be changed. Hence the data or ray measurements are inconsistent at any point in regard to a measurement of $\bar{\mu}$, because $\bar{\mu}$ will have been measured at different effective energies.

Beam hardening can be reduced, but not eliminated, by filtering the beam, that is, selectively removing the lower-energy components with aluminum or copper filtration. There is a practical limit to the amount of filtration that may be performed, however, because the total energy flux or x-ray output is reduced, and this increases noise. Also the loss of lower-energy photons reduces the contrast discrimination.

One artifact that can result from beam hardening is cupping. This describes the apparent increase in density of a uniform (constant density) object around its periphery. This happens because rays passing through the periphery of an object of uniform density will pass through a shorter tissue or material path than rays traveling through the center of the object. Therefore, these peripheral rays will be less attenuated and experience less hardening. Because they are less hard (i.e., have relatively more low energy photons), however, the amount of attenuation per unit path length will be greater than in central rays. Therefore, the attenuation coefficients through the object will appear to be greater in the periphery. This has been illustrated in Figures 2.49 and 2.50.

The cupping artifact is relatively correctable by the use of techniques described earlier (linearization) and is not usually seen clinically. This correction, however, must be changed with the energy spectrum, or, equivalently, the x-ray tube kilovoltage, and the filtration. This may be one reason why many manufacturers may limit the available selection of tube kVp and filtration.

Beam hardening has its most dramatic impact in bone. Unlike soft tissues, where the attenuation at the tube kilovoltages used in CT is almost entirely due to Compton scattering, there is a significant photoelectric absorption contribution to x-ray attenuation in bone. The linear attenuation coefficient for bone shows a much greater variation with energy for bone than for soft tissues, because of the presence of the photoelectric interaction in bone. The probability for the photoelectric effect to occur varies as the inverse cube of the photon energy (Equation 2.4), above the threshold energy necessary for the effect to take place. The linearizing function that is sufficient for soft tissues is inadequate for bone.

Bone artifacts are generally of two types: 1) some residual cupping of CT numbers just inside the skull, and 2) lucent streaks in tissues between pairs of bones. The former artifact may be especially prom-

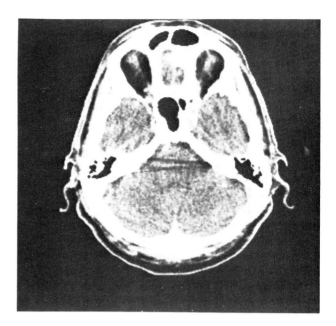

Figure A1.11. Interpetrous artifact. The lucent streaks between the petrous pyramids arise from beam hardening effects, although there may be other contributions such as edge gradient effects.

inent in the apex of the skull (DiChiro et al., 1978). The latter artifact is typified by the lucent artifacts seen between the ridges of the petrous pyramids (Figure A1.11).

Several approaches have been listed by Joseph (1981) to eliminate bone artifacts. In approximate order of decreasing difficulty, these include: 1) a modification of the line spread function of the algorithm, 2) the use of a water bath, 3) application of a postreconstruction correction algorithm, and 4) dual energy scanning, which has been described in Chapter 9.

PARTIAL VOLUME EFFECTS

Some description of partial volume effect has been given earlier in Chapter 2. These effects occur when the shape of an object changes within the thickness of the CT section or when an object occupies only a portion of the thickness of a section. Under either of these circumstances the attenuation coefficient or CT number of the object in that slice will be represented incorrectly. In fact, the representation will be an average of the object and the surrounding tissue in the voxel of interest. Even a small amount of bone or calcium intruding into or included within voxels in a slice will markedly increase the CT numbers of the affected voxels.

The partial volume effect may contribute to difficulties or errors in making accurate measurements of the size of an object, along with the point spread error described earlier. This may occur if the axis of the object is not perpendicular to the plane of the section, or if the dimensions of the object vary within the thickness of the section. In either case, the object does not completely fill a voxel. As an example, the curvilinear contour of the skull gives the false impression that the more cephalad portions of the skull, which are obliquely oriented relative to the scan planes, are thicker than the more caudad portions, which are more perpendicular to the scan sections (Figure A1.12).

Objects with sharp borders or edges oriented obliquely to the scan plane may suffer from the apparent loss of these sharp borders. For example, the borders of portions of the lateral ventricles are curved and obliquely oriented relative to the scan plane, so that there may appear to be a more gradual change in density between the ventricles and brain parenchyma on certain scans. Therefore, relatively abrupt borders or edges may be better appreciated on scans perpendicular to the borders, assuming that there are

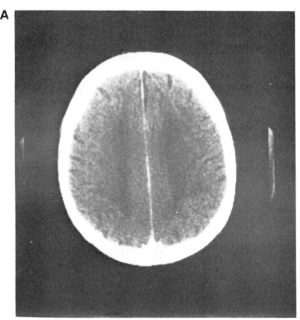

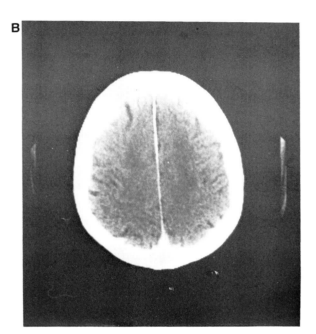

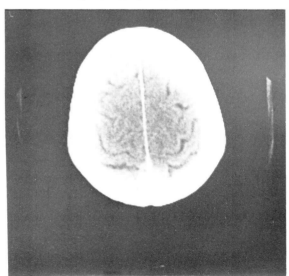

Figure A1.12. The skull appears thicker on successively more cephalad scans (*A* through *C*) because the orientation of the bone becomes more oblique and less perpendicular to the scan section.

not other artifacts associated with the borders. Usually, however, artifacts at sharp edges are more likely when bone or air are involved, rather than fluid and tissue. An analogy in conventional radiography occurs based on the law of tangents (Chapter 1), where border-forming shadows are identified by rays that are tangent to the borders.

The partial volume effect may also interfere with the accurate measurement of the CT number of an object if the voxel or voxels in which the measurement is made include other material or tissue. This may be particularly bothersome for smaller objects, which may not occupy the full thickness of a section.

This may occur if the dimension of the object along the direction perpendicular to the sections is less than the section thickness. It may also occur if the dimension of the object along this direction is greater than one section thickness but less than two section thicknesses, and the object lies partly in two adjacent sections. Partial volume effects on measurements of CT numbers may be minimized by the use of thin sections and by the selection for measurement of a section that lies in the center of the object. This is illustrated in Figure A1.13.

The Hounsfield partial volume effect discussed earlier in this appendix is a form of partial volume

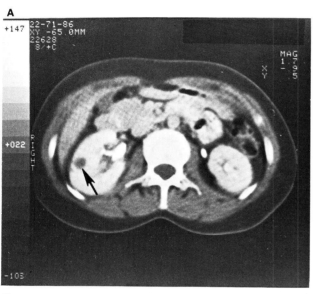
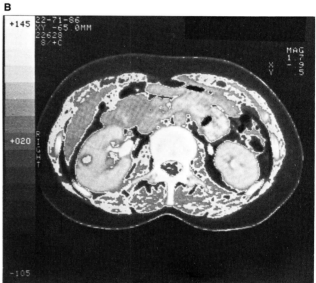
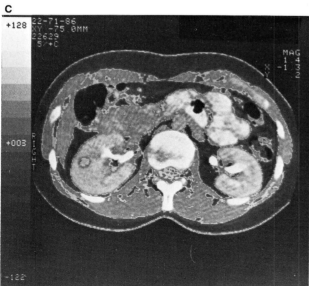

Figure A1.13. Partial volume effect. *A*, a small, apparently cystic mass (arrow) is present in the right kidney in a 1-cm thick scan. *B*, using the blinker function, the CT number is identified as +020 EMI units. *C*, a 0.5-cm thin scan through the middle of the cyst identifies the CT number of the cyst as +003.

effect occurring in 180° scanners, in which streaks are generated when the plane of the x-ray beam is not parallel to the plane of rotation. This is really a geometric artifact that can be eliminated by overscanning.

Joseph (1981) has also described a nonlinear partial volume effect which results in the occurrence of streaks in all scanners, including 360° scanners, as a result of attenuation measurements that are nonlinear. This nonlinear partial volume effect in a single bone will merely distribute an attenuation measurement error over different view angles. However, a pair of partial volume effects, as in the ridges of the petrous pyramids, results in an interactive effect. The nonlinear errors are superimposed in a synergistic fashion along the rays between the pair of partial bone volume effects, leading to streaks. This type of error probably contributes to the interpetrous lucency (Figure A1.11). The effect can be reduced by decreasing the number of bony structures that only partially occupy the scan section. This can be done by decreasing the section thickness.

VISUAL ILLUSIONS

The information on a CT image, or on a conventional radiograph, is displayed in the form of shapes or borders and in shades of gray. The viewer's perception of the specific level or shade of a gray tone is influenced by the surrounding background. Areas having the same gray tone level (or, equivalently, the identical density) may appear to be of different gray shades when their backgrounds are different.

There is a physiological reason for this phenomenon. It is based on the process of lateral inhibition produced by neural networks in the eye. In lateral inhibition, stimulation of a receptor in the retina of the eye lowers the rate of response of adjacent receptors.

There is an analogy to this phenomenon in conventional radiography. It is the Mach effect, originally described by the Viennese physicist Ernst Mach (1838–1916) in 1865. Mach described a visual phenomenon known now as Mach bands, which are caused by the presence of adjacent areas of different contrast. This effect is seen in conventional radiography as distinct narrow lines (often appearing lucent and simulating fracture lines) or edge enhancement and has been described by Lane et al. (1976).

In CT the phenomenon has been called the background contrast effect. The apparent gray tone of an object becomes dependent on the density of the adjacent or background structures. Thus, the shading of the object may appear altered. This effect in CT has been described by Daffner (1979).

REFERENCES AND SUGGESTED READINGS

Alfidi, R. J., MacIntyre, W. J., and Haaga, J. R. The effects of biological motion on CT resolution. American Journal of Roentgenology 127:11–15, 1976.

Brooks, R. A. and DicChiro, G. Beam hardening in x-ray reconstructive tomography. Physics in Medicine and Biology 21:390–398, 1976.

Brooks, R. A., Weiss, G. A., and Talbert, A. J. A new approach to interpolation in computed tomography. Journal of Computer Assisted Tomography 2:577–585, 1978.

Brooks, R. A., Glover, G. H., Talbert, A. J., Eisner, R. L., and DiBianca, F. A. Aliasing: A source of streaks in computed tomograms. Journal of Computer Assisted Tomography 3:511–518, 1979.

Bydder, G. M., and Kreel, L. Linear non-movement artifacts on an EMI CT 5005 body scanner. The Journal of Computed Tomography 4:29–36, 1980.

Chesler, D. A., and Riederer, S. J. Ripple suppression during reconstruction in transverse tomography. Physics in Medicine and Biology 20:632–636, 1975.

Daffner, R. H. Visual illusions in computed tomography: Phenomena related to Mach effect. American Journal of Roentgenology 134:261–264, 1980.

Di Chiro, G., Brooks, R. A., Dubal, L., and Chew, E. The optical artifact: Elevated attenuation values toward the apex of the skull. Journal of Computer Assisted Tomography 2:65–70, 1978.

Duerinckx, A. J., and Macovski, A. Polychromatic streak artifacts in computed tomography images. Journal of Computer Assisted Tomography 2:481–487, 1978.

Duerinckx, A. J., and Macovski, A. Nonlinear polychromatic and noise artifacts in x-ray computed tomography images. Journal of Computer Assisted Tomography 3:519–526, 1979.

Franklin, E., McCullough, E. C. and Frank, D. A. Fact or artifact: An analysis of artifact in high-resolution computed tomographic scanning of the sella. Radiology 140:109–113, 1981.

Gado, M., and Phelps, M. The peripheral zone of increased density in cranial computed tomography. Radiology 117:71–74, 1975.

Glover, G., and Pelc, N. Non-linear partial volume artifacts in x-ray computed tomography. Medical Physics 7:238–248, 1980.

Goodenough, D. J., Weaver, K. E., and Davis, D. O. Potential artifacts associated with the scanning pattern of the EMI scanner. Radiology 117:615–620, 1975.

Herman, G. T. Correction for beam hardening in computed tomography. Physics in Medicine and Biology 24:81–106, 1979.

Herman, G. T. Demonstration of beam hardening correction in computed tomography of the head. Journal of Computer Assisted Tomography 3:373–378, 1979.

Hounsfield, G. N. Picture quality of computed tomography. American Journal of Roentgenology 127:3–9, 1976.

Joseph, P. M., and Spital, R. D. A method for correcting bone induced artifacts in computed tomography scanners. Journal of Computer Assisted Tomography 2:100–108, 1978.

Joseph, P. M., Spital, R. D., and Stockham, C. D. The effects of sampling in CT images. Computerized Tomography 4:189–206, 1980.

Joseph, P. M., Hilal, S. K., Schulz, R. A., and Kelcz, F. Clinical and experimental investigation of a smoothed CT reconstruction algorithm. Radiology 134:507–516, 1980.

Joseph, P. M. Artifacts in computed tomography. In T. H. Newton and D. G. Potts, Eds., *Radiology of the Skull and Brain*, Part XVI, General Theory of Computed Tomography, Vol. 5, Technical Aspects of Computed Tomography, Chapter 114, pp. 3956–3992. C. V. Mosby, St. Louis, 1981.

Kijewski, P. K., and Bjarngard, B. E. Correction for beam hardening in computed tomography. Medical Physics 5:209–216, 1978.

Koehler, P. R., Anderson, R. E., and Baxter, B. The effect of computed tomography viewer controls on anatomical measurements. Radiology 130:189–194, 1979.

Kowalski, G., and Wagner, W. Artifacts in CT pictures. Medicamundi 22:13–17, 1977.

Kricheff, I. I., and Lin, J. P. Pitfalls in CT of the head. In P. Gerhardt and E. van Kaick, Eds., *Total Body Computerized Tomography, International Symposium, Heidelberg, 1977.* Georg Thieme, Stuttgart, pp. 46–52, 1979.

Lane, E. J., Proto, A. V., and Phillips, T. W. Mach bands and density perception. Radiology 12:9–17, 1976.

McCullough, E. C., Payne, J. T., Baker, H. L., Hattery, R. R., Sheedy, P. F., Stephens, D. H., and Gedgaudas, E. Performance evaluation and quality assurance of computed tomography scanners, with illustrations from the EMI, ACTA, and Delta scanners. Radiology 120:173–178, 1976.

McCullough, E. C. Factors affecting the use of quantitative information from a CT scanner. Radiology 124:99–107, 1977.

McDavid, W. D., Waggener, R. G., Payne, W. H., and Dennis, M. J. Correction for spectral artifacts in cross-sectional reconstruction from x-rays. Medical Physics 4:54–57, 1977.

Morin, R. L. and Raeside, D. E. A pattern recognition method for the removal of streaking artifact in computed tomography. Radiology 141:229–233, 1981.

New, P. F. J., and Scott, W. R. Physical considerations in computed tomography, *In Computed Tomography of the Brain and Orbit (EMI Scanning)*, Chapter 4, pp. 35–53, Williams & Wilkins, Baltimore, 1975.

Rao, P. S., and Alfidi, R. J. The environmental density artifact: A beam-hardening effect in computed tomography. Radiology 141:223–227, 1981.

Ruegsegger, P., Hangartner, T., Keller, H. U., and Hinderling, T. Standardization of computed tomographic images by means of a material-selective beam hardening correction. Journal of Computer Assisted Tomography 2:184–188, 1978.

Stockham, C. D. A simulation study of aliasing in computed tomography. Radiology 132:721–726, 1979.

Zatz, L. M. Image quality in cranial computed tomography. Journal of Computer Assisted Tomography 2:336–346, 1978.

APPENDIX II
MATHEMATICS OF RECONSTRUCTION

SIMPLE BACK-PROJECTION

ITERATIVE RECONSTRUCTION

ANALYTICAL RECONSTRUCTION
  Fourier Reconstruction
  Relationship to Simple Back-Projection
  Filtered Back-Projection
    Fourier Filtering
    Radon Filtering
    Convolution Filtering

REFERENCES AND SUGGESTED READINGS

The approach described below closely follows that of Brooks and Di Chiro (1976).

Every point of an object within a section to be reconstructed can be defined by its x,y coordinates in a Cartesian system. The contribution of every point to a detected signal is designated by the density function $f(x,y)$. For x-ray tomography, in particular transmission computed tomography, $f(x,y)$ represents the actual linear attenuation coefficient μ or $\mu(x,y)$. For radioisotope imaging, in particular emission computed tomography, $f(x,y)$ is proportional to the density or emissions of radioisotopes. The more general terminology employing the density function $f(x,y)$ is used in this appendix, where it is understood that in transmission computed tomography the density function $f(x,y)$ is the linear attenuation coefficient $\mu(x,y)$.

Each individual x-ray, or ray, is theoretically a line with no width or cross-sectional area. Each ray is best specified in terms of its own coordinate (r,ϕ), where the x-ray coordinate system is superimposed over the object's Cartesian system so that ϕ is the angle of the ray with respect to the y axis and r is its distance from the origin. This is illustrated in Figure A1.1. The s coordinate illustrated in Figure A2.1 represents distance along the ray. The path of each ray is designated as a ray-path.

The integral of $f(x,y)$ along a ray (r,ϕ) is called the ray-sum p:

$$p(r,\phi) = \int_{r,\phi} f(x,y)\, ds . \quad (A2.1)$$

The transmitted x-ray beam intensity I is given by:

$$I = I_0 \exp\left[- \int \mu(x,y)\, ds \right], \quad (A2.2)$$

where I_0 is the intensity of the incident beam. Substituting $\mu(x,y)$ for $f(x,y)$ in Equation A2.1:

$$p = -\ln\left(\frac{I}{I_0}\right) . \quad (A2.3)$$

Thus, the ray-sum is proportional to the logarithm of the detector signal.

A projection (view or profile) is the complete set of ray-sums at a particular angle (as defined for first and second generation units using a combined translational-rotational motion).

The x-ray coordinate system may be related to the object Cartesian coordinate system:

$$r = x \cos \phi + y \sin \phi . \quad (A2.4)$$

Theoretically, $f(x,y)$ is a continuously variable two-dimensional function, which requires an infinite number of projections for exact reconstruction. In practice, $f(x,y)$ is calculated for a finite number of

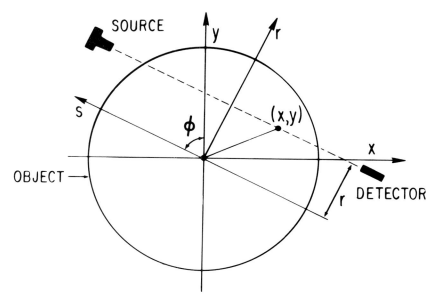

Figure A2.1. Coordinate systems. A point is designated by its coordinates (x,y) in a fixed Cartesian coordinate system. A ray, as indicated by a *dashed line*, is described by its angle, ϕ, with respect to the y-axis and its distance, r, from the origin. The coordinates indicate the distance along the ray.

discrete points from a limited number of projections. If reconstruction is limited to a circular region or domain of diameter d within the section and the points are regularly separated by a distance w, there are $n = d/w$ points along the diameter. The section may be divided squares, each of dimension w. The individual squares are picture elements for reconstruction, or pixels. A total of m projections can be assumed to be equally spaced from 0° to 180°, each projection consisting of n ray-sums at intervals w.

Purely rotational units will differ in their definition of a projection and in the manner in which data are collected.

SIMPLE BACK-PROJECTION

In simple back-projection, the relative reconstructed density $f(x,y)$, or the relative value of the linear attenuation coefficient $\mu(x,y)$ for any particular image point in relationship to its value at other image points, is the sum of all ray-sums passing through it (actually, each ray-sum is first divided by the number of elements or pixels in the corresponding ray, but no error will be introduced in using the above simplification).

This is described by the equation:

$$\hat{f}(x,y) = \sum_{j=1}^{m} p(r_j,\phi_j)\, \Delta\phi, \qquad (A2.5)$$

where ϕ_j is the jth projection angle, $\Delta\phi = \dfrac{\pi}{m}$ is the angular distance between projections, and the summation is performed over all m projections. The symbol $\hat{f}$ denotes the relative value of the density function, not its absolute or true value; that is, the relative value of $f(x_1,y_1)$ at the point (x_1,y_1) compared to $f(x_2,y_2)$ at the point (x_2,y_2).

Using Equation A2.4:

$$\hat{f}(x,y) = \sum_{j=1}^{m} p(x \cos \phi_j + y \sin \phi_j, \phi_j)\, \Delta\phi \qquad (A2.6)$$

The factor $x \cos \phi_j + y \sin \phi_j$ selects only those rays passing through the point (x,y) so that the back-projected value of f at each point is simply the sum of all ray-sums passing through the point. This is why back-projection is also called the summation method.

Simple back-projection was first used for medical imaging by Oldendorf (1961) and later by Kuhl and Edwards (1963).

ITERATIVE RECONSTRUCTION

The mathematical problem in image reconstruction is the solution of Equation A2.1 for the density function $f(x,y)$, expressed in transmission computed tomography as the linear attenuation coefficient $\mu(x,y)$.

Spatial resolution must be limited in the image reconstruction in order to avoid processing an infinite amount of data.

To limit the amount of projection data, each projection is divided into strips as shown in Figure A2.2. Each strip corresponds to a ray-path, but the strip has a finite width w, unlike the ray, which is ideally only a line or linear path. Practically, the term "ray" may be extended to include what is really a strip. Each projection is divided into $n = d/w$ strips, where d is the diameter of the area to be reconstructed. Each strip in the circular domain of reconstruction of diameter d has up to n square-shaped cells where $n = d/w$. The density function or linear attenuation coefficient of the ith cell is f_i.

The contribution of the ith cell to the jth ray is the weighting factor w_{ij}. Therefore, Equation A2.1 becomes:

$$p_j = \sum_{i=1}^{N} w_{ij} f_i, \qquad (A2.7)$$

where p_j is the jth ray-sum. This is the approach originally used by Hounsfield (1973). Most of the weighting factors are zero, since only a small number of cells contribute to a particular ray.

In iteration, a series of corrections are applied to an initial arbitrary set of values for the density functions to achieve a reasonable approximation to the measured values of the ray-sums in each projection.

The method works in the following way. First, an arbitrary set of initial values is chosen for the density functions, for example, a constant density "gray screen." By using these initial values, ray-sums are calculated and compared to the measured values. If a calculated ray-sum is smaller than the corresponding measured value, the density of each cell within that strip or ray can be decreased by the appropriate amount. After this has been performed for all the cells and all the rays, the first iteration is complete. This procedure can be repeated until a satisfactory agreement with the experimental data is obtained.

The process is described by the equation:

$$f_i^t = f_i^{t-1} + \sum_{j=1}^{M} \Delta f_{ij}^t, \qquad (A2.8)$$

where f_i^{t-1} is the ith coefficient before the iteration, f_i^t is the coefficient after iteration, and Δf_{ij}^t is the correction applied to the ith cell from the jth ray.

The difference between this method and that of simple back-projection is that the quantities being back-projected in Equation A2.8 are actually correction terms derived from the projections, not the projections themselves, and these corrections are added to the previous values.

If the initial set of density functions is made equal to 1, that is, a blank screen, the first iteration is identical to simple back-projection.

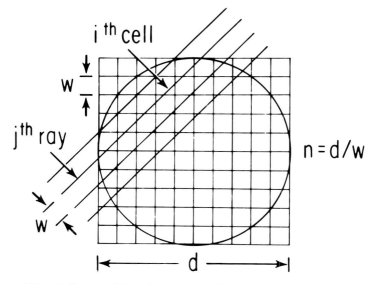

Figure A2.2. A diagram of the cellular array used in iteractive reconstruction. A circle with a diameter d lies within a square with width d. The large square is subdivided into square cells, each with width w. There are a total of $n = d/w$ cells along a diameter of the circle. The contribution of the ith cell to the jth ray is the weighting factor w_{ij}.

The iterative methods are classified by the sequence in which corrections are made and incorporated into an iteration. In the simplest approach, simultaneous correction, all projections are calculated at the beginning of the iteration and corrections are made simultaneously to all cells. The corrections are not incorporated until the end of the iteration. In a point-by-point correction, each point, or cell, is corrected for all rays passing through it. Other points are then handled the same way, except that corrections made during the iteration are included in successive calculations. In ray-by-ray correction (used by Hounsfield in the original version of the early EMI Mark I scanner), a given ray-sum is calculated and corrections are applied to all cells in the ray. This is repeated for successive strips or rays, including the previous correction in each new calculation.

ANALYTICAL RECONSTRUCTION

Analytical reconstruction is based on an exact solution of Equation A2.1. To do this, it is again necessary to limit the spatial resolution of the image. This is done by band limiting. The image will contain no spatial frequencies (wave numbers) greater than a maximum frequency $k_m = \dfrac{2\pi}{m}$.

There are three consequences of band limiting: 1) the image can be reconstructed on an array of cells with spacing w where

$$w = \tfrac{1}{2} k_m ; \qquad (A2.9)$$

2) the projections may be sampled at the same interval w; and 3) Fourier transforms may be replaced by discrete Fourier series. Band limiting is the only approximation that is required for analytical image reconstruction.

It was Cormack (1963) who performed the first analytical reconstruction of an x-ray image, although his particular method of analytical reconstruction is not the one currently used.

Fourier Reconstruction

The starting point for an analytical reconstruction is to express the density function (or linear attenuation coefficient) as a two-dimensional Fourier integral:

$$f(x,y) = \int_{-\infty}^{\infty} \int_{-\infty}^{\infty} F(k_x,k_y) \exp[2\pi i(k_x x + k_y y)] \, dk_x dk_y . \qquad (A2.10)$$

In this form, $f(x,y)$ is expressed as a superposition of sinusoidal and cosinusoidal waves, represented by the complex exponential whose real and imaginary parts are cosine and sine functions, respectively. The variables k_x and k_y are the wave numbers ($2\pi/\lambda$) in the x and y directions.

The Fourier coefficients $F(k_x,k_y)$ are defined by the Fourier transform:

$$F(k_x,k_y) = \int_{-\infty}^{\infty} \int_{-\infty}^{\infty} f(x,y) \exp[-2\pi i(k_x x + k_y y)] \, dx dy . \qquad (A2.11)$$

Rotating the (x,y) axes to new axes (r,s), shown in Figure A2.1, where the angle of rotation is:

$$\phi = \tan^{-1}(k_x/k_y) \qquad (A2.12)$$

and

$$k = (k_x^2 + k_y^2)^{1/2} \qquad (A2.13)$$

results in

$$F(k_x,k_y) = \int_{-\infty}^{\infty} \int_{-\infty}^{\infty} f(x,y) \exp[-2\pi i k r] \, dr ds . \qquad (A2.14)$$

Exchanging the order of integration, it can be seen that the s integral is just the ray-sum $p(r,\phi)$ given by Equation A2.1, so that:

$$F(k_x,k_y) = \int_{-\infty}^{\infty} p(r,\phi) \exp[-2\pi i k r] \, dr = P(k,\phi) , \qquad (A2.15)$$

where $P(k,\phi)$ is the Fourier transform of $p(r,\phi)$ with respect to r.

Equation A2.15 states that each Fourier coefficient or wave amplitude of the density function is equal to a corresponding Fourier coefficient of the projection taken at the same angle as the Fourier wave.

Interpolation is necessary because the Fourier coefficients obtained from the projections do not fall on a rectangular matrix, a requirement for the inverse two-dimensional transform. In theory, the interpolation can be done exactly with the sampling theorem; in practice, exact interpolation requires a great deal of computer time necessitating the use of alternative methods.

Relationship to Simple Back-Projection

The approximate reconstruction from simple back-projection may be related to the true image as follows. Equation A2.6 may be converted from a summation to an integral:

$$\hat{f}(x,y) = \int_{0}^{\pi} p(x \cos \phi + y \sin \phi, \phi) \, d\phi . \qquad (A2.16)$$

Replacing $p(x \cos \phi + y \sin \phi, \phi) = p(r,\phi)$ by its Fourier representation:

$$p(r,\phi) = \int_{-\infty}^{\infty} P(k,\phi) \exp(2\pi ikr)\, dk \quad (A2.17)$$

gives

$$\hat{f}(x,y) = \int_0^{\pi} \int_{-\infty}^{\infty} \frac{P(k,\phi)}{|k|} \exp[2\pi ik(x \cos \phi + y \sin \phi)] |k|\, dk d\phi, \quad (A2.18)$$

where the integrand has been multiplied and divided by $|k|$, the magnitude of the spatial frequency or the wave number, so that the right side is expressed in the form of a two-dimensional Fourier integral in polar coordinates. Taking the two-dimensional Fourier transform of Equation A2.18 and using Equation A2.15:

$$\hat{F}(k_x,k_y) = \frac{P(k,\phi)}{|k|} = \frac{F(k_x,k_y)}{|k|}, \quad (A2.19)$$

where $\hat{F}(k_x,k_y)$, the Fourier coefficients of the simple back-projections, are equal to the exact Fourier coefficients $F(k_x,k_y)$ of the true image divided by the magnitude of the spatial frequency $|k|$.

Filtered Back-Projection

A significant implication of Equation A2.19 is that back-projection may be feasible if the projections are modified appropriately, or filtered, prior to being back-projected. This is the basis for filtered back-projection. Three different but mathematically equivalent filter formulae have been used for filtered back-projection.

Fourier Filtering Equation A2.10 is rewritten in polar coordinates:

$$f(x,y) = \int_0^{\pi} \int_{-\infty}^{\infty} F(k_x,k_y) \exp[2\pi ik(x \cos \phi + y \sin \phi)] |k|\, dk d\phi, \quad (A2.20)$$

where ϕ and k have been defined in Equations A2.12 and A2.13, respectively. The value of k is allowed to range from $-\infty$ to ∞ so that the inner integral takes the form of a one-dimensional Fourier transform; ϕ must then have integration limits 0 to π. Using Equation A2.15 and replacing $F(k_x,k_y)$ with $P(k,\phi)$,

$$f(x,y) = \int_0^{\pi} P^*(x \cos \phi + y \sin \phi, \phi)\, d\phi, \quad (A2.21)$$

where

$$p^*(r,\phi) = \int_{-\infty}^{\infty} |k| P(k,\phi) \exp(2\pi ikr)\, dk. \quad (A2.22)$$

In practice, a summation is used.

$$f(x,y) = \sum_{j=1}^{m} p^*(x \cos \phi_j + y \sin \phi_j, \phi_j)\, \Delta\phi, \quad (A2.23)$$

where m is equal to the number of projections and $\Delta\phi$ is the interval between projections.

Equation A2.23 is similar to Equation A2.6, except that p^*, not p, is being back-projected. The use of p^* rather than p represents a filtering process by which the high frequency components are increased in proportion to their wave numbers. The result is a biphasic function with average value of zero. However p^*, unlike p, is not spatially bounded and cannot be expressed as a Fourier series.

Two approximations are needed to implement filtered back-projection. One is the substitution of a discrete sum for the integral over ϕ, that is, going from Equations A2.22 to A2.23. The other occurs because, for a specific projection angle, p^* is only calculated at a finite number of discrete points, not all along r. Approximate methods are generally used such as choosing the nearest value of p^* (nearest neighbor) or linear interpolation between the two closest values.

Radon Filtering There is a convolution theorem which states that the Fourier transform of a product is equal to the convolution of the individual Fourier transforms. Equation A2.22 represents the Fourier transform of the product of two functions $|k|$ and $P(k,\phi)$. The Fourier transform of $P(k,\phi)$ is $p(r,\phi)$; the Fourier transform of $|k|$ is $-1/(2\pi^2 r^2)$. Applying the convolution theorem to Equation A2.22, one obtains:

$$p^*(r,\phi) = -\frac{1}{2\pi^2} \int_{-\infty}^{\infty} \frac{p(r',\phi)}{(r-r')^2}\, dr'. \quad (A2.24)$$

This can be transformed into:

$$p^*(r,\phi) = \frac{1}{2\pi^2} \int_{-\infty}^{\infty} \frac{\partial p(r',\phi)/\partial r'}{r - r'}\, dr'. \quad (A2.25)$$

Equation A2.25 describes the filtering process as a single convolutional integral in which the derivatives of p are added together, weighted by the inverse distance from the point at which the filtered value is desired.

Equation A2.25, as well as Equation A2.21, were initially derived by Radon in order to solve gravitational problems.

Convolution Filtering There is a divergence in Equation A2.24 caused by the factor $|k|$ in Equation A2.22. The divergence can be avoided if $|k|$ is replaced by a function equal to $|k|$ for $|k| \leq k_m$ but

Appendix II   295

zero for $|k| > k_m$. The Fourier transform of the cutoff version of $|k|$ is

$$\int_{-k_m}^{k_m} |k| \exp(2\pi i k r)\, dk$$

$$= \frac{k_m}{\pi r} \sin(2\pi k_m r) - \frac{\sin^2(\pi k_m r)}{\pi^2 r^2}. \quad (A2.26)$$

Replacing $|k|$ in Equation A2.22 by its cutoff version and applying the convolution theorem,

$$p^*(r,\phi) = \int_{-\infty}^{\infty} p(r',\phi) \left(\frac{k_m \sin[2\pi k_m(r-r')]}{\pi(r-r')} - \frac{\sin^2[\pi k_m(r-r')]}{\pi^2(r-r')^2} \right) dr'. \quad (A2.27)$$

This may be simplified to:

$$p^*(r,\phi) = k_m p(r,\phi)$$
$$- \int_{-\infty}^{\infty} p(r',\phi) \left(\frac{\sin^2[k_m(r-r')]}{\pi^2(r-r')^2} \right) dr' \quad (A2.28)$$

where $p(r,\phi)$ is the measured profile, $p^*(r,\phi)$ is the modified profile, and k_m is the greatest spatial frequency or wave number present in the projection. Equation A2.28 has the form of a convolution integral, thus giving the name to this filter.

Equation A2.28 may be simplified for implementation. Because the integrand only contains frequencies up to k_m, it can be replaced by a summation with spacing of points at intervals $w = 1/2k_m$. Also, $\sin^2[\pi k_m(r-r')]$ is either zero or 1, depending upon whether $k_m(r-r')$ is an even or odd multiple of w. Therefore, Equation A2.28 can be rewritten as:

$$p^*(r_i) = \frac{p(r_i)}{4w} - \frac{1}{\pi^2 w} \sum_{j=1,\text{odd}}^{n} \frac{p(r_j)}{(i-j)^2}, \quad (A2.29)$$

with the summation performed over all j where $i - j$ is odd. This results in a relatively simple and fast computer program.

Convolution filtering is more accurate than Radon filtering and does not require derivatives. It is faster than Radon filtering, because only every other point is needed in the convolution integral, but not as fast as Fourier filtering.

The convolution method was first derived by Bracewell (1956). It was initially applied to radiological imaging by Ramachandran and Lakshminarayanan (1971) and later by Shepp and Logan (1974). It was used in the first body CT scanner, the ACTA, by Ledley et al. (1974). It is believed that most commercial CT units use this method.

REFERENCES AND SUGGESTED READINGS

Bracewell, R. N. Strip integration in radio astronomy. Australian Journal of Physics 9:198–217, 1956.

Brooks, R. A., and Di Chiro, G. Theory of image reconstruction in computed tomography. Radiology 117:561–572, 1975.

Brooks, R. A., and Di Chiro, G. Principles of computer assisted tomography (CAT) in radiographic and radioisotopic imaging. Physics in Medicine and Biology 21:689–732, 1976.

Cormack, A. M. Representation of a function by its line integrals, with some radiological applications. Journal of Applied Physics 34:2722–2727, 1963.

Herman, G. T. Advanced principles of reconstruction algorithms. In T. H. Newton and D. G. Potts (eds.), Radiology of the Skull and Brain: Technical Aspects of Computed Tomography, Vol. 5. Chap. 110. Part XVI. Sec. II. pp. 3888–3903. C. V. Mosby Company, St. Louis, 1981.

Hounsfield, G. N. Computerized transverse axial scanning (tomography): I. Description of system. British Journal of Radiology 46:1016–1022, 1973.

Kuhl, D. E., and Edwards, R. Q. Image separation radioisotope scanning. Radiology 80:653–661, 1963.

Ledley, R. S. Introduction to computerized tomography. Computers in Biology and Medicine 6:239–246, 1976.

Ledley, R. S., Di Chiro, G., Luessenhop, A. J., and Twigg, H. L. Computerized transaxial x-ray tomography of the human body. Science 186:207–212, 1974.

Macovski, A. Basic concepts of reconstruction algorithms. In T. H. Newton and D. G. Potts (eds.), Radiology of the Skull and Brain: Technical Aspects of Computed Tomography, Vol. 5, Chap. 110, Part XVI, Sect. I, pp. 3877–3887. C. V. Mosby Company, St. Louis, 1981.

Oldendorf, W. H. Isolated flying spot detection of radiodensity discontinuities—displaying the internal structural pattern of a complex object. IEEE Transactions on Biomedical Electronics, Vol. BMW 8:68–77, 1961.

Radon, J. On the determination of functions from their integrals along certain manifolds. Berichte über die Verhandlungen der königlich Sächsischen Gesellschaft der Wissenschaften zu Leipzig. Mathematisch-Physiche Klasse 69:262–277, 1917.

Ramachandran, G. N., and Lakshminarayanan, A. V. Three-dimensional reconstruction from radiographs and electron micrographs: Applications of convolutions instead of Fourier transforms. Proceedings of the National Academy of Science 68:2236–2240, 1971.

Shepp, L. A., and Logan, B. F. The Fourier reconstruction of a head section. IEEE Transactions on Nuclear Science NS-21 (3)21–43, 1974.

Appendix III
Comparative Features of CT Units

APPENDIX III
COMPARATIVE FEATURES

Company and model	Total body or head only	Generation of scan geometry[a]	Detector type; number	Scan time (s)	Image reconstruction time (s)	Gantry aperture diameter (cm)	Reconstruction diameter (cm)
ACTA 0100	Body	1	CaF_2 crystals with photomultiplier tubes (PMTs); 2 (1 per slice)	300–360	Head: both slices available immediately after scanning; Body: first slice available immediately after scanning; second slice available 300 s later	55	24 (head); 48 (body)
American Scientific and Engineering AS&E CT scanner (later Pfizer 0500)	Body	4	BGO crystals with photomultipliers; 600	5, 10, 20	60	65	24, 48
Compagnie Generale de Radiologie (CGR) CE 10000	Body	3	Xenon cells (26 atm pressure); 1,024 data + 11 reference	3.4, 6.8, 13.6	0.0 and 4.0 (256 matrix); 20.0, 40.0, and 80.0 (512 matrix)	52	52
Elscint Exel 905	Body	2	BGO crystals with photo multipliers; 52	5.3–50 with 2-s option	4 (head); 15 (body)	50	14.0–48.0
Exel 1002	Body	Combined 2 and 3	$CdWO_4$ with photodiodes; 280	1.8, 5, 10, 15, 22	4 (head); 15 (body)	50	14.0, 25.0, 33.0, 42.0, 48.0
EMI Mark I	Head	1	NaI crystals with PMTs; 2 data (1 per slice) + 1 reference	300, 390	30 s after scan (both slices)	23 (water box)	22.2
CT 1005	Head	2	NaI crystals with PMTs; 16 data (8 per slice) + 1 reference	60–240	35	25.6	24

CaF_2, calcium fluoride; BGO, bismuth germanate; NaI, sodium iodide; CsI, cesium iodide; $CdWO_4$, cadmium tungstate.

[a] Definitions of scan geometry generations are given in Chapters 2 and 3.

OF CT UNITS

Slice thickness (mm)	Gantry tilt (deg)	Views	Readings per view	Angle of rotation (deg)	Tube	Matrix	Slices per scan
7.5	+20 to −10	180	160, 320	180	Stationary anode, continuous	160 × 160 (head); 256 × 320 (body)	2
2–10	±20	600	255 (5 s), 511 (10 s), 1,023 (20 s)	400	Rotating anode, continuous	256 × 256; 512 × 512	1
5.0 or 10.0	±20	500+ at 3.4 s	1,024	360	Rotating anode, continuous	256 × 256; 512 × 512	1
5, 8, 12 at 3 or 1 mm resolution	Bed tilts +20 to −50; bed swivels on floor ±12; gantry tilt option for ±20	52 detectors × 5 translations or 260 views	512 (data samples per detector per translation, or per view)	180	Stationary anode, continuous	256	1
1.5, 3, 6, 10	Gantry tilts ±20; bed swivels ±12	1395 (2); 391 (3)		180	Stationary anode, continuous	256 × 256 (opt); 512 × 512; 340 × 340	1
8, 13	0	180, 225	160, 240	180, 225	Stationary anode, continuous	80 × 80; 160 × 160	2
8	0	480	480	180, 240	Stationary anode, continuous	160 × 160	2

Appendix III

Appendix III

(Continued)

Company and model	Total body or head only	Generation of scan geometry[a]	Detector type; number	Scan time (s)	Image reconstruction time (s)	Gantry aperture diameter (cm)	Reconstruction diameter (cm)
CT 1010	Head	2	NaI crystals with PMTs; 16 data (8 per slice) + 1 reference	60–240	24 (160 matrix); 270 (320 matrix)	25.6	21, 24
CT 5005	Body	2	NaI crystals with PMTs; 30 data + 1 reference	20–70	20 (160 matrix); 45 (320); 85 (320)	43	40, 32, 24, 16, 12 (opt)
CT 6000 (formerly Searle Pho/Trax 4000, now Omni 6000)	Body	3	Xenon cells (about 10 atm); 504	5, 10, 20, 40	<45 (360 views)	60	5–50 in increments of 1
EMI 7020	Body	2	NaI crystals with PMTs; 30 data + 1 reference	20, 60	20 (160); 45 (320); 85 (320)	43	12, 16, 24, 32, 40
EMI 7070 (Omni Quad I)	Body	4	CsI crystals with photodiodes; 1,088	3, 6, 9, 15, 30	<40 (320); <20 (160)	60	12, 25, 32, 40, 50
General Electric GE CT/T 7800	Body	3	Xenon cells (about 25 atm pressure); 289 data + 12 reference	4.8, 9.6	90–200	60	25, 35, 42
GE CT/T 8800	Body	3	Xenon cells (about 25 atm pressure); 511 data + 12 reference	2.8, 4.8, 5.7, 9.6	35	60	8–25, 35, 42
GE CT/T 8000 (7805)	Body	3	Xenon cells (about 25 atm pressure); 289 data + 12 reference	4.8, 9.6	35	60	8–25, 35, 42
GE CT/T 9800	Body	3	Xenon cells; 523	1.3–8	21–62	70	2.5–48
Interad WBS	Body	3	Xenon cells; 512	3, 6, 12	<60	62	5–50

CaF_2, calcium fluoride; BGO, bismuth germanate; NaI, sodium iodide; CsI, cesium iodide; $CdWO_4$, cadmium tungstate.

[a] Definitions of scan geometry generations are given in Chapters 2 and 3.

Slice thickness (mm)	Gantry tilt (deg)	Views	Readings per view	Angle of rotation (deg)	Tube	Matrix	Slices per scan
8, 4	0	480	480	180, 240	Stationary anode, continuous	160 × 160; 320 × 320	2
13, 5, 8 (opt)	0	540	600	180	Stationary anode, continuous	160 × 160; 320 × 320	1
3–12, in increments of 1	−10 to +20	360, 540	504	360	Stationary anode, continuous	256 × 256	1
5, 10, 13	NA	540	600	180	Stationary anode, continuous	160 × 160; 320 × 320	1
2–15, in increments of 1	+20 to −30; couch slew ±20°	1,088	1,324	360	Rotating anode, continuous	160 × 160; 320 × 320	1
1.5, 5, 10	±15	288 (4.8 s), 576 (9.6 s)	289	360	Rotating anode, pulsed	320 × 320	1
1.5, 5, 10	±15	288 (4.8 s), 576 (9.6 s), 342 (5.7 s)	511	360, 212	Rotating anode, pulsed	320 × 320	1
1.5, 5, 10	±15	288 (4.8 s), 576 (9.6 s)	289	360	Rotating anode, pulsed	320 × 320	1
1.5, 3, 5, 10	±20	1240–7880	742	360	Rotating anode, continuous	256 × 256; 320 × 320; 512 × 512	1
2, 5, 10	+15 to −25	360–720	512		Stationary anode, continuous	256 × 256	1

Appendix III

(Continued)

Company and model	Total body or head only	Generation of scan geometry[a]	Detector type; number	Scan time (s)	Image reconstruction time (s)	Gantry aperture diameter (cm)	Reconstruction diameter (cm)
Omni							
Omni 4001	Head	2	BGO crystals; 6 data (3 per slice) + 1 reference	120	5 s after scanning for 2 slices	33	25.6
Omni 6000 (formerly Searle Pho/Trax 4000 and EMI 6000, upgraded)	Body	3	Xenon cells; 504	5, 10, 20	45	60	5–50 in 1-cm increments
Omni Quad I (previously the EMI 7070)	Body	4 (nutating ring of detectors)	CsI crystals with photodiodes; 1,088	1.5, 3.0, 6.0	25	60	12, 22, 32, 45
Pfizer							
Pfizer 0200 FS	Body	2	CaF_2 crystals with PMTs; 30	19, 29	3–10	56	Nominal head, 25; body, 48 Variable, 7.5–48
Pfizer 0150: Repackage of ACTA 0100; updated gantry permitted ±20° tilt, mobile bed							
Pfizer/AS&E 0450	Body	4	BGO crystals with PMTs; 600	5, 10	35–60	66	Nominal head, 25; body, 48 Variable, 7.5–48
Pfizer PZ-2400	Body	4	$CdWO_4$ crystals; 2,400	2.5, 5, 10, 20	Variable to 60 s	68	Variable to 48 Nominal head, 25; body, 48
Philips							
Tomoscan 300	Body	3; Direct magnification (shift)	Xenon cells; 288	2.6, 4.2, 8.4	11, 21, 33	56	16, 24, 32, 40, 48
310	Body	3	Xenon cells; 576	3, 4.8, 9.6	10–45	56	3.0–48
Picker							
Synerview 120	Body	2	BGO crystals with PMTs; 41	12–60	15–25	44	25, 44

CaF_2, calcium fluoride; BGO, bismuth germanate; NaI, sodium iodide; CsI, cesium iodide; $CdWO_4$, cadmium tungstate.

[a] Definitions of scan geometry generations are given in Chapters 2 and 3.

Slice thickness (mm)	Gantry tilt (deg)	Views	Readings per view	Angle of rotation (deg)	Tube	Matrix	Slices per scan
4, 6, 8, 10	+10 to −15 and +5 to −20	60	1,530	180	Stationary anode, continuous	256 × 256	2
3–10 in 1-mm increments	−10 to +20	360, 540, 1,080	504	360	Stationary anode, continuous	256 × 256	1
2, 5, 10, 12	50 (from 30 to −20)	1,088	1,324	360	Rotating anode, continuous	320 × 320 (plus reconstruction zoom)	1
5, 8, 13	±20	270	256, 320 variable within a range of 160–488	180	Stationary anode, continuous	160 × 160; 256 × 256; 256 × 320	1
2–9, in increments of 1	±20 (bed)	600	599 (5 s); 1,199 (10 s)	360 + 11.25 overscan	Rotating anode, continuous	320 × 256; 256 × 256; 512 × 512; 640 × 512	1
2–10, increments of 1	+20 to −10	2,400	575–2,303 depending on mode	360 + 3 overscan	Rotating anode, continuous	512 × 512; 640 × 512	1
3, 6, 9, 12	±20	372 (2.6 s), 600 (4.2 s), 1,200 (8.4 s)	288	223 (2.6 s), 360 (4.2 s), 360 (8.4 s)	Rotating anode, pulsed	256 × 256	1
1.5, 3, 6, 9, 12	±20	370–1200	576		Rotating anode, pulsed	256 × 256	1
5, 10	0	40 detectors × 9 translations or 360 views	787 (data samples per detector per translation, or per view)	180	Stationary anode, continuous	256 × 256	1

Appendix III

(Continued)

Company and model	Total body or head only	Generation of scan geometry[a]	Detector type; number	Scan time (s)	Image reconstruction time (s)	Gantry aperture diameter (cm)	Reconstruction diameter (cm)
Synerview 300	Body	4	BGO crystals with PMTs; 360	1–20	30–45	60	24, 48, 5–48 in 1-cm increments
Synerview 600	Body	4	BGO crystals with PMTs; 600	1–20	30–45	60	24, 48, 5–48 in 1-cm increments
Synerview 600S	Body	4	CdWO$_4$ crystals with temperature-stabilized photodiodes; 600	1–20	12–25	60	12, 24, 48; 6–48 cm in 1-cm increments
Synerview 1200SX	Body	4	CdWO$_4$ crystals as in 600S; 1200	1–20	12–50	60	12, 24, 48; 6–48 cm in 1-cm increments
Searle Pho/Trax 4000 (see EMI CT 6000 and OMNI 6000)							
Shimadzu SCT-100N-2	Head	2	BGO crystals with PMTs; 16	40, 60, 100	1	29	25.6
SCT-200N	Head	2	BGO crystals with PMTs; 64	29, 55, 110	3	45	12.8–35.2
SCT-1000T	Body	3	Xenon cells; 549	2.4, 4, 8	30–40	60	24.0–44.0
Siemens Somatom 2	Body	3	CsI crystals with photodiodes; 512 data + 8 reference	3, 5, 10	0–6	54	Head: 5.4–27; Body: 5.4–54
DR2	Body	3	Solid-state crystals; 514	1.4, 2.1, 3.2, 4.7, 7, 12, 14	0–3	54	5.3 to 53, continuously variable
DR3	Body	3	Solid-state crystals; 514	1.4, 2.1, 3.2, 4.7, 7, 12, 14	0–3	54	5.3 to 53, continuously variable

CaF$_2$, calcium fluoride; BGO, bismuth germanate; NaI, sodium iodide; CsI, cesium iodide; CdWO$_4$, cadmium tungstate.

[a] Definitions of scan geometry generations are given in Chapters 2 and 3.

Slice thickness (mm)	Gantry tilt (deg)	Views	Readings per view	Angle of rotation (deg)	Tube	Matrix	Slices per scan
1–10 mm in 1-mm increments	±20	360	552	230, 360, 398	Rotating anode, continuous	256 × 256	1
1–10 mm in 1-mm increments	±20	600	552	230, 360, 398	Rotating anode, continuous	256 × 256; 512 × 512	1
1–10 mm in 1-mm increments	±20	600	512, 1024	230, 360, 398	Rotating anode, continuous	256 × 256; 512 × 512	1
1–10 mm in 1-mm increments	±20	1200	512, 1024	230, 360, 398	Rotating anode, continuous	256 × 256; 512 × 512	1
5, 10	±20	256–1024			Stationary anode, continuous	256 × 256	1
5, 8, 10	±20	1088–3904			Stationary anode, continuous	256 × 256; 256 × 320	1
2, 5, 10	±20	216–600	549		Rotating anode, pulsed	256 × 256; 256 × 320	1
2, 4, 8	±20	233, 360, 720	512	360	Rotating anode, pulsed	256 × 256	1
2, 4, 8	±20 to −20	240, 320 at 240°; 480, 720, 1440 at 360°	512	240 and 360	Rotating anode, pulsed	256 × 256	1
2, 4, 8	+20	240, 320 at 240°; 480, 720, 1440 at 360°	512	240 and 360	Rotating anode, pulsed	512 × 512	1

APPENDIX III

(*Continued*)

Company and model	Total body or head only	Generation of scan geometry[a]	Detector type; number	Scan time (s)	Image reconstruction time (s)	Gantry aperture diameter (cm)	Reconstruction diameter (cm)
Technicare (formerly Ohio Nuclear)							
Delta 50	Body	2	BGO crystals with PMTs; 6 data (3 for each slice) + 1 reference	Head: 120; body, 150	1 slice: 0; 2nd slice: 15 later	50	20, 30, 40, 45
Delta 50 FS	Body	2	BGO crystals with PMTs; 24 data (12 for each slice) + 1 reference	Head: 15, 25; body: 18, 34	1 slice: 15 after scan; 2nd slice: 30 later	50	Head, 25; body, 42,
Delta 25	Head	2	BGO crystals with PMTs; 14 data (7 for each slice) + 1 reference	80, 108, 172	1 slice: 0; 2nd slice: 10 later	30.5	25
Delta 2005	Body	4	BGO crystals with PMTs; 424 over 212°	5, 10, 15, 20	30	60	25, 40, 50
Delta 2010	Body	4	BGO crystals with PMTs; 424 over 212°	2, 4, 8, 16	30	60	25, 40, 50
Delta 2020	Body	4	BGO crystals with PMTs; 720 over 360°	2, 4, 8, 16	<55	60	25, 40, 50
Delta 2060	Body	4	Shaped-response crystals of BGO and CdWO$_4$; 720	2, 4, 8	10–40	60	12.5, 25, 40, 50
Delta 100 series	Head	2	BGO crystals with PMTs; 3 data + 1 reference; 6 data + 1 reference with dual slice	120	0; 2nd slice, 10 later	30.5	25
Toshiba							
TCT-35A	Head	2	BGO crystals w/ PMTs; 8 data + 1 reference	105	45 with 5-s option	28	24
TCT-65A	Body	3; Direct magnification (shift)	Xenon cells; 512 data + 1 reference	4.5, 9, 18	35	60	21, 25, 30, 35, 40

CaF_2, calcium fluoride; BGO, bismuth germanate; NaI, sodium iodide; CsI, cesium iodide; $CdWO_4$, cadmium tungstate.

[a] Definitions of scan geometry generations are given in Chapters 2 and 3.

Slice thickness (mm)	Gantry tilt (deg)	Views	Readings per view	Angle of rotation (deg)	Tube	Matrix	Slices per scan
8, 13	±20	180	256	180; 12 overscan	Stationary anode, continuous	256 × 256	2
8, 13	±20	180	256	180; 12 overscan	Stationary anode, continuous	256 × 256	2
5, 8, 13	+5 to −20	180	256	196	Stationary anode, continuous	256 × 256	2
4, 7, 10	±20	360	256	212	Rotating anode, continuous	256 × 256	1
4, 7, 10	±20	360	256	212	Rotating anode, continuous	256 × 256	1
2, 4, 7, 10	±20	720	512	360	Rotating anode, continuous	128 × 128; 256 × 256; 512 × 512	1
2, 5, 10	+20 to −20	720	512	360° plus fan angle of ~10°	Rotating anode, continuous	256 × 256; 512 × 512	1
10	0	180	256	186	Stationary anode, continuous	256 × 256	1 or 2
10	Tabletop tilts			186	Stationary anode, continuous	160 × 160; 240 × 240	1
2, 5, 10	+20 to −15	300, 600	512	360	Rotating anode, pulsed	160 × 160; 320 × 320	1

APPENDIX III

(Continued)

Company and model	Total body or head only	Generation of scan geometry[a]	Detector type; number	Scan time (s)	Image reconstruction time (s)	Gantry aperture diameter (cm)	Reconstruction diameter (cm)
TCT-80A	Body	3	Xenon cells; 320	2.7, 4.5, 9.0	<60	60	24–40
Varian V-360-3	Body	3	Xenon cells (about 6–8 atm pressure); 293 data + 8 reference	3 or 12	60 for 3-s scan, or 120 for 12-s scan	60	Variable from 1–47

CaF_2, calcium fluoride; BGO, bismuth germanate; NaI, sodium iodide; CsI, cesium iodide; $CdWO_4$, cadmium tungstate.

[a] Definitions of scan geometry generations are given in Chapters 2 and 3.

Slice thickness (mm)	Gantry tilt (deg)	Views	Readings per view	Angle of rotation (deg)	Tube	Matrix	Slices per scan
2, 5, 10	+15 to −20	181–600	320	360	Rotating anode, pulsed	320 × 320	1
Variable, 7.5 standard	0	360 for 3-s scan; 1,440 for 12-s scan. Each group of 360 views collected in one 360° rotation of a 12-s scan are offset from and independent of the views collected during other rotations.	301	Continuous rotation in one direction using slip rings; 360° for a 3-s scan; 1,440° for a 12-s scan	Rotating anode, pulsed	256 × 256	1

GLOSSARY

Absorption of X-Rays
> One of the two main processes by which diagnostic x-rays passing through an object are attenuated or reduced in their intensity. This occurs through the photoelectric effect. The other main process is Compton scattering. The absorbed x-rays are converted to lower-energy x-rays and to other forms of energy such as heat. See Compton Effect, Photoelectric Effect, Scattering.

Accuracy
> The degree to which a measurement or set of measurements represents the true value of a parameter. Accuracy indicates the degree of freedom from systematic error and is to be distinguished from precision.
> See Precision.

Acoustic
> Referring to sound or ultrasound.

Acoustic Impedance
> A description of the acoustic properties of a material. The acoustic impedance is the product of the density of the material and the velocity of sound in the material. Reflections or echoes occur at interfaces between materials of different acoustic impedance.

ACTA (ACTA Scanner)
> Automatic Computerized Transverse Axial Scanner. The first total body CT scanner, a first generation unit employing a single detector per image section.

Adder
> A digital electronic circuit which provides the function of addition of two binary numbers.

Address Bus (Data Bus)
> See Bus.

Afterglow.
> The continued emission of light by a scintillation crystal for a finite time following the termination of x-ray excitation. This is an undesirable effect in CT scanning. It may range from the order of microseconds up to minutes for different substances. Of the commonly used CT scintillation crystal detectors, afterglow has been most notable in sodium iodide.

Algorithm
> The sequential set of operations that provides the solution to a problem in a finite number of steps.

Aliasing
> An artifact that occurs when high frequencies that are cut out by band limiting reappear as lower frequencies. The artifact occurs when the sampling frequency is less than twice the highest frequency contained within the signals. Information in the signal at frequencies greater than one-half of the sampling frequency (the Nyquist frequency) appears superimposed on the signal information from lower frequencies. This results in distortion of the original signal. Aliasing is a basic problem which occurs as a result of an insufficient number of ray samples per beam width in the section.

Alpha Particle (α Particle)
> A particle emitted in a particular type of radioactive decay (alpha decay) which is identical to the nucleus of a helium atom with two protons and two neutrons.

Alphanumeric (A/N)
> A collection of letters, numbers, and other symbols. They are found on the input keyboard of a CT console and are also displayed visually on a CT monitor.

A-Mode (Amplitude Mode)
> An ultrasound display mode in which a single line of acoustic information is viewed along the line of sight of the ultrasound beam. The horizontal axis represents time or distance along the line of sight (the direction of the ultrasound beam); the vertical axis represents the magnitude of reflected echoes.

Amplifier
> An electronic device to amplify or increase the voltage, current, or power of an input signal.

Amplitude Mode
> See A-Mode.

Analog
> The coding of data in terms of the continuously variable amplitude of a signal.

Analog-to-Digital Converter (ADC)
A device for transforming information or data from an analog to a digital form.

AND
The binary equivalent of multiplication; all inputs must be "true" (equal to 1) to get an output which is "true" (1). One type of logic gate.

Angular Frequency (ω)
The frequency of oscillation or rotation defined in radians per second where 2π radians is equal to 360°; $\omega = 2\pi f$ where the frequency f is in Hertz (Hz) or cycles per second (cps).

Angular Momentum
A vector quantity which is a measure of the magnitude of a rotational motion. It is related to the mass of the rotating object, the radius of rotation, and the angular frequency of rotation. The rotation can be either about an axis outside the rotating object or about an axis within the object.

Annihilation Radiation
This occurs when a positron (arising from the radioactive decay of a nucleus with relatively too many protons compared to neutrons) encounters an electron. This encounter occurs within a few millimeters of the nucleus undergoing positron decay (the positron has only a very short path before stopping). The positron and electron are annihilated, with the formation of a pair of photons, each of 511 keV energy traveling in opposite directions. These can be detected by coincidental scintillations in scintillation detectors 180° apart intercepting the annihilation photons.

Annotation
Information, typically clinical or technical, that can be labeled or annotated on the CT image. This includes information, such as the patient's name and date, that is routinely and automatically added to each CT image, and information or labels added on at the discretion of the user.

Anode (Plate, Target)
The positive element or target in an x-ray tube which emits x-rays when bombarded by electrons. The electrons are emitted by the negative cathode and accelerated through a high electrical potential. The anode is usually composed almost entirely of tungsten because of its high melting temperature. Molybdenum and rhenium may be added to the tungsten. The anode may be stationary, with a small fixed target surface and limited heat capacity, or rotating, with a relatively larger ringlike target surface (permitting the heat to be spread over a larger area) and larger heat capacity.

Anode Heel Effect
See Heel Effect.

Aperture
See Detector Aperture, Gantry Aperture.

Applications Program
A computer software package generated by the user to perform a particular task.

Archive (Archival Storage)
A means of providing long-term storage of information. In CT this can be accomplished by storing the information on a magnetic tape or a floppy disk.

Arithmetic Logic Unit (ALU)
One of the two major components of the central processing unit, the other being the control unit. The ALU is responsible for the actual process of computation.

Array
See Detector Array.

Array Processor
A special purpose logical processing unit that is used to perform rapid image reconstruction. This is done in a pipeline fashion, with part of the algorithm executed during the actual scan as the raw data are being collected. The array processor actually constitutes a second computer and is controlled by the central processing unit.

Artifact
A distortion or error in an image that is unrelated to the subject being studied. In CT, artifacts may be produced by geometric effects or a machine peculiarity, an inadequacy in the reconstruction algorithm, an error in x-ray attenuation measurements, or as a result of alterations in the energy spectrum of the x-ray beam. Artifacts may be considered as a source of noise.

Assembler
A specialized form of compiler that converts or translates the assembly language version of the program, line by line, into the machine language program which is directly usable by the central processing unit.

Assembly Language
A computer language intermediate between machine language and higher language. Assembly language substitutes mnemonic equivalents for the machine language binary instructions on a one-for-one basis and allows the use of symbolic addresses.

Atomic Mass (Atomic Mass Number A)
: The mass A of an atom, approximated by the number of protons and neutrons it contains.

Atomic Number
: The number of protons (positively charged particles) in the nucleus of an atom. It is symbolized by Z and is an important factor in bremsstrahlung and the photoelectric effect.

Attenuation
: The term describing the decrease in the intensity of a transmitted x-ray beam due to the combined effects arising from the photoelectric absorption and the Compton scattering of the primary x-ray beam as it passes through an object.

Attenuation Coefficient
: See Linear Attenuation Coefficient, Mass Attenuation Coefficient.

Auxiliary Memory
: A form of computer memory that relies on a nonvolatile sequential storage of data. The information is generally loaded into or retrieved from auxiliary memory in the form of blocks rather than in individual words. Transfer to and from the main memory is under the control of the central processing unit.

Axial
: This refers to the long axis of an object or patient body. An axial cross-section is one that lies perpendicular to the body axis.

Back-Projection (Simple Back-Projection, Summation Method)
: The oldest and conceptually the simplest form of image reconstruction. It is based on the assumption that all the elements in a core of tissue through which x-rays pass contribute equally to the x-ray attenuation. The total measured x-ray attenuation for each successive core of tissue irradiated is back-projected onto the core and divided equally among all elements. The total attenuation value for any element is the summation of its back-projected contributions to all cores containing the element.

Back-Projection, Filtered
: See Filtered Back-Projection.

Band Limiting
: A limitation of the allowable frequencies within a signal band defined by a lower and upper limit. Frequencies outside the band are attenuated; that is, high and low spatial frequencies are lost when projections are sampled or digitized.

Bandwidth
: A range of frequencies, from the lowest to the highest, in a signal. The range of frequencies to which a device, for example, an amplifier, will respond.

Batch Processing
: A method of data handling in which the data and a set of instructions are submitted simultaneously, with no further interaction between the user and the central processing unit of the computer during the execution of the program.

Batch Reconstruction
: A process in which image data for multiple sequential scans are stored in the computer memory during scanning. Reconstruction is performed during and after scanning.

Beam Hardening
: The phenomenon by which a polychromatic x-ray beam traversing an absorbing medium becomes relatively richer in the higher energy x-rays because the lower energy x-rays or photons are preferentially absorbed by the material. Because higher energy x-rays will travel farther before being absorbed, the beam becomes relatively more penetrating, or "harder."

Beam Hardening Artifacts
: These may be manifested as streaks between bones and by spillover at bone edges or as cupping artifacts.
See Cupping Artifact.

Beta Particle (β Particle)
: An electron that is emitted by a radioactive nucleus undergoing beta decay.

Binary System
: Number system with base 2.

Binary Coded Decimal
: A form of representation of a binary number that allows easy conversion to and from a decimal number.

Binary Counter
: See Counter.

Bipolar Transistor
: See Transistor.

Bit
: An abbreviation for "binary digit," the smallest element of binary information expressed in the binary system of notation. A bit can have the values of 0 or 1.

Blinker Function
: A keyboard-controlled function by which all image elements or pixels within a range or band of CT numbers can be made to blink or flash on the display monitor at a set rate.

Blur (Blurring, Unsharpness)
: The "smearing out" or spreading of the image of a point as a result of the inability of an imaging system to form a perfect image of an object.
See Composite Blur (Total Blur), Focal Spot Blur (Geometric Blur), Motion Blur, Receptor Blur (Screen Blur), Parallax Blur.

B-Mode (Brightness Mode)
: An ultrasound display mode in which the magnitude of the reflected echo is represented as a dot of variable brightness on a monitor face at the corresponding distance along the horizontal axis, which represents the line of sight. Only a single acoustic line is shown. B-mode as such is not used in clinical practice but forms the basis for B-scan.
See B-scan.

Boltzmann Distribution
: The equilibrium distribution of atoms in different energy states.

Boolean Logic
: Switching logic or the algebra for manipulation of binary logic variables.

Bremsstrahlung
: X-rays emitted from the anode target of an x-ray tube as a result of the fundamental electrical interaction between the bombarding negative electrons from the cathode and the positive nuclei of the anode. It results from the rapid deceleration of the electrically charged electrons as they strike the anode target. The maximum x-ray energy produced in this process is equal to the maximum kinetic energy of the electrons. This in turn is equal to the product of the electron charge (e) times the maximum kilovoltage between the cathode and anode (i.e., the kVp). The energy spectrum of the bremsstrahlung is smooth or continuous, extending from 0 to ekVp. Bremsstrahlung accounts for the majority of the x-ray energy emitted by an x-ray tube, the remaining smaller portion being characteristic radiation.

Brightness Mode
: See B-Mode.

B-Scan
: The commonly used two-dimensional ultrasound display format. A cross-section based on ultrasound reflections is composed of multiple individual acoustic lines of information. It may be a static scan (formed by manual scanning) or a real time (dynamic) image.

Buffer (Buffer Memory)
: A small, conveniently located, relatively fast peripheral memory unit in which data or results are temporarily stored as input to or output from the central processing unit.

Bus (Bus Line, Bus System)
: A network of wires that allows communication between the various elements of a computer. One bus system supplies power to the computer components. A control bus relays information regarding the basic operation of the computer between the central processing unit and the other sections. Data is transmitted between and within sections of the computer along the data or address bus, as directed by the signal transmitted along the control bus.

Byte
: The smallest number of bits usually manipulated within the computer (typically 6 or 8 bits).

Calibration
: A process of assessing the accuracy and precision of a CT unit. Reference information can be collected by scanning specially constructed CT phantoms.

Calipers (Digital Calipers)
: A pair of cursors used to measure distance between two points in an image displayed on a monitor.

Cartesian Coordinate System
: A coordinate system for localizing a point in space by identifying its position with respect to three mutually perpendicular linear axes, usually specified as the x, y, and z axes. The three axes intersect at a common point, the origin.

Cathode
: The negative electrode of the x-ray tube that is heated to emit electrons, which are then accelerated through a high electrical potential to strike the positive anode target.

Cathode Ray Tube (CRT)
: The electronic basis for display monitors. A beam of electrons is directed to a photoemissive screen. The strength of the electron beam that strikes any point on the screen determines the amount of light emitted at that point by the photoemissive material.

Central Processing Unit (CPU)
: The "central nervous system" of the computer. The CPU performs the primary computer functions of carrying out rapid calculations and also directs the operations of the other major com-

puter components. The two major components of the CPU itself are the control unit and the arithmetic logic unit. The CPU also controls the bus system.

Characteristic Curve (Characteristic Film Curve)
A graph or plot of the film density as a function of the exposure or mAs. It is also called a Hunter and Driffield (H and D) curve after the first individuals to describe it.

Characteristic Radiation
Those x-ray photons emitted from the anode target of an x-ray tube that are related to the atomic properties of the target (usually made chiefly of tungsten). The energy spectrum of the emitted x-rays consists of characteristic spikes corresponding to transitions within the electron energy levels of the target atoms superimposed on the bremsstrahlung radiation.

Chemical Shift
A shift in the Larmor frequency in nuclear magnetic resonance which occurs because of the different magnetic fields seen by different nuclear magnetic moments as a result of variations in environment and chemical bonds (i.e., variations in electron shielding).

Circuit Breaker
A safety device which protects the equipment from extreme electrical surges by interrupting electrical contact.

Circular Artifact (Ring Artifact)
An artifact on the CT image consisting of a circle or concentric group of circles about the center of the field of view. This artifact may occur in third-generation CT units (rotating x-ray tube and detectors) as a result of the malfunction of a detector or group of detectors.

Coherent Scattering (Raleigh Scattering)
An interaction between a photon and matter which results in a change in the direction of the photon without any loss of energy of the photon. It is generally a minor cause of x-ray attenuation at diagnostic energies.

Coincidence
Simultaneous occurrence: In particular, the formation of two high-energy photons or gamma rays traveling at 180° with respect to each other following the annihilation of a positron. The principle of detection of coincident gamma rays is employed in positron emission computed tomography.

Collimator
An apparatus for shaping the x-ray beam, usually in CT in the form of a rectangular cross-section. The collimator reduces the x-ray beam to the required geometrical size.

Compiler
A software component that translates a higher language, for example, FORTRAN, into machine language. It translates symbolic instructions into an appropriate series of machine language instructions and assigns specific locations in memory to symbolic addresses. It also takes steps to improve the efficiency of the resulting machine language program.

Complement (Inverse, NOT)
Inverse function; a function that reverses the input. A "true" or 1 input becomes a 0 output; a "false" or 0 input becomes a 1 output. A type of logic gate.

Composite Blur (Total Blur)
The blur or unsharpness in a conventional radiograph arising from a composite of the different types of blur.

Compton Effect (Compton Interaction, Compton Scattering)
A fundamental interaction between electromagnetic radiation (e.g., x-rays) and matter. A photon is scattered by an electron, resulting in some energy transfer to the recoiling electron. The deflected photon has a lower energy (or frequency) following the interaction. Because only a portion of the photon energy is absorbed, the absorbed energy dose is relatively smaller than in the photoelectric effect.

Compton Electron
The recoiling or scattered electron in the Compton interaction.

Computed Angiotomography
See Dynamic Computed Tomography.

Computed Radiograph (Computed Digital Radiograph, Digital Computed Radiograph, Pilot Scan, Scout View)
The radiograph-like image reconstructed in the technique of computed radiography.

Computed Radiography
A technique for obtaining an image similar to a radiograph from a CT unit. As the patient is translated at constant speed through the gantry, the x-ray tube is activated, and the detector array measures the x-ray fan beam transmitted through the patient. The image may be commonly called

a scout view or pilot scan. The technique is an example of scanned projection radiography or slit beam radiography.

Computed Tomography
See Emission Computed Tomography, Transmission Computed Tomography.

Computer
An electronic device capable of rapidly processing data by following a set of instructions called a program. In CT the computer receives the data obtained by the detector array system, analyzes the data, and assigns mathematical values for the linear attenuation coefficient for each pixel.

Computer Card
See Hollerith Card.

Computer Graphics
The process of annotating and labeling CT images with alphanumerics, lines, traces, and so forth.

Continuous Wave
A continuous sine wave, which theoretically has no beginning or end, as opposed to a pulse or wave of finite duration.

Contrast
The difference between a signal or information and its background.
See Contrast Resolution, Film Contrast, Radiographic Contrast, Subject Contrast.

Contrast Resolution
The capability of an imaging system to distinguish small differences in contrast related to the differences in x-ray attenuation.

Control Bus
See Bus.

Control Programs (Control Systems)
The part of the operating system (the complete set of software available to the user as part of the initial computer system) that consists of the set of housekeeping instructions necessary for practical operation of the computer. It is also responsible for communication with the operator, particularly for those situations that cannot be controlled by the computer (e.g., changing a tape or disk pack).

Control Unit
The part of the central processing unit that directs the operation of the entire computer and is responsible for proper operation of each component of the computer. It is one of the two major components of the central processing unit, the other being the arithmetic logic unit.

Convolutional Integral, Convolutional Method
See Filtered Back Projection.

Coolidge Tube
See X-Ray Tube.

Core Memory
Computer memory using ferrite toroids (cores) for storing information in magnetic form. This is a relatively expensive form of memory that has the advantage of rapid retrieval; that is, it provides high-speed random access to information and is nonvolatile.

Coulomb
A unit of electrical charge. One coulomb is equal to the total charge of 6.3×10^{18} electrons. The unit is named after the French physicist Charles Augustin Coulomb (1736–1806).

Counter (Binary Counter)
A linear array of flip-flops which generates a binary number representing the number of input pulses received.

Crosstalk
Unwanted interference between adjacent electrical or electronic devices such as power lines, transmission lines, and cables.

CRT
See Cathode Ray Tube, Monitor.

CT Numbers
The numbers used to designate the x-ray attenuation in each picture element of the CT image. These are expressed in terms of old Hounsfield or EMI units (on a scale from -500 to $+500$) or new Hounsfield units (on a scale from $-1,000$ to $+1,000$).

Cupping Artifact
An artifact arising as a result of beam hardening. In imaging a homogeneous or uniform object by CT there will be an apparent or artificial decrease in the CT numbers (attenuation coefficients) about the center of the object unless an appropriate correction for beam hardening is made. Cupping is seen clinically in abdominal scans where there is relatively little bone. It may also be regarded as a tendency for the reconstructed image of a uniform object to demonstrate increased apparent density near the outer edges.

Curie
The unit for measuring radioactivity; the quantity of a radioactive isotope undergoing 37 billion (3.7×10^{10}) disintegrations per second. It is named after the Polish and French physicists Marie Curie (1867–1934) and Pierre Curie (1859–1906).

Current (Electrical Current)
: The rate of flow of electrical charge, usually measured in amperes, where 1 ampere is equal to a flow of 1 coulomb of charge per second.

Cursor
: An identifiable marker often in the form of a symbol, for example, crosshairs, a dot, a dash, a rectangle, or a circle, which may be moved over the surface of a cathode ray tube by a joystick, trackball, or light pen. The cursor can be used to alter, delete, or select instructions to the computer, to trace out areas, or measure distances. It thus allows communication of spatial information between an operator and a computer. A cursor may also be used to indicate the location on an alphanumeric monitor of the position of the next character to be typed.

Curvilinear Tomography
: See Linear Tomography.

Data Acquisition System (DAS)
: The components of a CT machine used to produce and collect the x-ray attenuation information: x-ray tube, detectors, and detector preamplifiers. These are mounted on the gantry.

Data Bus (Address Bus)
: See Bus.

Data Fan (Detector Fan)
: Another name for a view (profile or projection) in fourth generation CT units, that is, the set of discrete measurements recorded by each detector. The collection of rays seen by a detector, and constituting a view in the fourth generation, forms a fan with the apex at the detector.

Debugging
: An expression describing the process of removing or eliminating any errors or "bugs" in a computer program.

Decay
: Alteration of a radioactive nucleus by the emission of an alpha or beta particle, positron, or gamma ray.

Decimal
: Number system with base 10.

Decoder
: A device that converts binary information from one form to another (e.g., binary to binary coded decimal or binary to decimal).

Deconvolution
: A technique for multiplanar reconstruction in which contiguous thin transverse sections are derived from overlapping thicker sections.

Density
: A term frequently used to describe the relative CT number or x-ray attenuation of a tissue. Isodensity implies that a particular tissue has the same CT number as surrounding tissues. Hypodensity and hyperdensity imply a smaller or larger CT number than the surrounding tissue. Although CT numbers frequently are related to the density (in grams per cubic centimeter) of a material, they are actually an indication of the attenuation of x-rays by the material through a combination of Compton scattering and the photoelectric effect. Alternatively, density refers to the density of an x-ray film.
See Film Density.

Density Function
: A term used in image reconstruction theory to denote the contribution of each point to the detected signal. For transmission computed tomography it represents the linear attenuation coefficient; for emission computed tomography it is proportional to the radioisotope density or concentration.

Detector Angle (Detector Acceptance Angle)
: The solid angle with the detector at the apex which encompasses the paths of x-ray photons that will intercept the detector and be recorded as signals.

Detector Aperture
: The effective area or aperture of a detector intercepting an x-ray signal. The physical aperture is the area of the active part of the detector. The effective area or aperture may be increased along the direction of detector motion during scanning.

Detector Array
: A group of closely spaced detectors used for the rapid sampling of x-ray transmission data.

Digital
: A coding of data in terms of patterns equal amplitude pulses and spaces signifying the absence of pulses.

Digital Computed Radiography
: See Computed Radiography.

Digital-to-Analog Converter
: A device for transforming information or data from a digital to an analog form.

Digitization
: The process of converting a signal or information from an analog to a digital form.

Diode
: A two-element electronic vacuum tube or sem-

iconductor device which permits current flow in one direction only.

Disk
See Magnetic Disk.

Disk Pack
See Magnetic Disk Pack.

Display Console (Physician's Display Console, Physician's Diagnostic Console)
A console for viewing the scan information or CT images. It also incorporates features for image manipulation, annotation, and measurement.

Display Monitor
A television or cathode ray tube used to display the CT image. Monitors are therefore used in closed circuit applications. In both CT display monitors and television monitors the picture or annotation is formed by a series of horizontal lines resulting from a sequence of horizontal scans across the monitor face by the electron beam of a cathode.

Doppler Effect
When sound (ultrasound) is reflected from a moving target, the frequency f of the sound wave is shifted by an amount Δf equal to $v/c \cos \theta$, where v is the velocity of the moving target, c is the velocity of sound, and θ is the angle between the path of the wave and the direction of motion of the target. The effect is named after its discoverer, the Austrian physicist Christian Doppler (1803–1853).

Dose (Radiation Dose)
Radiation absorbed per unit of mass. It is usually expressed in rads, where 1 rad is equal to the absorption of 100 ergs of energy per gram of tissue.

Dose Efficiency
An indication of how well the radiation dosage to the patient is utilized in image formation.

Dose Equivalent
This quantity represents the radiation dose in rads multiplied by other factors which take into account other modifying factors such as the differing biological effectiveness of different types of radiation (x-rays, neutrons, etc.). It is measured in units of rems.
See Rem.

Dosimeter
A device such as a thermoluminescent device, ionization chamber, or film badge that measures the dose to a particular local region undergoing or exposed to radiation.

Dual Energy Scanning
A method for obtaining the average atomic number Z of a material by scanning at two different energies (kilovoltages). Alternatively, a detector system using a pair of detectors, one filtered and one unfiltered, may be used to separate energy components. The technique attempts to separate the total x-ray attenuation into its photoelectric absorption and Compton scattering components.

Duty Cycle
The fraction or percentage of the time during an exposure in which the x-ray tube is actively emitting x-rays.

Dynamic Computed Tomography (Rapid-Sequence CT Scanning)
A technique for performing multiple fast (typically 1–5 s) CT scans in rapid sequence. It can be used to perform a dynamic examination of one or more cross-sections. This permits visualization and quantitation of dynamic physiological functions such as blood flow and perfusion. Alternatively, the technique may be used to obtain an entire sequence of scans at different levels in a short time.

Dynamic Range
The range in signal magnitudes that can be detected and differentiated; alternatively, the range of signals that can be displayed discretely. It is often used in CT to describe the range of x-ray exposures at the detector to which the system can respond without saturation and produce satisfactory gray-scale images. The dynamic range may be expressed as a ratio of the magnitude of the largest signal measured to that of the lowest signal to be recognized.

Dynamic Spatial Reconstructor (DSR)
A multiple (28) x-ray tube source, high-speed (as short as 10 ms) transaxial imaging system, developed at the Mayo Clinic, for body scanning of a cylindrical volume.

Dynode
One of the multiple successive electrodes in a photomultiplier tube.
See Photomultiplier Tube.

Echo
A reflected sound (ultrasound) wave or pulse.

Edge Enhancement
A technique which emphasizes or enhances sharp discontinuities such as interfaces, boundaries, edges. It is usually incorporated into the algorithm.

Edge Gradient Streaks
Artifacts that occur as a mathematical effect arising from the finite width of the scanning beam. The artifacts are lucent streaks originating from the edges of denser objects with straight shapes or edges.

Edge Response Function
A description of the image of a straight boundary between adjacent regions of high and low x-ray transmission.

Electromechanical Printer
See Printer.

Electron Density
The number of electrons per unit volume. Compton scattering depends on the electron density.

Electron-Volt (eV)
The energy acquired by a particle with unit charge (1.602×10^{-19} coulombs), for example, an electron, as it is accelerated through an electrical potential of 1 volt. One electron-volt = 1.602×10^{-12} ergs = 1.602×10^{-19} joules.

Electronic Noise
Noise introduced by analog electronic circuits.

Electrostatic Printer
See Printer.

EMI
British company that developed and manufactured the first commercial CT unit.

EMI Units (Old Hounsfield Units)
A system of CT units based in the following relationship: EMI units = $(\mu - \mu_{H_2O})/\mu_{H_2O} \times 500$, where μ and μ_{H_2O} are the linear attenuation coefficients of the substance measured and of water, respectively.

Emission Computed Tomography (Emission CT)
A technique for obtaining cross-sectional images of the head or the body based on the detection of the geometric distribution of the emissions or activity of radionuclides. The emissions may be single photons (single photon emission CT) or coincidental photons arising from positron decay (position emission CT).

Enabling
The process of connecting a destination device (one which is to receive or respond to information being transmitted) to a bus line by a binary control signal transmitted ahead of the data.

ENIAC
Electronic Numerical Integrator and Calculator. The first electronic digital computer, completed at the University of Pennsylvania in 1946. It contained 18,000 electronic vacuum tubes.

Entrance Window (Entrance Slit)
A slit or aperture through which radiation can pass.

Erg
A unit of energy. One erg = 10^{-7} joule = 6.3×10^{11} electron-volts.

Exposure
The amount of radiation incident on an object. See Roentgen.

Extended CT Number Scale
A CT scale that has been extended to higher values than the usual +500 EMI or old Hounsfield units (+1,000 new Hounsfield units). Typically the extended scale will measure and display CT numbers up to +1,500 EMI units.

Fan Angle (Fan Beam Angle)
The angle subtended by a single detector or by the entire fan of detectors from the x-ray source in a fan beam scanner.

Fan Beam
An x-ray beam that diverges in the shape of a fan with a fixed thickness or depth.

Fatigue
The decrease in efficiency of a source or detector of electromagnetic radiation as a result of continued operation.

Field Effect Transistor (FET)
A transistor device that approximates a solid-state equivalent of an electron tube triode.

Field of View (FOV)
The size of the field within the gantry aperture selected for image reconstruction. It is usually expressed in terms of its diameter.

Filter
A technique for shaping the x-ray beam intensity. Filtration, typically in the form of an aluminum plate, is placed between the x-ray tube and the patient. Typically different filters are used for head scanning and body scanning. Alternatively, the modification of information in CT.
See Filter Function.

Filter Function
A mathematical function incorporated into the CT algorithm. Filter functions modify the spatial frequency content of the signal information by permitting selective removal or enhancement of information of different spatial frequencies.

Filtered Back-Projection (Integral Equation Method, Convolutional Method, Convolutional Integral)
: The mathematical process most commonly used in the reconstruction process for computed tomography. The profiles obtained in simple back-projection are modified or filtered prior to being back-projected, to correct for the background density that occurs in simple back-projection.

Film Contrast
: The contrast or difference in film density as a function of the exposure associated with the basic properties of the film. This is described for each film by its characteristic or Hunter and Driffield curve.
See Characteristic Curve.

Film Density
: A parameter used to describe the degree of opacification of a film (i.e., the film darkening).

Film Grain
: The basic graininess of x-ray film due to the individual silver halide crystals.

Flip-Flop
: A sequential logic circuit which maintains its output state indefinitely until instructed to change by a subsequent input pulse.

Floppy Disk
: A flexible magnetic memory disk in which the thin magnetic film is applied to a flexible Mylar backing, comparable to that used in magnetic tape but somewhat thicker. Typically a floppy disk can store from 250 kilobytes to 1 megabyte. Their inexpensive drive units and small size make them easier to handle than magnetic tapes or rigid disks. Floppy disks can also be used as archival storage.

Fluorescence
: A type of luminescence or process in which radiation, typically light, is emitted by a substance that has absorbed radiation from an external course. The emitted radiation is generally of lower energy than the absorbed energy. In contrast to phosphorescence (the other type of luminescence), the emission occurs and terminates very rapidly (typically within 10^{-8} s or less) after the energy absorption.

Fluorescent Screen
: A two-dimensional device for converting the transmitted x-ray beam into an optical image.

Flux
: The quantity of flow of a physical substance across a two-dimensional surface, generally defined perpendicular to the surface per unit surface area.

Focal Spot
: The area of the anode or target of the x-ray tube that is bombarded by high-energy electrons and from which x-rays are generated.

Focal Spot Blur (Geometric Blur)
: Blur or unsharpness in conventional radiography arising because of the finite size of the x-ray tube focus.

FORTRAN
: One of the oldest of the higher computer languages, designed for scientific and engineering applications. The name is derived from FORmula TRANslation.

Fourier Reconstruction
: A mathematical technique for image reconstruction using a Fourier transform theory.

Fourier Transform
: A mathematical process for changing the description of a function by giving its value in terms of its frequency components instead of its spatial coordinates (or vice versa). It is named after the French mathematician Jean Baptiste Joseph Fourier (1768–1830) who developed it.

Free Induction Decay
: The decay of the nuclear induction NMR signal following application of the radiofrequency pulse. It is described as "free" because the nuclei precess freely without an applied radiofrequency field.

Frequency
: The rate of variation, in time or space, of a physical parameter. It is the reciprocal of the period, the duration in time or space, of a single cycle.

Fulcrum
: The pivotal point about which rotation occurs in conventional tomography. It determines the position of the focal plane.

Full Width at Half-Maximum (FWHM)
: The width of a pulse; a distribution or a function measured between the two points at which the amplitude has dropped to one-half its maximum value.

Gain
: A measure of the increase or amplification of the magnitude of a signal from an amplification stage.

Gamma Emission Computed Tomography (Gamma ECT, Single Emission Computed Tomography (SECT))
: The form of emission computed tomography in which the image of a head or body cross-section

is reconstructed by detecting the gamma rays emitted directly by decaying radionuclides.

Gamma Rays (Gamma Particles, γ Rays, γ Particles)
Electromagnetic radiation emitted during a particular type of radioactive nuclear decay or in a nuclear transition.

Gantry
The movable frame on a CT machine that holds the x-ray tube, collimators, and the detectors.

Gantry Aperture
The central opening in the gantry in which the patient is placed. It is usually described in terms of its diameter or circumference.

Gas Detector (High-Pressure Gas Detector)
An x-ray detection system using high-pressure inert gas (typically xenon) ionization chambers. It has been the most commonly used detector system in CT systems with a rotating tube and detectors.

Gate (Logic Gate)
Logic switching element; a mechanical or electrical device that generates a digital output, either 0 or 1, depending on input signals. Also the electrical or mechanical equivalent of a logic function.

Gated Computed Tomography
A process for sychronizing scanning or data collection with some physiological process. A technique for imaging accurately the heart in different phases of the cardiac cycle by accumulating data for discrete portions of the cardiac cycle (typically 100 ms) over many cycles. The cardiac cycle is gated on the basis of the electrocardiogram.

Gauss
A unit of magnetic field strength. It is generally used for magnetic fields of lower magnitude. As an example, the magnetic field of the earth is about 0.6 gauss. 1 gauss = .0001 tesla. It is named after the German mathematician Carl Friedrich Gauss (1777–1855).

Gaussian
A mathematical function that describes the probability distribution of random errors. It is peaked at the center and falls to zero at either end. Deviation from the center is expressed in terms of standard deviations.

Generation
A term used to classify CT units by the geometry of the scanning motion, the detector system, shape of the x-ray beam, and scanning time. Also, a computer term indicating the historical changes in the construction of digital electronic computers from electron vacuum tubes through transistors to progressively more complex integrated circuits.

Geometric Blur
See Focal Spot Blur.

Geometric Misalignment Artifacts
These occur because of mechanical misalignment in the detectors or x-ray source. They are typically manifested as streaks originating from high-density objects.

Gradient
A variation in the value of some quantity (e.g., magnetic field) with distance along a particular direction.

Grain (Picture Grain)
Picture grain is caused by an insufficiency of photons arriving in the detectors after penetrating the body; this limits the accuracy to which each picture point can be calculated within the matrix. The random variation of the amplitude of the matrix points to the picture grain, which can be expressed in terms of amplitude and coarseness.

Gray (Gy)
The unit of absorbed dose. It is defined as the absorption of 1 joule of energy per kilogram of material, or, equivalently, 10,000 ergs per gram of material. Therefore, 1 Gy = 100 rads.

Gray Scale Bar
A linear bar, typically in either a vertical or horizontal position along the edge of an image, in which the gray scale is displayed from white to black, and the shades of gray are related to the corresponding CT numbers.

Gray Scale Ultrasound
An ultrasound B-scan display in which the variable magnitudes of the ultrasound reflections or echoes are displayed in terms of different shades of gray.

Grid
Two sets of mutually perpendicular lines, one set parallel to the x axis, the second parallel to the y axis. The lines in each set are equally spaced at fixed distances. Individual 1-cm coordinates are usually located along the x and y axes. A grid can be superimposed on a CT image. Alternatively, the third or middle electrode in a vacuum tube triode.

Gyromagnetic Ratio (γ, Magnetogyric Ratio)
A physical constant for a particular magnetic nucleus that relates the resonant frequency (cor-

responding to the energy difference between two magnetic states) or precession frequency and the external magnetic field. For atomic nuclei (as opposed to electrons or other particles) it may also be referred to as the magnetogyric ratio.

Half-Life ($t_{1/2}$)

The time for a quantity or parameter (e.g., a sample of radionuclides) which decays exponentially to decrease by a factor of two.

Hard Copy

A permanent copy format for image visual display, usually radiographic or Polaroid film, in contrast to monitor images or magnetic tape or disk storage.

Hardware

The electrical devices or individual physical components of a computer, for example, the central processing unit, memory, and input and output devices.

Hardwiring

A technique in which all or part of a program or set of instructions for a computer are actually wired onto circuit boards. Alterations in the program entail changing one or more of the hardwired circuit boards. For convenience in making changes the boards may be designed to be plugged in or pulled out manually from a particular location.

Heat Capacity

See X-Ray Tube Heat Capacity.

Heel Effect (Anode Heel Effect, X-Ray Tube Heel Effect)

The absorption of X-rays by the anode. This effect increases with smaller anode angles and occurs predominantly in the anode side of the x-ray beam.

Herring Bone Artifact

See Streak Artifact.

Hertz (Hz)

A cycle per second. The standard unit of frequency, it is named after Heinrich Hertz (1857–1894).

Hexadecimal

Number system with base 16.

Higher Language

The language that a user utilizes in programming. It is a means of communication between the user and the computer, the latter being able ultimately to respond only to a series of electrical pulses.

Hollerith Card

A computer batch device consisting of a card in which data are entered as holes punched in 80 columns of 12 rows. Each column can thus store 12 binary or 4 octal digits. It is named after Herman Hollerith (1860–1929), the inventor of a tabulating machine that was a precursor of the electronic computer.

Hounsfield Partial Volume Effect

This is an artifact occurring only in first and second generation translational-rotational scanners with a 180° scanning angle. The artifacts are manifested as vertical streaks from high-density objects that extend only partly into the scan section.

Hounsfield Units (New Hounsfield Units)

A system of CT units based on the following relationship: $HU = (\mu - \mu_{H_2O})/\mu_{H_2O} \times 1000$, where μ and μ_{H_2O} are the linear attenuation coefficients of the substance measured and water, respectively. This system utilizes a constant factor of 1,000, in contrast to the factor of 500 used in EMI or old Hounsfield units.

Hysteresis

This is a phenomenon in which the output of a detector depends on its history of previous radiation exposure as well as the present level of incident radiation.

Image Intensifier

An electronic vacuum tube device for increasing the intensity of a two-dimensional light image from a fluoroscopic screen. The incident x-ray beam pattern is converted into light by a fluoroscopic screen. The light then strikes a photocathode surface, ejecting electrons that are focused and accelerated toward a second phosphor screen where an intensified optical image is produced.

Image Manipulation

Operations that modify an image to enhance useful information relative to noise.

Incrementation

The movement of the CT table relative to the gantry by a given increment in order to position the patient for the next scan.

Infrared

Electromagnetic radiation with a photon energy or frequency between light and high-frequency microwaves. Detection of the naturally occurring body emission of infrared is the basis of imaging by thermography. The frequency range of infrared is about 10^{11} to 10^{14} Hz; the corresponding range in wavelength is from about 1 to .001 mm.

Integral Dose
This the total amount of energy absorbed by the body. The basic unit of integral dose is the gram-rad, which is equivalent to 100 ergs of energy. The integral dose is the product of the dose (in rads) times the amount of tissue (in grams).

Integral Equation
See Filtered Back-Projection.

Integrated Circuit
A device containing a large number of solid-state elements housed in a single package. It is composed of a semiconducting substrate upon which various layers of insulators and conducting and semiconducting materials are deposited and etched into specific patterns. These then function as substitutes for assemblies of discrete transistors, resistors, capacitors, and diodes. The use of integrated circuits to fabricate logic circuits characterizes third and fourth generation electronic digital computers.

Integration Time
The time during which an electrical signal, in the form of a cumulative x-ray detection, is measured, the instantaneous signal being summated over the integration time.

Intensity
The energy per unit area per unit time incident on or flowing through a two-dimensional surface.

Interactive Processing (Interactive Mode)
A method of data handling in which the user is in constant communication with the central processing unit of the computer throughout execution of the program.

Interpolation
A term referring to a process of estimating the value of a data point lying between two known data points. It is required in filtered back-projection and in two-dimensional Fourier reconstruction.

Inverse (Inverse Function)
See Complement.

Ionization
A process in which an electrically neutral atom acquires charge by gaining or losing electron(s).

Ionization Chamber
A device or chamber which measures the ionization produced by a radiation.

Isocenter
In a third generation CT system the center of rotation of the x-ray tube and detector array.

Isotope
Any one of two or more species of atoms of a particular chemical element having the same atomic number Z (corresponding to a number of protons equal to Z) but different numbers of neutrons, and hence a different atomic mass or mass number A.

Iteration (Iterative Reconstruction)
A mathematical technique for image reconstruction which relies on repetitive operations. It is based on the principle of successive approximations, utilizing the computational capabilities of the computer to derive successively better approximations to the value of the attenuation coefficient in each voxel. An arbitrary starting point or value may be chosen for each voxel. Corrections are then applied to these arbitrary values to bring them into better agreement with measured projections. The process is repeated with successively corrected values until a satisfactory agreement with measured data is obtained. There are three methods of applying the corrections: simultaneous, point-by-point, and ray-by-ray.

Iteration with Point-by-Point Correction
A form of iterative correction in which the correction is made sequentially, point-by-point (pixel-by-pixel) for each element. Each correction is incorporated into successive corrections.

Iteration with Ray-by-Ray Correction
A form of iterative correction in which the correction is made for each element in a single ray. This is then done sequentially for each ray in each projection, always incorporating the previous corrections into new ones.

Iteration, Simultaneous
A form of iterative correction in which the corrections are made simultaneously for each element or pixel in the matrix at the end of the iteration.

Joule
A unit of energy named after the British physicist James Prescott Joule (1818–1889). It is the unit of energy in the Système Internationale and is defined as 1 kg-m^2/s^2. 1 joule = 10^7 ergs = 6.3×10^{18} electron-volts.

Joystick
A stick that is freely moveable about a pivot on an operator or display console or keyboard that allows the user to move a cursor over a cathode ray tube. The track of the cursor may also be traced out as a continuous line (as to outline an

area). It is similar in function to a light pen or trackball.

Junction-Type Transistor
See Transistor.

Keyboard
A device permitting a user to interact with a computer. It is similar in layout to a conventional typewriter keyboard but includes both alphanumeric symbols and special functions.

kVp
The kilovoltage peak of a ray tube. The maximum energy of the x-rays produced by the tube is equal to ekVp.

Large-Scale Integrated Circuits (LSI)
Sophisticated integrated circuits containing in excess of 10,000 active elements, fabricated on a single chip of silicon several millimeters in size. Fourth generation computers are characterized by their use of LSIs.

Larmor Equation
The equation describing the fundamental principle of NMR: $\omega_0 = \gamma H_0$ where ω_0 is the angular frequency of precession, γ is the gyromagnetic ratio, and H_0 is the strength of the magnetic field.

Larmor Precession Frequency
The frequency of the precession or rotation of the net magnetic moment or magnetization of a collection of magnetic nuclei (or atoms) about an external magnetic field at the resonant frequency. It also corresponds to the difference in energy states that the magnetic moment may assume in the magnetic field.

Laser
The name is derived from light amplification through the stimulated emission of radiation. A highly collimated, monochromatic beam of light used in CT for localization of the patient within the gantry.

Law of Tangents
This law states that the radiographic image is determined primarily by the portions of the x-ray beam that pass tangentially or nearly tangentially along the borders between objects of different densities and thicknesses.

Leakage Current
Any current from the output of a detector when there is no radiation input to the detector.

Level
See Window Level.

Light
The relatively narrow visual or optical portion of the electromagnetic spectrum. It ranges from red light, with a wavelength of 640 mμ (10^{-9} m) and a frequency of 4.7×10^{14} Hz, to blue light, which has a wavelength of 480 mμ and a frequency of 6.3×10^{14} Hz.

Light Pen
A device for communication between a user and computer via a cathode ray tube. The light from the pen is detected by the cathode ray tube and is used for such purposes as selecting or altering instructions, moving a cursor, or tracing areas. It is similar in function to a joystick or trackball.

Line Printer
See Printer.

Line Spread Function
A transfer function that measures the response of an imaging system to an input consisting of a line.

Linear Attenuation Coefficient
A quantitative measure of x-ray attenuation per centimeter of material. The logarithm of the ratio of intensity of the incident x-ray beam to that of the transmitted beam is equal to the linear attenuation coefficient times the thickness of the attenuating material. The coefficient is dependent upon the x-ray energy (kV) and the material itself. It is usually expressed in units of inverse centimeters and represented by the symbol μ. It is essentially the linear attenuation coefficient that is calculated for each voxel in computed tomography and expressed in terms of CT numbers (old or new Hounsfield units).

Linear Energy Transfer (LET)
The amount of energy deposited by a photon or particle per unit length of travel, expressed in keV per micron.

Linear Tomography (Unidirectional Tomography)
A form of conventional tomography in which the x-ray tube and film move synchronously so that the central ray of the x-ray beam moves in a single plane. Rectilinear motion implies that the x-ray tube and film each move in a straight line. For curvilinear motion the x-ray tube and film both move in an arc within a given plane.

Linearity
A property of a detector characterized by an output electrical current that is exactly linearly proportional to the input radiation incident on the detector.

Linearization
A mathematical technique incorporated into an algorithm to offset effects of both beam hard-

ening and detector nonlinearity. Beam hardening introduces nonlinearity in x-ray absorption, which then is "linearized" with a software correction.

Logarithm
See Natural Logarithm.

Longitudinal Relaxation Time
See Spin-Lattice Relaxation Time (T_1).

Luminescence
A general term describing the emission of light by a substance after a stimulation (e.g., a radiation absorption). If the emission is instantaneous (less than 10^{-8} s), it is called fluorescence. If it is not instantaneous, it is called phosphorescence.

LSI
See Large-Scale Integrated Circuits.

Machine Language
A computer language in which each instruction to the computer consists of a binary number, which is converted by the read-only memory within the central processing unit into a more detailed set of instructions that is actually executed by the central processing unit. It is the lowest language level accessible to the user.

Magnet
See Magnetic Dipole.

Magnetic Dipole
A magnet, or source of a magnetic field, may be conceptualized as a pair of magnetic poles of strength $+m$ and $-m$ separated by a finite distance. The individual poles or monopoles are equivalent to electric charges (electric monopoles). The combination of the two magnetic poles is a dipole. An individual magnetic monopole may not exist in nature, however, and thus is an abstract concept. A magnetic dipole has an associated magnetic moment.

Magnetic Disk
A form of memory using a thin film of ferrite material on a disk. This form is intermediate between magnetic tape and random access memory in both speed and cost per word of memory.

Magnetic Disk Pack
A stack of individual magnetic disks all of which can be addressed simultaneously. This permits a significant expansion of the storage capacity compared to a single disk.

Magnetic Field
A vector field that originates from magnetic moments, a magnetized material, or from moving electrical charges (electrical current). A magnetic field induces or exerts a force on a moving electrical charge.

Magnetic Moment
A fundamental vector quantity associated with a magnetic dipole. The magnetic moment is a measure of the torque exerted on the magnetic dipole by an external magnetic field. Elementary particles, including nucleons and electrons, possess characteristic magnetic moments and spins.

Magnetic Tape
A peripheral or auxiliary memory of the sequential storage type using a tape containing ferrite material. It is the oldest and cheapest form of peripheral memory.

Magnetic Tape Drive
A computer hardware device for transferring data back and forth between magnetic tape and a magnetic disk.

Magnetogyric Ratio
See Gyromagnetic Ratio.

Magnification
Enlargement of a portion of an image without any improvement in resolution. Alternatively, the term may be used to describe a mode of scanning in which only a limited field of view is reconstructed from the scan data, resulting in a larger image of the area with improved resolution. Also, in some third generation scanners, a geometric magnification with better resolution is obtained by shifting the center of rotation closer to the x-ray tube.

Main Memory
This refers to storage locations, invariably of the random access type, that are used by the central processing unit exclusively during the execution of a program.

Mainframe
A term sometimes used (to some extent incorrectly) to describe either a computer or a central processing unit.

Mark I
The first transmission CT system, a dedicated head unit employing a combined translational-rotational motion. It was designed by Godfrey N. Hounsfield and built by the EMI Company. Initial clinical trials were performed in 1971–1972. Also the name of the first successful digital computer, which utilized electromagnetic relays. This electromechanical predecessor to later electronic digital computers was used at Harvard University from 1935–1944. It was also described as the Automated Sequence Con-

trolled Calculator. An early gamma-ray emission CT unit, designed by David Kuhl and Ray Edwards, was also designated the Mark I.

Mass Attenuation Coefficient

This is an attenuation coefficient originated to quantitate the x-ray attenuation of materials independently of their physical state as a solid, liquid, or gas. For example, water, ice and steam (three different physical states of H_2O) all have the same mass attenuation coefficient. It is obtained by dividing the linear attenuation coefficient μ of a material by its density ρ (in units of grams per cubic centimeter) and is represented as μ/ρ. It is expressed in units of grams per square centimeter.

Matrix

An array of numbers composed of rows and columns; each number corresponds to an element of the matrix.

Memory

A device for storing digital information.
See Auxiliary Memory, Main Memory, Nonvolatile Memory, Random Access Memory, Read-Only Memory, Refresh Memory, Sequential Storage Memory, Volatile Memory.

Microcomputer

A computer made from large-scale integrated circuits and composed entirely of a microprocessor of 4- to 8-bit capacity and an extremely limited set of basic functions. There is usually only limited, if any, addressable memory. Connections to peripheral devices and software modifications are extremely limited.

Microinstructions

The lowest level of language or instruction within a computer.

Microprocessor

A single large-scale integrated circuit consisting of an arithmetic logic unit as well as a control unit, including timing circuits, bus control circuits, and several registers of memory. It requires only the addition of memory and appropriate input and output devices to form a complete computer. It is essentially a central processing unit on a single chip.

Microwaves

A form of electromagnetic energy whose energy (or frequency) is intermediate between radiowaves and infrared. Their wavelength is of the order of millimeters and centimeters and their frequencies of the order of 10^9 to 10^{11} Hz.

Minicomputer

A computer made from large-scale integrated circuits which has one or more microprocessors, each with a capacity for direct manipulation of 8- to 16-bit words. It has a more extensive set of instructions than a microcomputer. There is usually a 4- to 64-kbyte random access memory. Peripheral supports usually include a cathode ray tube display and typewriter keyboard; a printer and floppy or rigid disk drives may also be included. A limited number of input and output devices may be supported.

Modulation Transfer Function (MTF)

A measurement of the relative spatial frequency response of a system. Quantitatively, it is the ratio of the amplitude of the output of a system to the amplitude of the input at a specific spatial frequency. This ratio can then be measured for different frequencies. It may also be derived by a Fourier transformation of the line spread function of the system, since the modulation transfer function is the representation in terms of spatial frequencies of the line spread function.

Monitor (CRT Monitor, Display Monitor, Television Monitor, Viewing Monitor, Video Monitor)

A cathode ray tube used to display an image, which is viewed on the face of the tube. The image is displayed using a television or video format. Monitors are used for direct viewing of the image and in photographing hard copy.

Monochromatic

X-rays characterized by a single energy or wavelength.

Motion Artifacts

These occur as a result of inconsistency in the attenuation measurements because of patient motion. Frequently these are manifested as long streaks connected to air or high-contrast objects.

Motion Blur

Blur or unsharpness in conventional radiography arising from patient motion.

Multiformat Camera

A popular hard copy device for displaying CT images on radiographic film. The camera uses single-emulsion film (film in which the photographic emulsion is on only one side of the film base). Typically four to nine images can be displayed on an 8 × 10 sheet of film, or four to 20 images on a 14 × 17 inch sheet. Multiformat cameras may move the film over a single lens, move a single lens over the film, or use multiple lenses in obtaining separate exposures.

Multiplexer
: A device with multiple inputs, one of which is connected to the output when the appropriate binary signal is applied to the select line of this device.

NAND
: Inverse of the AND function. The most versatile and widely used logic gate.

Natural Logarithm (log, ln)
: For a given positive number, the natural logarithm is the exponent to which the base 2.71828 ... (designated by the letter e) must be raised so that the expression equals the given positive number. It is also known as the Napierian logarithm, after its originator, John Napier, who also introduced the decimal point.

Negative Mode
: A white-on-black display mode; the image is shown as white and shades of gray on a black or dark background.

New Hounsfield Units
: See Hounsfield Units.

NMR
: See Nuclear Magnetic Resonance.

Noise
: A part of the signal that does not contain information. Noise may be due to fundamental quantum limitations or to system limitations. See Artifact, Electronic Noise, Film Grain, Quantum Mottle (Photon Fluctuation), Roundoff Errors, Statistical (Quantum) Noise.

Noise Power Spectrum (Wiener Spectrum)
: A graph or plot of the frequency distribution of the noise in an image. The noise power is plotted as a function of the noise frequency.

Nonlinear Attenuation Errors
: Artifacts that occur because of erroneous attenuation measurements caused by nonlinear detector performance or scatter detection.

Nonlinear Partial Volume Effect
: This arises because of objects, especially dense bones, extending only partly into the scan section. The effect is usually manifested by lucent streaks appearing between pairs of high density objects (e.g., bones, surgical clips). They can be reduced by using thinner sections.

Nonvolatile Memory
: Memory in which energy is not required for maintenance of stored information.

NOR
: Inverse of the OR function. A type of logic gate.

Normalization
: A process of measuring and correcting the errors, offsets, and sensitivities of individual detectors in order to achieve uniform relative measurements.

NOT
: See Complement.

Nuclear Magnetic Resonance (NMR)
: A resonance phenomenon in which there is absorption and emission of resonant radiofrequency energy by naturally occurring nuclear magnetic moments or magnets in tissue when the body is placed in a static external magnetic field. These intrinsic magnetic moments have a naturally occurring or resonant frequency (Larmor precession frequency) when placed in a magnetic field. The phenomenon of NMR occurs when an external radiofrequency magnetic field identical to the Larmor precession frequency is applied perpendicular to the static magnetic field.

Nuclear Magnetic Resonance Imaging
: A method of obtaining cross-sectional head or body images in any arbitrary orientation by the use of NMR techniques to map out parameters such as the density of magnetic moments and magnetic relaxation times.

Nutation
: A wobbling or slight rotational motion in which the axis of a structure or vector quantity nods up and down.

Nyquist Theorem
: This states that faithful reproduction of a spatially varying object requires a spatial sampling frequency that is twice the highest spatial frequency or rate of change within the object.

Octal
: Number system with base 8.

Old Hounsfield Units
: See EMI Units.

Operating System
: The complete set of software available to the user as part of the initial computer system. It is the software that comes with computer. It is composed of a control system and a processing system.

OR
: Binary equivalent of addition. If at least one input is "true" (equal to 1), then the output is "true" (1). A type of logic gate.

Orthochromatic Film
: Film that is sensitive to green light. Many films

used in conjunction with fast rare earth screens are orthochromatic, whereas other medical or radiographic film is usually sensitive to blue light (which is emitted by conventional x-ray screens).

Overscan
The collection of additional scanning views beyond the minimum number required for image formation as a means of reducing motion artifacts in processing.

Pair Production
The production of an electron and a positron (a positively charged electron) resulting from the interaction of a high-energy photon with the nucleus of an atom. Because the minimum photon energy for pair production is 1.02 MeV, this process does not contribute to the attenuation of x-rays in the diagnostic energy range. However, it does assume importance in attenuation of x-rays in megavoltage beam therapy.

Paper Tape
A device for batch data input to a computer utilizing sequences of holes punched in tape to represent data for processing. It is similar to that formerly seen in teletype machines.

Parallax Blur
Blur or unsharpness arising in conventional radiography from the fact that two images are present in double-emulsion films, each separated by the thickness or width of the film base.

Paramagnetic
Atoms or ions that slightly increase a magnetic field when placed within it are called paramagnetic. They have an odd number of electrons and a partially filled inner shell, such as found in transition elements, rare earths, and actinides; they also occur in a few compounds with an even number of electrons (most notably molecular oxygen) and some metals.

Parasitic Streaks
The streaks or residual lines seen in conventional linear tomography as a result of the incomplete or poor blurring of structures whose longitudinal axes are parallel to the direction of x-ray tub movement.

Partial Volume Effect
When a voxel is occupied by two different tissues, its CT numbers will be an average of the CT numbers of the two tissues, weighted by their relative partial volumes within the voxel. This is most significant when a small object lies entirely within a thick slice, or at the edge of adjacent slices.

PECT
See Positron Emission Computed Tomography.

Pencil Beam
A small sharply collimated x-ray beam with a cross-section that is typically rectangular.

Period
The temporal or spatial duration of one cycle of a periodic wave or function.

Peripherals (Peripheral Devices)
Accessory devices such as terminals, printers, magnetic disks, and tape drives that communicate with the central processing unit for transferring and storing information.

Phantom
A physical object used to measure the response of the CT system. A particular phantom is chosen to simulate certain characteristics of the objects that ultimately will be measured on the machine. Typically the calibration of a CT unit involves the use of different phantoms that vary in their shape and material.

Phantom Images
Artifacts produced in conventional tomography by the blurred margins of structures outside of the focal plane.

Phosphorescence
A process in which radiation, typically light, is emitted by a substance that has absorbed radiation from an external source. The emitted radiation is generally of lower energy than the absorbed energy. In contrast to fluorescence, the emission is slower (greater than 10^{-8} s) after absorption and will continue after excitation ceases.

Photoelectric Effect
Fundamental interaction between electromagnetic radiation (e.g., x-rays) and matter. The photon is entirely absorbed by the atom with expulsion of a photoelectron. The atom becomes ionized and characteristic radiation is emitted. The absorbed energy dose is relatively high.

Photoelectron
The electron that is liberated from an atom in the photoelectric effect. The kinetic energy of this electron is equal to the energy of the incident x-ray photon minus the initial binding energy of the electron in the atom.

Photomultiplier
An electronic vacuum tube that transforms incident light photons or optical energy into electrical energy in the form of an electron current

that is amplified through successive stages involving electrodes called dynodes.

Photon

A discrete unit or quanta of electromagnetic radiation; in CT (and conventional radiography) high-energy or "hard" x-ray photons are employed. Light photons are of a lower energy than x-ray photons.

Photon Fluctuation

See Quantum Mottle.

Piezoelectricity (Piezoelectric Effect, Pressure Electricity)

A property of certain naturally occurring crystalline materials and polycrystalline ceramics. When an electrical voltage is applied across the faces of the crystal or ceramic, the thickness of the crystal is altered (deformed). Conversely, when mechanical pressure is applied to deform the crystal, an electrical voltage is produced between the faces of the crystal.

Pilot Scan

See Computed Radiograph.

Pipeline Reconstruction.

A technique for scanning and image reconstruction in which the data from a scan are processed and reconstructed as an image before another scan is initiated; that is, a new scan cannot be performed until the previous scan has been reconstructed as an image.

Pixel

An abbreviation for "picture element cell." The pixel is a two-dimensional representation of the volume element on the display in the form of a square. The average linear attenuation coefficient, expressed in terms of a CT number, of a voxel is assigned to a pixel representing the cross-sectional area of the three-dimensional voxel. The CT number assigned to the pixel is then expressed in terms of a shade of gray.

Plate

See Anode.

Pluridirectional Tomography

A form of conventional tomography in which the x-ray tube and film synchronously undergo a complex tomographic motion (e.g., circular, ellipsoidal, hypocycloidal, spiral).

Point Spread Effect

This is a problem or artifact in which high contrast objects seem to be larger or smaller than they are. It arises because of the width of the point spread function. The apparent size of the object can be changed by varying the window settings.

Point Spread Function

A transfer function which depicts the output of a device or system to a high-amplitude point input.

Polar Coordinate System

A coordinate system in which the location of a point is specified by its distance or radius from the origin of the coordinate system and the angles of this radius with the vertical and a horizontal axis of the Cartesian coordinate system.

Polarity

Image display as either black-on-white (positive) or white-on-black (negative). The customary display is in the negative mode, although the positive mode is often used for displaying bone.

Polychromatic

An x-ray beam with components of different energies or wavelengths.

Positive Mode

A black-on-white mode; that is, the image is shown as black and shades of gray on a white or light background.

Positron

The antiparticle of the electron. A fundamental atomic particle with the mass of an electron but with a positive charge. Radioactive nuclei which decay with the emission of a positron are used in one type of emission computed tomography.

Positron Emission Computed Tomography (Positron Emission CT, PECT)

A form of emission computed tomography in which the image of a head or body cross-section is reconstructed by detecting the annihilation radiation resulting from the decay of positron emitters. This is done by using arrays of detectors operating in a coincidence mode, that is, arrays arranged at 180° to each other. The image is a map of the cross-sectional distribution of positron-emitting nuclei.

Power

The temporal rate at which energy is generated or used; the rate of performing work.

Precession

A rotation about an external axis analogous to the way in which a spinning top rotates about a vertical axis.

See Larmor Precession Frequency.

Precision

Self-consistency of a set of measurements; freedom from random error (to be distinguished from accuracy). An experiment that measures the freezing point of H_2O as 23.456°F ± 0.0001°F is very precise but not accurate.

Printer (Electromechanical Printer, Electrostatic Printer, Line Printer)

An electromechanical or electrostatic device that converts the computer's binary digital output to printed form as alphanumeric characters. Line printers can print an entire line of as many as 132 characters of output from a computer simultaneously on paper at speeds of 100–300 lines per minute. A printer is a batch output device. It is generally supplied as an optional piece of equipment in a CT system.

Processing System

The part of the operating system that provides a number of software packages which simplify the task of generating applications programs. Processing system can be divided into two broad areas, compilers and utility programs.

Profile (Projection, View)

The plot of detector readings versus position made during a linear traverse of the scanning gantry, that is, the complete set of ray sums at any given angle. The equivalent in a continuous rotation (purely rotational) multielement detector CT system.

Quantum

A photon or discrete particle-like unit of radiation.

Quantum Mottle (Photon Fluctuation)

The principle source of noise in conventional radiography due to the random variation in the number of photons absorbed by the intensifying screens.

Quantum Noise

See Statistical Noise.

Rad (Radiation Absorbed Dose)

A measurement of the quantity of radiation absorbed per unit of mass. One rad represents the absorption of 100 ergs of energy per gram of material.

Radiographic Contrast

The difference in the film density or darkening in different regions of the radiograph.

Radionuclides

Unstable atomic nuclei which undergo decay or disintegration with the emission of gamma rays, electrons, or positrons.

Radiotherapy Treatment Planning (RTP)

A software capability which permits the user to determine external outlines, a target outline, and internal inhomogeneity outlines on the CT image. It also enables the user to assign tissue densities, plan the position(s) of the therapy beam(s), and calculate the depth dose. The isodose contours with the doses and beam or patient data may be displayed, either alone or superimposed on the CT image.

Radiowaves (RF)

That portion of the electromagnetic spectrum characterized by relatively longer wavelengths (of the order of meters) and shorter frequencies (of the order of 10^5 to 10^9 Hz). Radiowaves are not currently used directly in diagnostic imaging.

Ramtek

The computer component that handles most of the CT system's display capabilities.

Random Access Memory (RAM)

A form of memory in which each word can be immediately retrieved for processing by specifying its location in the memory unit. It has the advantage of speed in retrieval but is relatively expensive to construct.

Range of Interest (ROI)

A technique for selecting a region on a CT image and obtaining parameters such as its area and average CT number.

Rapid-Sequence Computed Tomography

See Dynamic Computed Tomography.

Raster

A video or television format consisting of a series of horizontal lines scanned repetitively at a specific frame rate.

Raw Data (Scan Data, X-Ray Data)

The data or information representing the intensity of x-rays entering the detectors after digitization.

Ray

Theoretically, a straight line path through an object. Practically, a ray may be defined as a bundle of paths from the source to a small region of a given shape on the projection; alternatively, a ray indicates the portion of the x-ray beam that interacts with a single detector.

Ray Path

The straight line path that a ray follows.

Ray-Sum (Ray-Projection)

Theoretically, the mathematical integral of the density function or linear attenuation coefficient along the ray. Practically or experimentally, it is the measured total density (x-ray attenuation) within a ray, that is, an estimate of the total density of the object contained in the bundle of paths defining the ray.

Read-Only Memory (ROM)
A form of memory that allows the reading of information stored in the memory with the same ease and speed as in random access memory (RAM) but without the option of changing the information in the memory.

Receptor Blur (Screen Blur)
Blur or unsharpness in conventional radiography arising from the finite or nonzero thickness of the x-ray screens, which results in light diffusion in the fluorescent layer.

Reconstruction
An estimate of the density distribution or variation in the x-ray attenuation. A finite dimensional approximation of the x-ray attenuation distribution in a transverse section of the patient.

Reconstruction, Sagittal and Coronal
See Reformatted Images.

Rectilinear Tomography
See Linear Tomography.

Reference Signal
The x-ray signal measured by a detector placed near the x-ray tube, but not in the path of the primary beam.

Reformatted Images
Reconstructed images of cross-sections in planes other than transverse axial or original scan cross-sections. The data is reformatted to give an image of a cross-section that may be in a plane at any arbitrary orientation or obliquity to the original, usually transverse sections. Initially the reformatted images were restricted to sagittal or coronal planes.

Refresh Memory
A memory used to modulate the intensity of the electron beam of the CRT at a high repetition rate, in order to refresh the image on the face of the CRT or display monitor.

Register
A group of flip-flops arranged to hold an entire binary word of information.

Register, Parallel Load
A register with a separate input and output line for each flip-flop in the register, allowing each bit to be loaded or transmitted to a new location simultaneously on receiving the appropriate instruction.

Register, Shift
A register in which each bit is loaded sequentially from a single input line.

Relative Biological Effectiveness (RBE)
A quantity used to express the impact of a radiation in producing a specific biological effect, rather than general biological damage. Its unit is the rem, the same as for the dose equivalent.

Relaxation Time
See Spin-Lattice Relaxation Time (T_1), Spin-Spin Relaxation Time (T_2).

Rem
The unit for measuring the dose equivalent. The rem is essentially the dose of any form of radiation that will produce the same biological effect or damage as 1 rad of x-rays. By definition it is the amount of ionizing radiation that results in the same damage to humans as 1 roentgen of 200 KeV x-rays.

Resolution
See Contrast Resolution, Spatial Resolution.

Resonance (Resonant Frequency)
The response of a system in terms of its resonant frequency to an appropriate stimulus. The resonant frequency is the natural frequency of a system in terms of energy vibration or rotation. In NMR resonance is the energy difference between two different magnetic states or the precession frequency of the net tissue magnetization about the external magnetic field. In ultrasound resonance refers to the natural vibrational frequency of a particular crystal transducer.

Ring Artifact
See Circular Artifact.

Roentgen
Unit for measuring radiation exposure. It is expressed in terms of the total ionization charge produced by radiation in a unit mass of air. By definition, 1 roentgen is 2.58×10^{-4} coulombs of electrical charge per kilogram of air. The roentgen is named after the discoverer of x-rays, the German physicist William Conrad Roentgen (1845–1923).

Roundoff Errors
Errors or noise introduced as a result of the limited number of bits used to represent numbers in a digital computer.

Sampling (Sampling Frequency)
The spatial frequency or rate with which data or rays are obtained, that is, how close together individual data measurements are made. Alternatively, the temporal rate or frequency at which data are collected.

Saturation
The situation in which a detector is incapable of any further increase in its output current above

a certain level (the saturation level) as the input radiation intensity is increased.

Scan
The mechanical motion required to produce a CT image. This may be a combination of translation and rotation of the x-ray tube and detector(s), or it may be a single rotational motion. In some units a single scan can give rise to two images.

Scan Data
See Raw Data.

Scanned Projection Radiography
An imaging technique that uses a detector system which images only one small portion of the patient at any time. The detector sequentially scans the region to be imaged by mechanically translating the patient or the x-ray source and detector. Computed radiography is an example of this technique.

Scanning Electron Beam Systems
A purely electronic (i.e., nonmechanical) approach to ultrafast scanning. It involves the replacement of the conventional Coolidge x-ray tube(s) by a large device in which an electron beam is magnetically deflected along a circular anode ring or target surrounding the patient.

Scattering (Compton Scattering)
One of the two ways in which x-ray beam intensity is diminished in passing through an object. Scattering takes place by collision with the atomic constituents of the object. The x-rays are scattered in a direction different from the original beam direction. Such scattered x-rays falling on the detector do not add to the production of the image but rather reduce the contrast in that image, and so steps are usually taken to eliminate the scattered radiation from the detector.

Scintillation Crystal
A crystal detector that converts x-ray energy into light energy. The scintillation crystal is interfaced to a photomultiplier tube for signal amplification. This was the first CT detection system and continues to be in major use. Crystals employed have included sodium iodide, calcium fluoride, bismuth germanate, and cesium iodide.

Scout View
See Computed Radiograph.

Screen Blur
See Receptor Blur.

Screen Structure Mottle
Mottle or noise in conventional radiography arising from variations in the crystals of the intensifying screens.

Semiconductor
A solid material with properties intermediate between those of a conductor and an insulator.

Sequential Storage Memory
A form of memory in which the memory must be examined word by word until the required piece of information is located. It is slower in retrieval than random access memory but relatively cheaper.

Sharpness
The capability of an imaging system to define an edge.

Signal-to-Noise Ratio (SNR, S/N)
The ratio of the amplitude of a signal to the amplitude of the background noise.

Simulation
The representation of one system by a physical or mathematical analog.

Single Emission Computed Tomography (SECT)
See Gamma Emission Computed Tomography.

Slice
The cross-sectional portion of the body that is scanned for the production of the CT image.
See also Tomographic Plane.

Slit Beam Radiography
Any imaging technique that utilizes a slitlike detector, in contrast to the large area used in conventional radiography.

Smoothing
The selective removal of high-frequency detail from an image.

Software
The set of instructions that controls the operation of a computer.

Sonar
From Sound Navigation and Ranging.
See Ultrasound.

Spatial Frequency
A sinusoidal variation of a spatial quantity; a periodic repetition of a parameter in space.

Spatial Resolution
This refers to the capability of an imaging system to record a distinct image of two or more closely spaced high-contrast objects.

Spatial Uniformity
The capability of a CT scanner to measure the same CT number of an object or substance regardless of its position within the scan section.
See also Uniformity.

Spectral Sensitivity (Film Spectral Sensitivity)
The sensitivity of medical imaging or radiographic film as a function of the color of light used in exposing the film. In conventional radiography the light arises from screens pressed against the film which convert x-ray energy into light energy. In CT the light arises from the CRT camera monitor on which the image is displayed for photography.

Spectral Shift
A change in frequency.
See Beam Hardening.

Spectrum
The arrangement of the intensity of the x-rays (or any other electromagnetic radiation) according to wavelength, frequency, or energy, which are fundamentally equivalent quantities.

Spectrum
The distribution of the energy of a signal among its different frequency components.

Spin
Individual protons and neutrons (nucleons) can be considered as moving in orbit around the nucleus, and so possess angular momentum. These nucleons also rotate about their axes and thus also have a spin or intrinsic angular momentum just like electrons. Pairs of neutrons or protons align so that their spins cancel out. A nucleus with an odd number of neutrons and/or protons will have a net rotational component characterized by an integer or half-integer quantum number called the spin of the nucleus. Spin may be regarded as the intrinsic angular momentum that a particle has as a result of internal rotation (rotation about its own axis).
See Angular Momentum.

Spin Density
The number of nuclei resonating within a unit volume.

Spin Echo
Under certain irradiation conditions, nuclei can be made to resonate so that the axes of their spins point in the same direction at repeated, fixed intervals in time, producing a strong signal called the spin echo.

Spin-Lattice Relaxation Time (T_1, Longitudinal Relaxation Time)
The exponential time constant at which the component of magnetization parallel to the external magnetic field grows or decays; in other words, a measure of the time needed for the nuclear magnetic moments to reach equilibrium with their environment.

Spin-Spin Relaxation Time (T_2, Transverse Relaxation Time)
The exponential time constant at which the component of magnetization perpendicular to the external magnetic field decays; in other words, a measure of the time needed for the nuclear magnetic moments to reach equilibrium with each other.

Standard Deviation
An index of the distribution of a sample about the mean. For a Gaussian distribution, 95% of the sample lies within the range of 2 standard deviations of the mean.

Statistical Noise (Quantum Noise)
In general, any noise that arises as the result of the random variation in the number of the x-ray photons detected.

Step Response Function
See Edge Response Function.

Storage Capacity
Capacity of the computer for data storage, expressed in terms of millions of bytes of information.

Streak Artifact
Straight lines projecting across the field of view in the form of an arc converging to a common point. This common point or source of the artifact may be related to an object lying within or outside of the field of view. Streak artifacts may arise from a number of different sources and are the most common way in which artifacts are manifested in CT.

Subject Contrast
The "natural" contrast in the subject or patient being imaged. This is determined by the differences in thickness, mass density, atomic number, and x-ray photon energy (or kVp) associated with the different structures or parts within the subject.

Summation Method
See Back-Projection.

Surface Integral Exposure (SIE)
This is a measure of the total amount of radiation delivered to a surface area. It is the product of the exposure in roentgens and the surface area involved and is expressed in $R \times cm^2$.

Symbolic Address
The association of an address in memory with an alphanumeric mnemonic.

Table (CT Table)
: The bed or portion of the CT unit on which the patient is placed. The patient remains stationary relative to the table, which is then periodically moved or incremented into or out of the gantry so that a new cross-section of the patient is centered in the gantry for imaging.

Tape
: See Magnetic Tape, Paper Tape.

Target
: See Anode.

Target Scan
: A high spatial resolution CT image obtained by reconstructing the raw data of a scan on smaller pixels.

Teletype
: See Typewriter Keyboard.

Tesla
: A unit of magnetic field strength used to describe relatively stronger magnetic fields. One tesla = 10^4 gauss. It is named after the physicist Nikola Tesla (1856–1943).

Thermography
: An imaging technique based on the detection of the naturally occurring body emission of infrared radiation.

Thermoluminescent Dosimeter (TLD)
: A crystalline substance that traps electrons excited by radiation at impurity sites within the crystal. After heating, the trapped electrons are released, with the emission of light which can be measured. This provides an estimate of the exposure or absorbed dose.

Tomographic Plane
: A section of the body imaged by the tomographic process. Although in CT the tomographic plane or slice is displayed as a two-dimensional image, it should be remembered that there is a certain finite width associated with the plane.

Tomography
: From the Greek "to write" and "a slice or section". The process of imaging a particular body cross-section or slice.

Torque
: A change in angular momentum as a result of a force changing the rotation; a force that produces or tends to produce rotation.

Total Blur
: See Composite Blur.

Trace
: A closed outline of arbitrary size and contour traced over the CT image with a cursor.

Trackball
: A freely rotatable ball whose center is fixed in position on an operator console or keyboard which allows a user to move a cursor over a cathode ray tube. It is similar in function to a joystick or light pen.

Transducer
: A device that transforms energy from one form into another. An example is an ultrasound transducer, which can transform electrical energy into mechanical energy, or vice versa, by the piezoelectric effect.

Transfer Function
: A function that describes the response or output of a device or system to a particular input.

Transistor (Bipolar Transistor, Junction-Type Transistor)
: A three-element semiconductor device, which is the simplest form of solid-state device capable of amplification. The use of transistors to fabricate logic circuits characterized second generation electronic digital computers.

Transistor-Transistor Logic
: An integrated circuit device in which bipolar transistors are directly coupled to each other. This circumvents the problems associated with the use of poorly miniaturized intervening resistors.

Transmission Computed Tomography (Computed Tomography, Computerized Transverse Axial Tomography, Computer Assisted Tomography, Computerized Tomography, Reconstruction Tomography, Transverse Axial Tomography)
: The presentation of anatomical information in a body cross-section or slice by computer synthesis or reconstruction of an image from x-ray transmission data obtained by passing a finely collimated x-ray beam through the cross-section in multiple different directions.

Transverse Relaxation Time (T_2)
: See Spin-Spin Relaxation Time (T_2).

Traversal (Translation, Traverse)
: In translational-rotational CT units, a complete linear movement of the x-ray tube and detector(s) in synchrony across the subject.

Triode
: A three-element electronic vacuum tube, which is the simplest form of electronic tube capable of amplification.

Truth Table
   The relationship between the input and the output for a given logic function.
Tube
   See X-Ray Tube.
Typewriter Keyboard (Teletype)
   A device used for communication between a user and the computer. Instructions or data entered into the keyboard are displayed on a cathode ray tube, where they can be checked for accuracy before transmission to the central processing unit. It is similar in layout to a conventional typewriter except that only capital letters are customarily used.
Ultrasound (Sonar)
   Sound (mechanical or pressure wave) with a frequency above 20 kHz. A tomographic technique using high-frequency (1–10 MHz) nonionizing sound waves to produce cross-sectional images of soft tissues.
Ultraviolet
   That portion of the electromagnetic spectrum lying between light and x-rays with a frequency range of about 10^{15} to 10^{17} Hz. The corresponding range of wavelengths is of the order of .1–.001 microns (1 micron = 10^{-6} m). Ultraviolet radiation is not currently used for diagnostic imaging.
Unidirectional Tomography
   See Linear Tomography.
Uniformity
   A measurement of spatial independence or variation of CT numbers. It can be measured by use of a phantom. Nonuniformity may occur secondary to detector response (nonlinearities), beam hardening, algorithm (polar to Cartesian coordinate system conversion for large field of view), geometrical considerations related to using a fan beam, and afterglow effects in sodium iodide detectors.
UNIVAC
   The first commercially available electronic digital computer, which appeared about 1950.
Utility Program
   A program that is part of the operating system (the software that comes with the computer), but which also provides many software functions that would otherwise be part of many applications programs. As opposed to an applications program, a utility program is supplied to the user as part of the initial computer system. Within the framework of the operating system a utility program is part of the processing system (in distinction to the control system).
Vacuum Tube
   An early electronic device with two or more electrodes enclosed in a vacuum tube. Features include rectification (allowing electrical current to pass in only one direction) and amplification. The use of vacuum tubes to fabricate logic circuits characterized first generation electronic digital computers.
Vector
   A quantity that has directional properties as well as those of magnitude. For example, velocity indicates not only the speed of a motion but its direction as well.
Video
   A television display system in which the image consists of multiple horizontal scan lines in a raster format. The image is changed or refreshed at a specific frame rate (e.g., 30 per s) and displayed on a cathode ray tube monitor.
View
   See Profile.
Volatile Memory
   Memory in which energy is required for maintenance of stored information.
Voxel (Volume Element)
   The basic volume unit of the CT reconstruction. The depth is equal to the thickness of the slice. The cross-sectional area is equal to the pixel area and is determined by the reconstruction algorithm.
Water Bag
   This was used in early CT scanners to avoid abrupt changes in x-ray beam attenuation on either side of the skull at the beginning and end of a linear traversal. The water also hardens the x-ray beam, making it more monochromatic, and provides a direct measurement of the attenuation coefficient of water as a standard.
Wave
   A periodic alteration or vibration in time and/or space of a physical parameter. A wave is characterized by velocity, frequency, and wavelength.
Wave Number
   The inverse of the wavelength ($\frac{1}{\lambda}$, where λ is the wavelength). It is expressed in units of inverse centimeters (cm^{-1}).
Wavelength
   The distance between corresponding points of a wave, that is, the distance between successive

peaks or troughs (or corresponding points) of a wave.

White Noise
A type of noise characterized by a fairly uniform or constant distribution of the noise power with frequency.

Width
See Window Width.

Wiener Spectrum
See Noise Power Spectrum.

Window Level
The center of the window of CT numbers to be displayed, that is, the CT number of the middle of the gray scale.

Window Width
The range of CT numbers encompassed in between black and white for display, that is, the range of the CT numbers in the gray scale.

Word
The largest group of bytes or bits that can be accessed and processed by a computer as a single functional unit.

X-Ray
Electromagnetic radiation employed in diagnostic and therapeutic radiology. Typical energies employed in diagnostic radiology are 40–140 keV.

X-Ray Data
See Raw Data.

X-Ray Dose
See Dose, Rad.

X-Ray Exposure
See Exposure, Roentgen.

X-Ray Tube (X-Ray Source, Coolidge Tube)
A vacuum tube device in which electrons emitted from a hot cathode are accelerated through a high electrical potential (typically 40–140 keV) striking an anode target (typically of tungsten). The electron bombardment of the anode target results in the production of x-rays, which are directed out of the tube. The present form of the x-ray tube is the invention of the American physicist William D. Coolidge.

X-Ray Tube Heat Capacity
The amount of energy, expressed in heat units, that can be safely stored in the x-ray tube without damage to the tube.

Xenon
A heavy (atomic number Z of 54 and average atomic weight of 131.3), colorless, inert gas, easily ionized by x-rays. At high pressure it is used as a detector in many third generation CT systems.

Zoom
A feature incorporated into many CT systems that permits magnification of a portion of a CT image on a monitor, either for direct viewing or photography. Usually no additional resolution is achieved, only image enlargement. Alternatively, in some CT systems the term is used to describe a higher resolution, usually performed for a smaller field of view.

INDEX

Absorption blur, 177
Accuracy, of CT numbers, 205
Acoustic impedance, 251
ADD command, 95, 96
Adders, 81
Address bus, 84, 85
Address field, 94, 95
Afterglow, 284
Algebraic reconstruction technique (ART), 111–114, 122
Algorithm, 25, 64, 107
   artifacts, 281–282
Aliasing, 119, 188, 280
   artifacts, 279
Ambient conditions, 172
American Association of Physicists in Medicine (AAPM), 192, 206
Amplitude mode (A-mode), 252
Analog computers, 70
Analog-to-digital converter, 43
Analytical reconstruction, 116–122, 294–296
   evaluation of, 118–120
   filtered back-projection, 116–118, 119–120, 149, 295–296
   Fourier analysis, 116, 119, 294
AND gate, 73, 75, 76, 79
Anger camera, 243
Angiotomography, computed, 217, 220
Angular sampling, 280
Anisotropic function, 178
Annihilation, 244
Annihilation coincidence detection (ACD), 241
Annotation, 144
Anode tubes; see X-ray
Antimatter, 244
Antineutrino, 244
Apertures, 28, 29
   detector, 34, 185–188
Application programs, 99, 100–101
Arithmetic logic unit (ALU), 84, 85–86
Array processor, 165
Artifacts, 51, 176, 194, 275–290
   algorithm, 281–282
   from attenuation measurement errors
      nonlinearity and, 284–285
      scanner geometry and, 282–284
   beam hardening and, 285–286
   geometric, 276–281
      aliasing, 279
      edge gradient streaks, 280–281
      motion, 277–279
      sampling inadequacy and, 280
   partial volume effects, 281, 286–289
   streaks, 275–277, 280
   visual illusions, 289
ASCII system, 89
Assembler, 94, 98
Assembly language, 97–98
Asynchronous flip-flop circuit, 79
Atomic number, 22, 181
Attenuation, x-ray; see X-ray
Automated scanning, 256
Automatic Computerized Transverse Axial (ACTA) scanner, 16, 29, 33, 34, 36–37
Auxiliary memory, 89–91
Average gradient, 182
Axial transverse tomography, 9, 10

Background contrast effect, 289
Back-projection
   filtered, 116–118, 119–120, 149, 295–296
   simple, 108–110, 188, 189, 292, 294–295
Band limiting, 119, 121
Base, 77
   color, 154
BASIC, 99
Batch devices, 91–92
Beam hardening, 33, 44–45
   artifacts, 285–286
Bell Telephone Laboratories, 77
Beta emitters, 243–244
Biliary contrast, 148
Binary coded decimal (BCD), 72
Binary counters, 81
Binary digit (bit), 79, 80, 90
Binary states, 73–77
Binary system, 71, 72
Biodynamic Research Unit (Mayo Clinic), 237
Bismuth germanate (BGO), 62, 246
Blinker function, 144–145
Blur, 177–178
Body section radiography, 1
Boltzmann distribution, 258
Bone, 44
Boolean logic, 72–73
Bowel, 147
   peristalsis, 51
"Bow tie" filtering, 285
Bremsstrahlung, 32
Brightness mode (B-mode), 252

British Department of Health, 15
B-scanning, 252–256
Buffer, 74, 91
Bureau of Radiological Health, 192, 206
Bus system, 84–85
Byte, 80

Cadmium tungstate ($CdWO_4$), 62
Calcification, 43
Calcium tungstate, 177
Calculator, 70
Calibration, 285
Capture efficiency, 35–36
Cardiovascular CT (CVCT) scanner, 240
Cathode ray tube (CRT), 92, 127–128
Central processing unit (CPU), 82, 83, 84–86, 164, 169
   arithmetic logic unit (ALU), 84, 85–86
   control unit (CU), 84, 86
Cesium fluoride (CsF), 246
Cesium iodide (CsI) crystals, 62, 63
CGR Benelux Company, 3
CGR Ce 10000, 32, 53
Characteristic radiation, 22
Chemical shift, 262
Cleon-710 Brain Imager, 243
COBOL, 99
Coincidence, random, 245–246
Collector, 77
Collimation, 163–164, 184
   contrast resolution and, 193
   entrance, 42
   in purely rotational systems, 56, 61–62
   in translational-rotational systems, 33–34, 48
Collimator, 162, 163
Color display, 142
Compiler, 94, 98, 99
Complementary metal-oxide-semiconductor (CMOS), 78, 79
Complex integrated circuits, 79–82
Composite blue, 177–178
Composite phantom, 206
Compton effect, 22–23, 199, 228, 236
Computed angiotomography, 217, 220
Computed tomography (CT) units,

337

Computed tomography (CT) units, (*Cont.*)
  comparative features of, 298–309
Computerized transverse axial tomography, 11
Computers, 69–105
  analog, 70
  application programs, 99, 100–101
  applications in CT, 101–105
  background and development, 70
  binary states and, 73–77
  Boolean logic, 72–73
  central processing unit (CPU), 84–86
  digital, 70
  graphics, 143–144
  hardware installation, 103–105
  input and output (I/O) devices, 91–93
  integrated circuits, 78–83
  languages
    assembly, 97–98
    FORTRAN, 98–99
    machine, 93–97
    other types of, 99
  memory, 82, 86–91
  number systems, 70–72
  operating systems, 99–100
  organization of, 83–84
  programming levels, 94
  reconstruction using, 42–43
  transistors in, 77–78
  virtual, 94
Contrast, 10, 46, 176, 177, 289
  enhancement of, 23, 147–149
  film, 153, 181–182
  resolution, 192–196, 218
    defined, 192
    factors determining, 192–193
    noise and, 193–196
    in radiography, 180–183
Contrast transfer function (CTF), 191
Control bus, 84, 85
Control program, 99
Control system, 100
Control unit (CU), 84, 86
Conventional tomography, 1–11
  history and development, 1–3
  principles of, 3–8
  types of, 8–11
Convergence, 121
Convolution, 116–117, 180, 192
  algorithms, 64
  divergent beam and, 122–123
  filtering, 108, 295–296
  kernel, 188–189
Crystal-photodiode system, 58, 62, 63
Crystal-photomultiplier systems, 34–36, 58, 62, 64, 66–67
CT number, 43–44
  definitions of, 205–206
  linear attenuation coefficient as, 43, 204–205

measuring, 144–147
  scale, 128–129
    extended, 134–136
  see also Gray scale window
Cupping, 44, 286
Cursor, 140, 143
  box, 145–146
Cyclotron, 247
Cystografin, 148

Data acquisition system (DAS), 159, 163–164
Data processing system, 164–165
Data samples, 39–40, 42
Dead time, 60–61
Decimal system, 70
Decoders, 81
Deconvolution, 219
Delta 100, 30
De Morgan's theorem, 73
Density, 181–182
Detail, 177
Detection systems, 34–36, 38, 188
  crystal-photodiodes, 58, 62, 63
  crystal-photomultiplier, 34–36, 58, 62, 64, 66–67
  gas, 56–58, 59, 64, 66–67, 163
  multicrystal, 242–243
  for positron ECT, 246
  sensitivity of, 193
Detectors, 25, 38, 59
  aperture, 34, 185–188
  faulty, 283
  fixed, 60–67
  patient dosage and, 201–202
  rotating, 51–60
  in rotational systems, 56–58, 59, 62–63
  spacing of, 56, 61–62
  in translational-rotational systems, 34–36, 38
Diagnostic display console (DDC), 228
Digital computers, 70
Direct magnification, 58–59
Disk drives, 90
Disk unit, 164, 169
Display, image; *see* Image display
Display resolution, 66
Display terminals, 165–167
Divergent beam, 122, 123
  see also Fan beam
DNA, 264
Do loop, 98
Doppler effect, 248, 256
Dosage, patient, 197
  measurement, 203–204
  parameters affecting, 200–203
  radiation exposure and, 198–200
Dose phantoms, 208
Dosimeters, 203–204
Dual energy scanning, 236–237
Duty cycle, 170
Dynamic B-scanning, 253–256

Dynamic computed tomography, 219–227
Dynamic range, 218, 285
Dynamic scanning, 217
Dynamic Spatial Reconstructor (DSR), 237–239, 240
Dynode, 35

Echocardiography, 249
Echoes, 251
Edge
  enhancement, 151, 281–282
  gradient, 177
    streaks, 280–281
  response function, 190
Electrical gates, 73
Electric lens, 127
Electromagnetic radiation, 20–21
  see also X-ray
Electronic noise, 194
Electronic Numerical Integrator and Calculator (ENIAC), 76
Electron paramagnetic resonance (EPR), 256
Electron spin resonance (ESR), 256–257
Elscint Exel scanners, 30, 38, 59
EMI scanners, 15–16, 29, 34, 36–37, 38, 54, 107, 112, 122, 137, 243
Emission computed tomography (ECT), 11, 13, 240–248
  gamma ray, 242–243
  general description, 240–242
  positron, 241, 243–248
Emitter, 77
  beta, 243–244
Emitter coupled logic (ECL), 80
Environment, patient, 171–173
Exponential attenuation, 23–25
Exposure, 170–171
E-Z-CAT, 147

Fan beam, 29–30, 58–59, 122
  see also Divergent beam
Fat, 43, 196–197
Field, 94, 95, 127
  of view, 28, 121–122, 171
Field effect transistor (FET), 78
Film, 47
  contrast, 153, 181–182
  grain, 183
  positive print, 151
  as radiation measurement device, 204
  speed, 153–154
  transilluminated, 151, 152–154
Filtered back-projection, 116–118, 119–120, 149, 295–296
  algorithms, 64
  "bow tie," 285
  convolution, 108, 295–296
  Fourier, 108, 118, 295

image display, 149–151
noise, 194
Radon, 108, 118, 295
Filtration, 163–164
Flip-flops, 79–80
Floor space, 171
Floppy disk, 90–91
Fluorescence, 177
Focal plane, 4
Focal spot
 blur, 177
 size, 184
Focused nuclear resonance (FONAR), 263
FONAR Corporation, 257
FORTRAN, 98–99
Fourier analysis, 116, 119, 294
Fourier filtering, 108, 118, 295
Fourier transformation, 180, 191, 295
Fraunhofer zone, 250, 251
Frequency, 20–21
Fresnel zone, 250, 251
Fulcrum, 3, 4
Full width at half-maximum (FWHM), 190

Gamma camera, 243
Gamma ray, 21
Gamma ray emission computed tomography, 242–243
Gamma value, 182
Gantry, 28, 29, 159–164, 169
 X-ray tube and, 55–56
Gas detection systems, 56–58, 59, 64, 66–67, 163
Gastrografin, 147
Gated scanning, 234–236
Gauss units, 259
General Electric CT/T scanners
 7800 model, 53, 159, 162, 164, 170
 8800 model, 58, 123, 159, 162, 164, 165, 168, 170, 171, 218, 233, 280
 9800 model, 59, 163, 164
General Electric Gray/White Phantom Mod III, 206–208
Generation, 60
 defined, 29
Geometric artifacts, 276–281
 aliasing, 279
 edge gradient streaks, 280–281
 motion, 277–279
 sampling inadequacy and, 280
Geometric blur, 177
Geometric scale factor, 184–186
Grain, 150, 183, 196–197
Graphics, 143–144
Gray scale imaging, 253
Gray scale window, 46–47
Grid, 76, 77, 144

Half-adder, 81

HALT command, 95
Handshake, 85
Hard copy, 151–154
Hardware, 77–83
 installation of, 103–105
 integrated circuits in, 78–83
 transistors in, 77–78
Hard x-rays, 21
Hexadecimal system, 71
High resolution computed tomography, 233–234
Hollerith card, 91–92
Hounsfield partial volume effect, 281, 288
Hysteresis, 284

IF statement, 98
Image, synthesized, 126–127, 189
Image clarity; see Contrast; Noise; Spatial resolution
Image display, 47–49, 127–154, 193
 cathode ray tube (CRT), 127–128
 color, 142
 computer graphics, 143–144
 contrast enhancement and, 147–149
 CT number scale and, 128–129, 134–136
 filtering, 149–151
 hard copy, 151–154
 magnification, 139–140
 measurements, 144–147
 multiple, 140–142
 reversals of, 136–139
 window settings, 129–136
Image manipulation, 218–219
Impedance, 251
Inaccuracy, 197
Independent physician display console (IPDC), 167
Infarction, 226
Infrared radiation, 21
Inherent contrast, 192
Input and output (I/O) devices, 91–93
Integral dose (ID), 200
Integral equation method, 116
Integrated circuits, 78–83
Intel Corporation, 82
Interactive devices, 92–93, 143–144
Interpetrous artifacts, 286
Interpolation, 119–120, 121
Intrathecal contrast, 148
Intravenous contrast, 147–148
Ionization chambers, 203
Isotropic function, 178
Iterative least-squares technique (ILST), 111, 122
Iterative reconstruction, 110–116, 120–122, 292–294

Joystick, 93, 143
JUMP command, 85, 95, 96

Keyboard, 92, 143
Keypunch, 92
Kinetic energy, 22
K shell, 22

Laminagraphy, 1
Language, computer, 93–99
 assembly, 97–98
 FORTRAN, 98–99
 machine, 93–97
Large scale integrated circuit (LSI), 82–83
Larmor precession frequency, 259–260
Latch, 79
Law of tangents, 5–6
Leakage current, 284
Lens, 127
Light pen, 93, 143
Light radiation, 21
Line, 143–144
Linear attenuation coefficient, 24, 25, 128, 129, 285, 291
 as CT number, 43, 204–205
 voxel and, 40, 41
Linear energy transfer (LET), 200, 244
Linearity, 205
Linear tomography, 8
Line printer, 165
Line spread function, 178–179, 190
LISP, 99
Lock-in current, 74
Logic functions, 72, 73
Logic gate, 72–73, 77
Logic inverter, 74
L shell, 22
LSI-II microprocessor, 94
Luminescence, 177
Lung tissue, 43–44

Mach effect, 289
Machine language, 93–97
Magnetic lens, 127
Magnetic moment, 258, 260
Magnetic storage devices, 87, 89–90, 164–165, 169
Magnets, 263–264
Magnification, 6–8, 58–59, 139–140
Mainframe, 164
Matrix, 26–28
Maxiray x-ray tubes, 159–163
Mayo Clinic, 237
Measure function, 145
Mechanical calculators, 70
Memory, computer, 86–91
 auxiliary, 89–91
 random access, 82, 86, 87–89
Metal-oxide-semiconductor (MOS), 78, 79
Microcomputer, 82–83
Microprocessor, 86, 94
Microwave computed tomography, 264

Index 339

Microwaves, 21
Minicomputer, 82–83
Modulation transfer function (MTF), 179–180, 190–192
Momentum, 258
Monochromaticity, 24
Motion
   mode (M-mode), 252
   of patient, 51
      artifacts due to, 277–279
      blur due to, 177
Mottle, 183–184
Multicrystal detector systems, 242–243
Multiformat camera, 152–154, 167–168, 169
Multiplanar reconstruction, 219
Multiple images, 140–142
Multiplexers, 81

NAND gate, 73, 74, 75, 79, 80
National Acoustic Laboratories, 249
Neutrino, 244
Noise, 122, 150, 176
   contrast resolution and, 193–196
   in conventional radiography, 183–184
   picture grain, 196–197
   power spectrum, 194–195
Noncomputed tomography, 1
Nonlinearity, in measurements, 284–285
Nonvolatile memory, 87, 89
NOR gate, 73, 74, 79, 80
Nuclear magnetic resonance (NMR) imaging, 11, 256–264
   basic principles, 257–260
   biological effects, 264
   parameters of, 260–262
   techniques, 262–264
Number systems, computer, 70–72
Nutation, 63
Nyquist sampling theorem, 188, 279

Octal system, 71
Omni scanners, 38, 53, 54, 58, 59
Operating systems, computer, 99–100
Operation field, 94, 95
Operator's display console (ODC), 167, 169
Optic radiation, 21
Oral contrast, 147
OR gate, 75, 76, 79
Overscanning, 278–279

Pantomography, 2
Paper tape, 92
Parallax blur, 177
Parallel load register, 80–81
Parasitic shadows, 5
Parity bit, 90

Partial volume effect, 47, 281, 286–289
Pencil beam, 33–34
Penumbra, 177, 201
Peristalsis, bowel, 51
Pfizer scanners, 32, 38, 62, 63, 123
Phantom images, 9
Phantoms, 191–192, 206–208, 281
Philips Tomoscan 300, 30–32, 53
Phosphorescence, 177
Photodiodes, 58, 62, 63
Photoelectric effect, 21–22, 181, 236
Photoelectron, 22
Photomultipliers, 34, 35, 36, 62
Photon, 20–21, 21
   fluctuation, 183–184
   transmission, 40
Pho/Trax 4000, 54
Picker Synerview scanners, 32, 38, 62, 220
Picture elements; *see* Pixels
Picture grain, 196–197
Piezoelectric effect, 248, 249
Pin phantom, 281
Pixels, 27, 28, 292
Planck's constant, 20
Planigraphy, 1
PL/1, 99
Pluridirectional tomography, 8–9
Point-by-point correction, 111, 114, 122
Point spread function, 178, 190, 281
Polarity, image, 136–137
Polaroid film, 48, 151
Polychromaticity, 24, 32
Polytome, 3
Positive print film, 151
Positron cameras, 246
Positron emission computed tomography, 241, 243–248
Positron emission transaxial tomography (PETT), 247
Precision, of CT numbers, 205
Processing system, 99–100
Profile, 39, 42, 291
Programmable read-only memory (PROM), 88, 89
Projection, 291
Pulse bias tank, 162
Pulse-echo technique, 248
Pulse width code (PWC), 170
Pulsing, 54

Quality assurance phantoms, 208
Quantum mottle, 183–184
Quantum noise, 194–196

Rad, 199
Radiation, 20–22
   exposure, 198–200
   intensity, 24
   quality, 181

   scatter, 182–183, 283
   therapy, 227–233
Radiographic film, 34
Radiography
   body section, 1
   computed, 214–219
      clinical applications of, 216–218
   conventional, 176–184
      blur in, 177–178
      contrast in, 180–183
      noise in, 183–184
      sharpness in, 176–177, 178
      spatial resolution in, 176–177, 178–180
Radiowaves, 21
Radon filtering, 108, 118, 295
Ramtek, 165
Random access memory (RAM), 82, 86, 87–89
Random coincidence, 245–246
Rapid sequence CT scanning, 219–227
Raster, 127
Ray, 20, 39, 41, 53, 61, 65
   aliasing, 280
Ray-by-ray correction, 111–114, 122, 294
Rayleigh criterion, 178
Ray-sum, 40, 46, 65, 291
   as total x-ray attenuation, 39, 42
Read-only memory (ROM), 86, 88, 89
Real time scanning, 253–256
Receptor blur, 177
Reconstruction, 107–123, 291–296
   analytical, 116–122, 294–296
      evaluation of, 118–120
      filtered back-projection, 116–118, 119–120, 149, 295–296
      Fourier analysis, 116, 119, 294
   computers and, 42–43
   for divergent beams, 122–123
   field of view for, 171
   iterative, 110–116, 120–122, 292–294
      evaluation of, 115–116
      point-by-point correction, 111, 114, 122
      ray-by-ray correction, 111–114, 122, 294
      simultaneous correction, 111, 122
   multiplanar, 219
   simple back-projection, 108–110, 188, 189, 292, 294–295
   spatial resolution and, 188–189
Reconstruction tomography, 11
Refresh memory, 128
Registers, 80–81
Relative biological effectiveness (RBE), 200
Renografin-60, 147
Reno-M-Drip, 147
Repeat field scanning, 127, 128

Resolution, contrast, 192–196, 218
  defined, 192
  factors determining, 192–193
  noise and, 193–196
  in radiography, 180–183
Resolution, display, 66
Respiration, 51
Reversals, image, 136–139
Roentgen unit (R), 198, 199
Root-mean-square deviation (RMS), of statistical noise, 195–196
Rotational isocentric therapy, 231
Rotational scanning systems, 51–68, 188
  collimation in, 56, 61–62
  detector, 56–58, 59, 62–63
  sampling and, 63, 61
  variations in, 58–60, 63–64
  x-ray tube in, 53–56, 59, 61
Rotor controller, 162

Sampling, 45, 279, 280
  data, 39–40, 42
  rotational scanning systems and, 61, 63
  spatial resolution and, 188
Saturation, 284
Scale factor, 43, 128
Scanned projection radiography, 215
Scanners, 59–60
  accuracy and speed of, 189
  generations of, 29–32
  geometry, 200, 282–284
  see also Rotational scanning systems; Translational-rotational systems; specific models
Scanning, 36–37, 39
  B-, 252–256
  dual energy, 236–237
  dynamic, 217
  electron beam systems, 239–240
  gated, 234–236
  parameters, 168–171
  plane, 28
  real time, 253–256
  repeat field, 127, 128
  time, 200
  ultrafast transmission, 237–240
Scatter radiation, 23, 182–183, 283
  reduction of, 193
Scintillation crystals, 34–36, 58, 62
Scout view, 214
Screen blur, 177
Screen mottle, 183
Section thickness, 197
Shadows, 5
Sharpness, 176–177, 178
Siemens Somatom 2, 32, 53
Signal processing, 193
Simple back-projection, 292, 294–295
Simulated phantoms, 208
Simultaneous correction, 111, 122

Simultaneous iterative reconstruction technique (SIRT), 111, 114, 122
Single-photon counting (SPC), 241
Single-photon emission computed tomography (SPECT), 241
Single-sensitive-point method, 263
Skin-surface-dose (SSD), 231
Slip-rings, 59
Smoothing, 149–150
SNOBOL 4, 99
Sodium iodide (NaI(T1)), 246
Software, 76, 93–101, 165
  application programs, 99, 100–101
  defined, 93
  languages
    assembly, 97–98
    FORTRAN, 98–99
    machine, 93–97
    other types of, 99
  operating systems, 99–100
Soft x-rays, 21
Sonar, 248
Source program, 100
Spatial resolution, 64, 66, 178–180, 184–192, 218
  display parameters, 188
  geometric limitations, 184–188
  grain and, 197
  image reconstruction and, 188–189
  measurement of, 190–192
  mechanical factors and, 189
  in radiography, 176–177, 178–180
  sampling and, 188
Spatial uniformity, 205–206
Spectral sensitivity, 154
Spin, 258, 260–261
  density, 260
  mapping, 263
Standard deviation, 195–196
Static B-scanning, 252–253
Statistical noise, 194–196
Stator coils, 160
Step response function, 190
Storage system, 164–165
Stratigraphy, 1
Stratomatic, 3
Streaks, 275–277, 280
Subject contrast, 180–181, 192
Suite design, 171–172
Summation method, see Back-projection
Surface integral exposure (SIE), 200
Switching logic, 72–73
Synchronous flip-flop circuit, 79
System display console (SDC), 165–167, 168, 169
Systéme Internationale (SI), 199

Table, patient, 28, 29, 158–159, 169
Tangents, law of, 5–6
Target reconstruction, 189
Technicare Delta scanners, 30, 38

Temporal resolution, 218
Terminals, 165–167
Tesla unit (T), 259
Thermoluminescent dosimeters (TLDs), 203, 204
Tomoscopy, 1
Toshiba TCT-35A, 38
Trace, 144
Tracer, 146
Trackball, 93, 143
Transaxial tomography, see Emission computed tomography
Transducer, 249–250, 253–255
Transformer, high voltage, 162
Transilluminated film, 151, 152–154
Transistors, 77–78
Transistor-transistor-logic (TTL) circuits, 79
Translational-rotational systems, 32–39, 188
  collimation in, 33–34, 38
  detector, 34–36, 38
  water bag, 36
  x-ray tube, 32–33, 38
Transverse axial tomography, 10, 11
True phantoms, 208
Truth table, 72
Tube current, 170
Turnkey operation, 93

Ultrasonography, 48
Ultrasound, 136, 248–256
  B-scanning, 252–256
  Doppler techniques, 256
  general principles, 249–252
  historical background, 248–249
Ultraviolet rays, 21
Union Carbide Imaging Systems, 243
UNIVAC, 77
Utility program, 100

Varian V-360-3, 59
View, 53, 64–65, 280, 291
  aliasing, 280
  overscan, 61
  of a projection, 39
Virtual computer, 94
Volatile memory, 87, 89
Volume averaging, 47
Volume elements, see Voxels
Voxels, 27–28, 29, 40, 41

Water bag, 36
Wave, 20–21
Weighting factors, 114, 115
White noise, 195
Wiener spectrum, 194–195
Window settings, 129–136

Xenon, 56–58, 226
  gas detectors, 163

X-ray, 20–25
  attenuation, 23–25, 35, 236
    contrast resolution and, 192
    ray-sum and, 39, 42
  beam geometry, 200–201
  Compton effect and, 22–23, 199, 228, 236
  generator, 164, 169
  monoenergetic, 44
  photoelectric effect, 21–22, 181, 236
  polychromaticity, 24, 32
  properties of, 20–21
  source variations, 284
  tube, 59, 159–163
    gantry and, 55–56
    pulsed, 53, 168–171
  in rotational systems, 53–56, 59, 61
  in translational-rotational systems, 32–33, 38

Z80 microprocessor, 94
Zonography, 1